A Primer on Complete Denture Prosthodontics

K. Chandrasekharan Nair
Purushotham Manvi
S. Srividya

aph

AHUJA PUBLISHING HOUSE
New Delhi (India)

A Primer on Complete Denture Prosthodontics

K. Chandrasekharan Nair
Purushotham Manvi
S. Srividya

Published by Tarun Ahuja
For **AHUJA PUBLISHING HOUSE**

Regd. Office C-8/124B Lawrence Road
Delhi - 110 035. India

Distributed by Ahuja Book Company Pvt. Ltd.
1438/4C, Ansari Road,
Darya Ganj, New Delhi - 110 002. India
Phone: 91-11-23276564, 23245859, 23289999
e-mails: info@ahujabooks.com, ahujabookcompany@gmail.com
Fax: 91-11-23281514
shop online: www.ahujabooks.com

BRANCH OFFICE:

BENGALURU No. 616, 4th Main, Pipeline
Srinagar, Bengaluru – 560 050. India
Telephone : 91 – 80 – 26670322, 26670323
Telefax : 91 – 80 – 26670321
e-mail: blr@ahujabooks.com, bengaluru@ahujabooks.com

KOCHI No.41/2897, First Floor,
St. Vincent road, Kochi – 682 018. India
Telephone : 91 – 484 – 4031078
e-mail: kochi@ahujabooks.com

First Edition: 2013

ISBN : 978-93-80316-25-3

Typeset by
Suman Graphics, Trivandrum
sumangfx@gmail.com

Printed at: Saras Graphics Pvt. Ltd. (India)

A Primer on Complete Denture Prosthodontics

Dedication

To all our Teachers and Students of Prosthodontics

Acknowledgements

Making of this book on Complete dentures has taken a few years of our life. Many masterly books on the subject were already available and hence we thought of adapting the content to suit the Indian conditions. Our vision was ably moulded by many of our teachers, colleagues and friends. Prof. E. Muniratnam Naidu gave this book a valuable foreword and we are deeply touched. We wish to acknowledge Prof. Jacob Hyson, Prof. N. George Paulose, Prof. K.N. Velayudhan Nair, Prof. T. Mohan Kumar, Prof. Jaykar Shetty, Prof. Oommen Aju Jacob, Prof. C.K. Chandrasekhar, Prof. P.A. Murukan, Prof. Pradeep Dathan, Prof. Vidyasree Nandini, Prof. Ravindra C. Savadi, Dr. Rajmohan, Prof. Vahini Reddy, Prof. Divya Hegde, Prof. M. Lovely, Dr. Senthil Nathan, Prof. K. Jyothindrakumar, Prof. K. Nandakumar, Prof. T. Sreelal, Prof. Harshakumar, Prof. Sameer Karachivala Prof. Srinivasa Raju Datla, Dr. Priya, Sri. Venkatesh and Prof. Harish for the interest taken during the different stages of development of this book. Our former students Dr. Ashish, Dr. Mohit Dudani, Dr. Sushma and Dr. Sadhvi have made significant photographic contributions.

Our family members have sacrificed a lot and allowed us to pursue the task of making this book. We are ever indebted to them for the soulful support provided during trying times. Our knowledge on Prosthodontics has been converted to wisdom when we discussed the subject with many of our postgraduate students. We are thankful to them for being the subject of our intellectual experiments. We would like to mention the names of a few of our colleagues – Dr. Suphala Shetty, Dr. Chiranjeevi Reddy and Dr. Lakshmikanth for the love and affection shown while preparing the manuscript.

When we started writing this book, sourcing the knowledge content was difficult. But technology, the internet has opened up a wide world of information which we have profusely made use of. We are ever thankful to the known and unknown contributors of the internet.

Shri. Sudheerkumar of Suman Graphics, Trivandrum has designed the beautiful layout and patiently sat through long hours of correction sessions. His suggestions were valuable and we are thankful to him.

Shri. Venkatraman, our publisher has been a great source of inspiration. We thank him personally and his publishing firm.

God has been kind to us otherwise how to become authors in a subject which we have learned. If any part of the book is felt useful in the clinical practice, we do not take the credit but it is God's grace.

K. Chandrasekharan Nair
Purushotham Manvi
S. Srividya

Foreword

The curricular requirements of complete denture prosthodontic education, are undergoing drastic reformation in view of the changes reflected in the treatment needs of the society. Clinical and technological aspects of complete denture fabrication were once considered as the backbone of prosthodontic education. Complete dentures offered blanket treatment solutions to most of the dental diseases. But the recent past has witnessed the emergence of speciality treatment methods which have limited the scope of complete dentures as the blanket treatment option. Once the demand for complete denture treatment got reduced, the instructional importance of complete dentures followed a similar course. However, the treatment process has become more complex because most of the edentulous patients required repeated fabrication of dentures due to the increased expectancy of life. Fabrication of a third denture for an edentulous individual has become very common but this treatment demands the highest form of clinical acumen. Slowly the complete denture treatment is transforming into a highly skilled speciality. This transformation, I fear, might ultimately deprive the graduate dentist from learning the art and science of complete dentures. Perhaps this realization might have made the authors of this book to modify the feel of the subject. It is titled, a primer of complete denture prosthodontics –may be a primer for both undergraduates and postgraduates. Multiple techniques have been logically avoided and elaboration has been limited to the most appropriate, befitting to the Indian conditions. This book contains a well thought out strategy for complete denture teaching and which will ensure its place in the undergraduate as well as postgraduate curriculum in the times to come. This will also provide ways to achieve clinical competence for a graduate avoiding the necessity for a specialist to provide complete denture treatment. The thought process of the authors will stimulate many young brains to find creative solutions for complete denture problems which are very special to India. One who reads this book will definitely become optimistic on the future relevance of complete denture prosthodontics.

Dr. E. Munirathnam Naidu, M.D.S.
Former Vice-Chancellor
Meenakshi Academy of
Higher Education and Research
Chennai – 600 092

Preface

Complete denture prosthodontics has been questioned for its relevance in the recent past. Dental health has improved beyond our imaginations and perhaps that might have built an over confidence to think that complete dentures can be dispensed with. Hence a palpable deterioration has taken place in taking particular interest in complete denture prosthodontics. Decrease in the number of patients requiring complete denture service is greatly compensated by the higher expectancy of life. In India, the average age of a patient requiring complete dentures and that too the third and the fourth dentures, is crossing seventy. The need for complete denture service has not yet reduced but the process has become more complicated. The present day dentist in fact do not relish making complete dentures because many of our techniques are old, time consuming and not user friendly. Patients have also started disliking the crude time consuming methods. While we started writing this book, these were the thoughts that came across and we have tried our best to simplify the clinical methods without limiting the desired quality envisaged by the founders of our profession. Allow us to take pride in claiming a better user friendliness of the clinical methods described in this book. We do not claim a space that is occupied by the standard text books which are followed by the Indian Universities. But while reading, you will be tempted to experiment with many of the techniques explained which are very easy to follow because of the user friendly materials. We invite your suggestions to modify the contents so that the next edition will be a better product. The authors are grateful to Professor Muniratnam Naidu who was kind enough to provide this book with a foreword. We sincerely thank the contributors who have added tremendously to the quality of this book. The authors sincerely urge the teachers, practising professionals and the students to give a kind and critical perusal of this book.

K. Chandrasekharan Nair
Purushotham Manvi
S. Srividya

Authors

K. Chandrasekharan Nair, MDS
Professor of Prosthodontics
AECS Maaruti College of Dental Sciences and Research Centre
Bangalore

Formerly, Professor of Prosthodontics
M.R. Ambedkar Dental College
Bangalore

Formerly, Associate Professor of Prosthodontics
Govt. Dental College, Trivandrum
e-mail: chandrasekharannair.drk@gmail.com

Purushotham Manvi, MDS
Principal
Professor of Prosthodontics
Best Dental Science College, Madurai
Formerly, Professor & HOD, Prosthodontics
Maharanapratap Dental College, Gwalior, M.P.
Formerly, Professor of Prosthodontics
ACES Maaruti College of Dental Sciences and Research Centre
Bangalore
e-mail: manvipurush@gmail.com

S. Srividya, MDS
Senior Lecturer in Prosthodontics
AECS Maaruti College of Dental Sciences and Research Centre
Bangalore
e-mail: drsrividya5@gmail.com

Contributors

M. Shivashanker, MDS
Professor of Prosthodontics
Krishnadevaraya College of Dental Sciences, Bangalore

G. Viswanath, MDS
Assistant Professor, Department of Restorative Dentistry
Libyan International Medical University
Kairawan St., Al-Fwaihat, Benghazi, Libya.
Formerly Professor of Prosthodontics
ACES Maaruti College of Dental Sciences and Research Centre
Bangalore

Contents

1

Dentist-patient relationship Competencies for the dental graduate

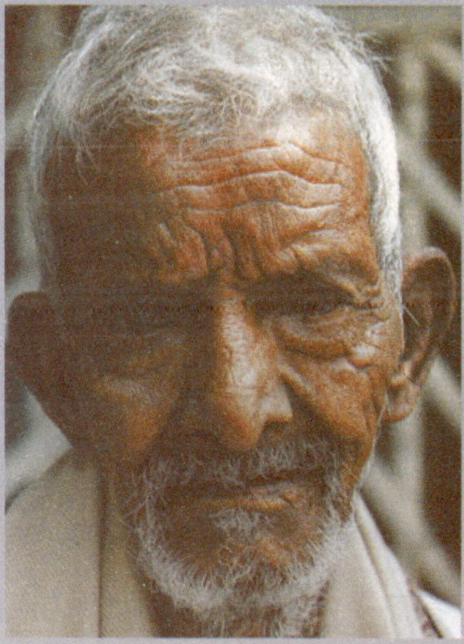

The relationship between dentist and complete denture patient cannot be considered as formal but it is the beginning of a long lasting relationship evolving into an exemplary story of human bondage

Welcoming the patient

It is very important to greet the patients and look at them in the eyes while doing so. Dentist must introduce himself and make the patient feel welcome and the patients should feel that the dentist is genuinely happy that they are there. Always refer to a patient by respectfully calling the name. In Indian context it is better to address Sir or Madam. It is discourteous to point a patient to the dental chair and start working.

The dentist must feel confident of himself and project that feeling to the patient. Dentist must feel and act happy to take care of the patient. Patients will sense the anxiety and will notice a frown because people are frightened enough when they walk in and are hyper-alert. They are looking for verbal and nonverbal clues about what to expect. It is critically important that the words and behavior of the dentist make the patient feel comfortable.

Why are patients so afraid of dentists? Because they deal with teeth and face which are extremely sensitive. A particularly sensitive part of the human body is combined with possibly a few bad prior experiences and the result is a patient who clings to every potential clue about whether the dentist will hurt. Students should learn on the behaviour by role playing during the course.

Listen to the Complaint

Lack of communication is one of the biggest complaints patients have about their dentist. One must be a good listener if he wants to become a good dentist. After the patient is seated, look at the new patient in the eyes and ask, "Why are you here?" and then write down the response, making a list if necessary. No patient will reply, "I'm here for a full mouth radiographs, study models, head and neck exam, periodontal probing, charting of decayed, missing and filled teeth and then to be checked off by possibly five different instructors." They usually reply, "I broke a tooth in the back," or "I'm here for a check-up." Patients are happy to see the dentist listening, and writing down, what the patient says.

The first component of record-making will focus on whether the concern is functional, cosmetic and/ or painful. Also discuss the patient's medical history and make notations in the chart, and then list any medical condition. It is preferable to write "medical condition discussed" because it is inadequate medico-legally to just review a patient's medical history without actually discussing it with them to ensure that they understood the questions. Notice again how important it is that patient's actually understand all that you are doing.

Then ask the patient when he last went to the dentist and for what reason. Note in the record, for example-past dental history-one year ago for a prophylaxis and then inquire why he did not return to the previous dentist. This can give you a lot of insight into the patient's emotional needs. Sometimes patients may tell that they have not been to the dentist for many years or they get agitated sitting in the chair. The most common reasons for not visiting the previous dentist are lack of time, lack of money, indifference, or fear.

It is very common among people to get so caught up with work and family leaving little time to complete their necessary dental treatment. For such patients the dental treatment should be completed quickly and with a high level of skill. A lot of people ignore the need for dental treatment without understanding that by ignoring a problem they usually create the need for more complex, costlier work later. Taking care of any problem earlier will always save money in the end. If lack of money is a barrier to receive proper dental care, it may be considered while discussing treatment options.

Fear is frequently a large component of why people don't seek dental care. It is generally found that the more powerful an individual, either physically or professionally, the more uncomfortable they are in going to a dentist. Though initially ironic, this is quite logical. A frail old lady is rarely afraid of dentistry because they are relatively powerless in controlling their outside environment. On the other hand, a physically strong athlete or a successful executive might have got used to sensing a certain level of control over their environment. These people have the most difficulty giving up control and therefore experience the most fear of dentistry. The way dentists help fearful patients cope with their dental treatment is by giving them control by explaining what we do, when we do it, how we do it, how much it will cost, what it will look like and how it will function. We also give them control over the potential of pain with a variety of medications both during and after any procedure.

Getting back to the actual chief complaint, determine whether it is functional, aesthetic and/or painful. One needs to also learn the degree of this concern for example how painful is the tooth. Next determine to what extent the patient's medical history and past dental history will have an impact on the treatment. Then determine what must be accomplished during this first visit to adequately (not necessarily completely, nor permanently) treat the patient's chief complaint. Lastly, make the appropriate records for treating the chief complaint only.

The dentist must first give the patient what he wants. Then, attempt to teach him to want what he needs. Before making records, repeat from the written notes the patient's chief complaint and convince patient that the dentist has understood specifically why the patient has come.

Presenting the case to the patient

Case presentation is the communication of both the diagnosis and treatment plans in a manner a patient can understand so that they are able to personally choose what is best for them. The patient's choice is usually determined by budget, time available for treatment, esthetic concerns, functional demands and overall tolerance of dental procedures.

The dental student must be able to verbally and/or graphically explain different treatment plans to a patient in a manner easily understood by the patient. The choice of words used in conversation, including dental terminology, and graphics may need to vary tremendously from patient to patient. Keep the explanations short and sweet. Be empathetic and confident during the discussion.

While explaining whether a patient should extract a tooth or have root canal therapy they will probably want to know for each procedure how long will it take, what will it feel like during the procedure and afterwards, how much will it cost and how will chewing be affected. They do not want to learn the differences between internal hex or external hex of an implant. Focus on the differences in the benefits of the procedures not the technicalities

Records of the patient

Making records of a patient could include radiographs (full mouth series, panorex and/or cephalometric), study models, head and neck exam, and a clinical exam (including charting of decayed, missing, and filled teeth, and prosthesis; malpositioned wisdom teeth, full periodontal charting and occlusal analysis, including potential orthodontic needs).

If a patient presents for a first visit seeking a check-up, then a set of x-rays, head and neck examination and complete clinical examination would be indicated. If a patient presents with a broken filling of a tooth as his chief complaint then the records necessary to make a proper diagnosis must be made.

It is a common mistake among students to be so overly thorough at first that even after several visits the patient may still not have the chief complaint, the reason for which the patient reported, properly addressed and treated. It is also not advisable to hurriedly treat the patient's chief complaint and miss an important part of a diagnosis either. A master clinician understands the importance of timing in patient care.

If the patient is in pain, it is our duty to give him/her relief before he/she leaves the clinic.

Competencies for the Dental Graduates

1. Graduates must be competent in patient assessment and diagnosis for the child, adolescent, adult and geriatric patient.
2. Graduates must be competent in treatment planning and case presentation for the child, adolescent, adult and geriatric patient.
3. Graduates must be competent to communicate and collaborate with groups and individuals to promote oral and general health and select strategies, resources and interventions appropriate for the prevention of oral disease in the community.
4. Graduates must be competent in control of pain and anxiety, clinical pharmacology, inhalation sedation techniques, and management of related problems.
5. Graduates must be competent in the prevention and management of dental and medical emergencies.
6. Graduates must be competent in the restoration of defective and/or missing teeth to form, function and esthetics in the child patient.
7. Graduates must be competent in the diagnosis and restoration of defective teeth to form, function and esthetics in the adolescent, adult and geriatric patient.
8. Graduates must be competent in the fixed replacement of missing teeth to form, function and esthetics in the uncomplicated adolescent, adult and geriatric patient.
9. Graduates must be competent in treating uncomplicated partially edentulous patients with removable partial dentures to restore and maintain oral function, health, comfort and appearance.
10. Graduates must be competent in treating uncomplicated edentulous patients with complete dentures to restore and maintain oral function, health, comfort and appearance.
11. Graduates must be competent in the diagnosis and management of periodontal disorders.
12. Graduates must be competent in the prevention, diagnosis and management of pulpal and periradicular diseases.
13. Graduates must be competent in the diagnosis and management of oral mucosal disorders.
14. Graduates must be competent to collect and assess diagnostic information to plan for and perform uncomplicated oral surgical procedures.
15. Graduates must be competent to recognize malocclusion in the primary, mixed and permanent dentition and to identify from an acceptable problem list an uncomplicated case with limited developmental/acquired abnormality.
16. Graduates must be competent in describing the indications, contraindications, advantages and disadvantages of space maintainers, and demonstrating the basic skills in making simple orthodontics appliances and space maintainers.
17. Graduates must be competent in discerning and managing ethical issues and problems in dental practice.
18. Graduates must be competent in the understanding and application of the appropriate codes, rules, laws and regulations that govern dental practice.
19. Graduates must be competent in behavioral patient management and interpersonal skills.
20. Graduates must be competent in understanding the fundamental elements of managing a dental practice.
21. Graduates must be competent in performing and supervising infection control procedures to prevent transmission of infectious diseases to patients, the dentist, the staff and dental laboratory technicians.

22. Graduates must be competent to critically evaluate and incorporate new dental procedures/ therapies into their practices when these procedures/therapies have proven scientifically efficacious.
23. Graduates must have the ability to recognize the role of lifelong learning and self-assessment to maintain competency.
24. Graduates must be competent in the use of information technology resources.
25. Graduates must be competent in detection, diagnosis, risk assessment, prevention, and management of dental caries.

Suggested reading

1. Jeremy Jacquot, *Trust in the Dentist-Patient Relationship:* A Review, Journal of young investigators 2005; 12(6):
2. Yamalik Nermin, *Dentist-patient relationship and quality care 2.* Trust, Int Dent Journal, 2005; 55(3): 168–170.
3. Yamalik N, *Dentist-patient relationship and quality care 3. Communication,* Int Dent J. 2005;55(4):254-6
4. Corah NL, O'Shea RM, Bissell GD. *The dentist-patient relationship: perceptions by patients of dentist behavior in relation to satisfaction and anxiety.* J Am Dent Assoc. 1985 Sep; 111(3):443-6
5. Ruth Freeman, *The psychology of dental patient care: A psychodynamic understanding of the dentist–patient interaction,* Br Dent J 1999;186: 503 - 506
6. Ayer WA, *The dentist-patient relationship,* Int Dent J. 1982 Mar; 32(1):56-64.

2

Evaluation of the patient

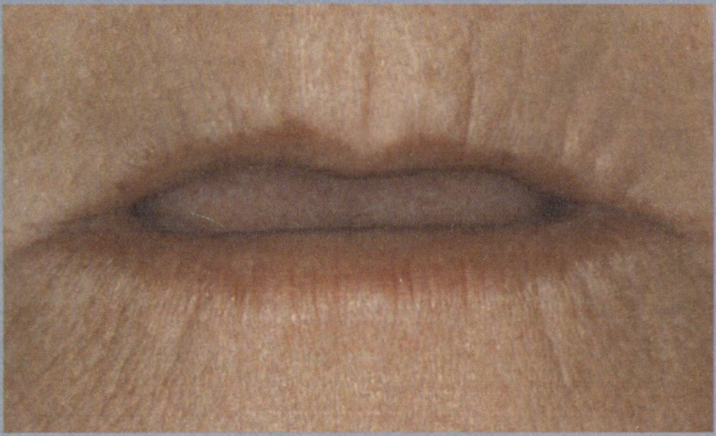

Success of complete denture treatment depends greatly on clear understanding of the possibilities and the limitations

A thorough, systematic examination of all the conditions of the mouth and of the patient is essential because success or failure of complete dentures will greatly depend on clear understanding of the limitations and possibilities of each case. The following outline will aid in systematizing the evaluation of a patient.

I. Patient data

1. Age

Whenever possible chronological age must be recorded and if the exact information is unobtainable, an estimate may be made and age is recorded as "under 40", "40 to 60 years", and "over 60 years". General appearance and gait for the normal age are also to be observed. The significance of ascertaining the age from the dentist's point of view is in evaluating the ability of a patient to wear dentures successfully for two reasons:

Adaptability: It is generally believed that young people adapt themselves with greater ease and therefore are more likely to have successful denture experiences. Preservation of tissues is of vast importance in advancing age. Mental attitudes must also be considered along with.

Physiologic condition of supporting structures: Residual ridges always change but metabolism or the rate of interchange of nutritious elements for bone formation is better in young people. Under normal conditions, the process of aging would imply poor calcification of bones. The role of the endocrine glands in this connection is now better understood, especially the influence of the sex glands on calcium metabolism. In older people, when sex hormones are at a minimum or entirely absent, the quality of the bone becomes poor and more unfavorable experiences in wearing dentures may be anticipated. The overlying mucosa is also affected in a manner qualitatively similar to the bone.

2. Sex

Sex has a bearing on denture treatment because of esthetics and of the influence of sex hormones on the supporting structures. Women can be more demanding and are usually more concerned with their appearance than men. Unlike men, women may regard appearance as more important than the efficient functioning of dentures. There is a drastic change in the physiologic functions when women undergo menopause. The withdrawal of some or most of the ovarian secretion affects the alveolar ridge adversely; both the bone and the overlying mucosa. Often, mental instability of varying degrees accompanies the menopause and this may make wearing of the dentures difficult.

3. Race

Race can be critical factor in characterization of dentures (i.e. choice of denture base shade, placement of denture base stains etc)

4. Occupation

Occupation of an individual demands special attention in view of the esthetic, phonetic, or functional considerations. People who make public appearances, such as artists, actors, salesmen, public speakers, singers, teachers, etc., are particularly concerned with the appearance and phonetics while tradesmen, mechanics, or labourers, etc., are more concerned with functional efficiency. Occupational considerations are also important because of the possible detrimental effects on health as in occupational metal poisoning or bronchial irritation. Beauticians, who open bobby pins with their teeth might place leverage on the front teeth and which may cause unseating of dentures.

II. Chief complaint

Patient's chief complaint has to noted down in his own words. Patients can be desirous of obtaining complete denture for reasons of esthetics or mastication. According to De Van, 'the dentist should meet the mind of the patient before he meets the mouth of the patient". Hence the dentist must determine the reason the patient is seeking prosthodontic treatment. The patient should be questioned regarding his or her chief complaint. There are several reasons for seeking this information.

1. If this is not done the chief complaint may be overlooked during therapy
2. The response allows the practitioner to assess whether the patients expectations are realistic or attainable.
3. Finally the response provides information regarding the patients psychological classification (for House's personality classification)

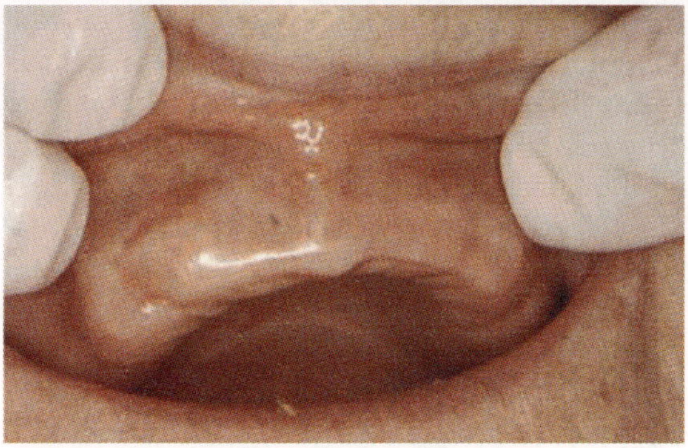

Fig. 2.1 Dry mouth in diabetes mellitus

III. Systemic status

Patients who come for complete dentures are generally in an age group where health deficiencies of varying degrees are expected. Healthy patients can make a better adjustment than the ill, tense, or nervous patient. Many chronic, debilitating diseases offer a poor prognosis and have early oral manifestations. Symptoms patients present may be subjective, as pain or burning sensation or they may be objective really involving tissue changes in both bone and overlying tissues. Some of the diseases causing pain or burning sensations may be anemia, diabetes, aclorhydria, estrogen privia and other endocrine and nutritional disorders. Psychological disturbances resulting from financial troubles, family worries, or maladjusted sex relations may also be explored. Diseases causing considerable tissue changes are syphilis, tuberculosis, blood dyscrasias, diabetes, endocrinopathies, neoplasms and osteodystrophies. Caution should be exercised while making dentures on patients who have undergone radiation therapy in the region of the jaws because of the inability of tissues to repair and because of the increased susceptibility to infection following injury. The following is a list of some of the diseases frequently encountered in prosthodontic practice and the considerations that must be made by the dentist:

Diabetes (Fig 2.1)

The disease must be controlled by medical treatment. Impression technique must be physiologically compatible. Masticatory load applied to the supporting tissues should be controlled.Careful occlusal corrections should be accomplished to remove all interferences. The food table should be small and the patient should be given detailed instructions on eating habits and oral hygiene. Frequent evaluation of the dentures is necessary.

Hypertension

Hypertensive patients may have xerostomia induced by antihypertensive drugs. They may also be prone to orthostatic hypotension. As dental treatment is considered a stressful appointment, scheduling these patients early can be helpful.

Other CVS diseases

It is always advisable to consult the patient's cardiologist before commencing treatment. Cardiac patients will require shorter appointments.

Arthritis (Fig 2.2)

The limited movement of the mandible during impression making may necessitate modification of trays and techniques. It may be difficult to get proper jaw relation registrations. Occlusal corrections must be made often because of arthritic changes in the tempromandibular joint.

Anemia

The condition should be treated medically. Dentures

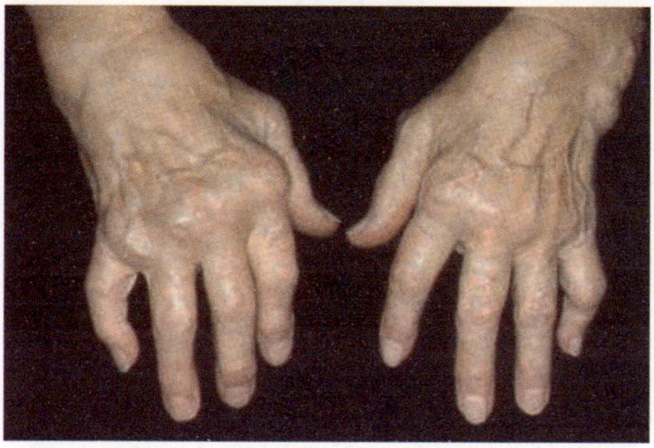

Fig. 2.2 Rheumatoid arthritis

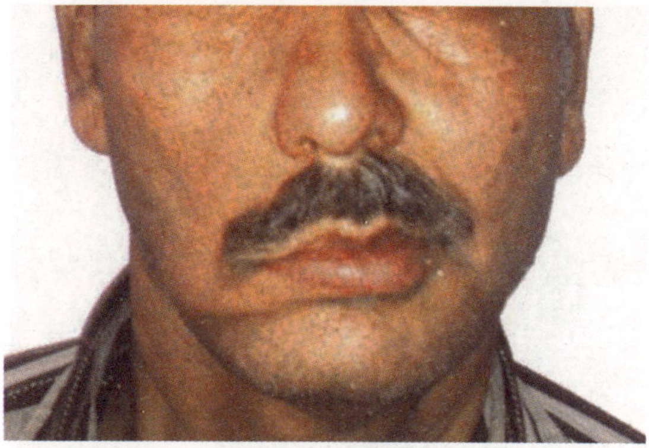

Fig.2.3 Bells palsy

should improve masticatory efficiency since diet is an important part of the medical treatment. A small food table with maximum coverage of supporting area is desirable to keep the supporting tissue from being over stressed. Careful patient instruction should be given for good oral hygiene.

Allergy

Patient has to be asked if he has had allergic reaction to any drugs taken in the past or if he is a previous denture wearer his reaction to denture base resin. If not known, but the patient gives a history that he is allergic to many commonly used drugs or medications, materials, then a subcutaneous test for the response to denture base resin has to be done.

Bells palsy (Fig 2.3)

Retention is difficult or often hard to achieve and denture adhesive may be necessary. Paralysed musculature can affect both function and aesthetics Limitations of denture should be explained to the patient. The patient should be educated in mastication and in oral hygiene.

Parkinsons disease (Fig 2.4)

Control of the patient movements during fabrication of the denture can be accomplished with sedatives. Retention is difficult, and an adhesive may be necessary. It may be wise to remove dentures when they are not in use. This will add to the comfort of the patient and eliminate the danger of accidental swallowing of dentures.

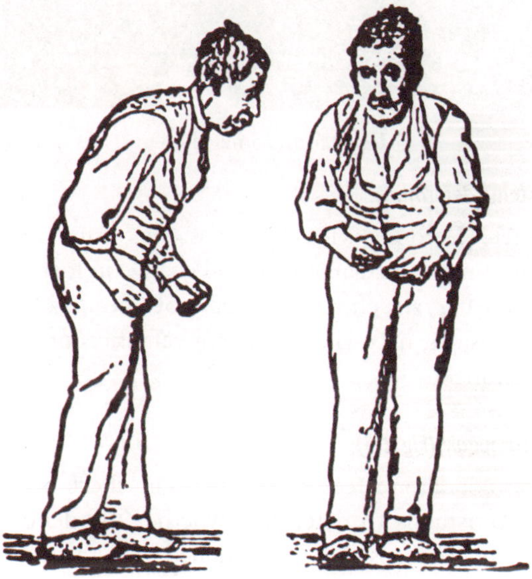

Fig.2.4 Parkinsonism

Radiation

If dentures are to be made, it is imperative that abrasion and irritation to supporting tissues are to be eliminated. An open lesion may be the start of a serious condition, namely osteonecrosis. It is best not to use dentures at all, over irradiated tissues but if dentures are necessary, they should not be used until at least two years after radiotherapy.

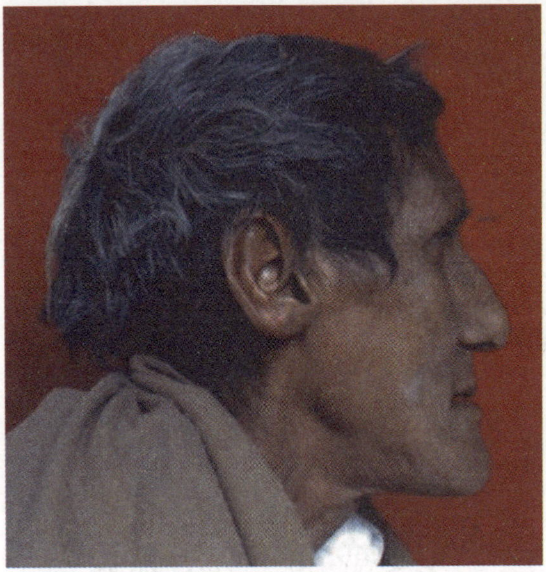

Fig.2.5 Acromegaly

Osteitis deformans

Osteitis Deformans is a chronic osseous disturbance. The continued enlargement and change in form of supporting structures, especially of the maxillary tuberosities, necessitate frequent refabrication and adjustments.

Acromegaly (Fig 2.5)

This condition necessitates a periodic check up of the prosthesis to determine whether the denture requires changes due to continued growth of the mandible and maxilla.

IV. Personal history

a. Diet

According to studies, one in five older people reported that oral condition prevented them from eating the foods they would choose, 15% took longer time to complete their meal and their enjoyment of food was limited by oral condition, 5% avoided eating certain foods because of chewing problems. In addition, a poor diet coupled with a sedentary lifestyle are known to be risk factors for life- threatening chronic diseases viz heart disease, stroke, hypertension, diabetes and some forms of cancer and death. Tissue dehydration – xerostomia caused by polypharmacy , calcium deficiency and osteoporosis in postmenopausal women, fragility of oral mucosa resulting in frictional trauma during denture wearing and muscle weakness and loss of tonicity – resulting from diet low in protein and poor digestion and absorption are all direct or indirect results of inadequate nutrition. These factors should be identified and patient and caretakers be educated about the importance of adequate nutrition and its role in general well being as well as success of any dental rehabilitation.

b. Habits

Patients should be questioned if they have habit of smoking, consume alcohol or were clenching or bruxing their teeth when they had their natural teeth. The number of cigarettes/ beedis they smoke per day and frequency of smoking also should be noted. A positive history of tobacco consumption should alert the dentist about any premalignant lesions such as leukoplakia, OSMF resulting in restricted mouth opening. The patient has to be educated regarding the ill effects of such habits and advised to refrain from doing so.

Nicotinic stomatitis: (Fig 2.6)

Nicotinic Stomatitis is a form of chemical injury to the oral mucosa and mucous glands. The area may be covered with a denture. Even in patients with natural dentition, the area is covered as part of the

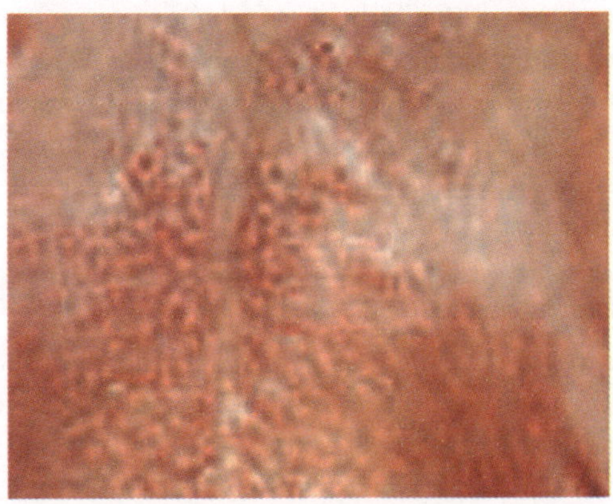

Fig. 2.6 Nicotina palatinus

treatment. Secretion from the mucous glands, may affect the surface details of impression.

V. Dental history

i. History of dental extraction

Years edentulous - Responses to this question provide information about bone resorption patterns and progressions, as well as the timing of the tooth loss. The patient should be questioned regarding the reasons for tooth loss (example – periodontal disease, gross caries, trauma etc)

Expectations - The patient should be asked about his and her expectations. The dentist should evaluate the patient's expectations and classify them as realistic or attainable and unrealistic.

Period of Edentulousness - This data gives information about the amount and pattern of bone resorption. The cause for the tooth loss should be enquired (caries, periodontitis, etc.)

Pre-treatment Records - Pre-treatment records include information about the previous denture, existing denture, pre-extraction records and diagnostic casts.

ii. Previous denture

It denotes the dentures, which were worn before the current denture. The reason for the failure of the prosthesis should be enquired with the patient. The patients who keep changing dentures in a short period of time are difficult to satisfy and are risky to deal with.

iii. Examination of existing denture

Existing Dentures should be evaluated to determine physical, esthetic and anatomic characteristics. Shade, mold, and material should be recorded for both anterior and posterior teeth. If the mold cannot be determined, the general shape of the teeth should be recorded (E.g., Square, Square-tapering, tapering, ovoid, etc)

Esthetics, Phonetics, retention, stability, extensions and contours: Existing esthetics, phonetics, retention, stability, extensions and contours should be evaluated. These attributes should be rated 1. Good 2. Fair 3. Poor.

Centric Relation and Vertical Dimension of Occlusion: Centric Relation and Vertical Dimension of Occlusion should be assessed and rated " acceptable" or "unacceptable". If unacceptable it should be noted whether the existing VDO is "inadequate" or " excessive".

Occlusal Pane Orientation: The Orientation of the occlusal plane should be noted. Improper orientation as a result of tooth setting or changes in bony architecture often creates a " reverse smile line". This condition is characterized by teeth that slope downward as one progresses posteriorly. Consequently, the anterior teeth assume a curvature that does not follow the arc of the lower lip.

Palate: The palate of the existing maxillary denture should be examined. The denture base material and thickness should be noted. Anatomic features should be assessed. The practitioner should note the presence or absence of rugae on the cameo surface of the denture base. Denture wearers may have become accustomed to a particular palatal form, and may resist change. The practitioner should listen to speech patterns, and determine whether appropriate "valving" is taking place. Placement of rugae or a change in thickness may affect pronunciation.

Post dam: The posterior border of the maxillary denture should be examined. Like wise, soft tissues in the vicinity of the ' vibrating line' should be observed. The seal of the existing maxillary denture may be traced to improper post damming. The post dam should be rated "acceptable" or " unacceptable".

Base Adaptation: The fit of maxillary and mandibular bases should be assessed using an appropriate disclosing medium. Adaptation should be rated " acceptable" or " unacceptable"

Midline: Maxillary and mandibular midlines should be observed. Although discrepancies between maxillary and mandibular midlines may be present, it is critical that the maxillary midline coincide with the facial midline. Discrepancies in midline should be evaluated using intraoral (Eg incisive papilla) and extraoral landmarks (Eg., nasion, filtrum, middle of the chain). The midline should be rated " acceptable" or " unacceptable". Deviations of the maxillary midline should be recorded by direction and amount (eg., maxillary midline 2mm to the right of the facial midline)

Buccal Vestibule: The buccal vestibule is an important esthetic and functional component in complete denture service. Consequently this space should be assessed carefully. The Buccal vestibule should be judged "acceptable" or " unacceptable". Corrective actions should be proposed.

Crossbite: The presence of a unilateral or bilateral cross bite often presents a challenging situation. Cross bites should be noted and their effects on tooth placement anticipated. This information may be entered into the dialogistic record using the categories " none", "unilateral" or " bilateral".

Characterization: Characterization or staining of existing dentures bases should be evaluated and recorded. Existing denture bases may be classified as "characterized " or " uncharacterized".

Comfort: The patient should be questioned regarding the comfort of maxillary and mandibular dentures. Comfort for the respective arches should be classified as " acceptable" or "unacceptable". Patients should who experience discomfort should be questioned to determine the nature and source of the discomfort.

Hygiene: The patient's ability and motivation to clean the dentures should be assesses during clinical evaluation. The patient also should be questioned about his her denture cleansing regimen. These factors may affect denture-base contouring (eg., closed interdental contours versus open interdental contours) and tooth arrangements (eg., presence or absence of diastemata). Hygiene should be classified as 1) minimal, 2) moderate, or 3) severe.

Wear: Wear often is an indicator of Para functional habits or an abrasive diet. The wear process must be assessed with respect to time. With these factors in mind, wear should be classified as 1) minimal, 2) moderate or 3) severe.

Attachments and Hardware: Attachments are hardware usually are limited to over dentures situations. When working under these constraints, it is important to know the specific system in use and the availabity of components.

iv. Pre-extraction Records

Pre-extraction records records are desirable for all patients. These records will serve as guides in the construction of the proposed new dentures and will also be of importance for any subsequent dentures. Preoperative records can provide information about the shape, form, color, and position of the natural teeth, the vertical dimension of occlusion, the support of the lips, and the relationship of the teeth to the lips. These records may consist of photographs, diagnostic casts, tattooing of intraoral structures, measurements of extraoral structures, charts of remaining teeth, and radiographs.

Photographs: A series of photographs made prior to removal of the remaining teeth should show the patient in a relaxed state and with a smile, both from the front and profile. Close-ups should be made of the individual teeth, dental arches, and occlusion.

Diagnostic Casts: If teeth remain, diagnostic casts should always be made to serve as guides for the placement of the artificial teeth and an indication of the vertical dimension of occlusion.

VI. Mental attitude

Complete denture diagnosis based only on oral biophysical condition is incomplete unless the psychological factor is also evaluated. Patients anticipate denture use with some of preconceived ideas about their nature and the cost in time and money. The patient's ideas may be faulty but in any event they are faced with social, functional and phonetic problems to which each will react differently. Overcoming difficulties is at least as important to success as is the excellence in denture fabrication. Personality difficulties become exaggerated under the influence of ill health, old age, menopause or flair up because of unfavorable social or business environment or the state of dominating or being dominated by others. The method of acquiring the necessary information to evaluate this factor is the empirical procedure of exploratory conversation as no valid question and answer routine has been developed. The classification established will depend upon the interrogative and analytical ability of the dentist and upon the truthfulness and completeness of the patient's responses. Many failures are blamed on uncooperative, biased or neurotic patients. It is as imprudent to abuse the privilege of blaming someone else for failure as it is to expect that the routine pursuit of a set standard of scientific procedure will always produce a successful result. Mental attitudes are divided into four classes according to M M House

Class I - Philosophical

a. Those who have presented themselves prior to the extraction of their teeth, have had no experience in wearing artificial dentures, and do not anticipate any special difficulties in that regard.

b. Those who have worn satisfactory dentures, are in good health, are a well-balanced type, and are in need of further denture service. These patients will have an equanimous approach to life.

Class II - Exacting

a. Those while suffering from poor oral health, are seriously concerned about appearance and efficiency of artificial dentures. They are reluctant to accept the advicc of the physician and the dentist and are unwilling to submit to the removal of their artificial teeth.

b. Those wearing artificial dentures unsatisfactory in appearance and usefulness, and who so doubt the ability of the operator to render a service which will be satisfactory that they often insist on a written guarantee or expect the dentist to make repeated attempts to please them.

Class III - Hysterical

a. Those in bad health with long neglected pathological mouth conditions who dread dental service and submit to the removal of their teeth as a last resort and who are positive in their minds that they can never wear artificial dentures.

b. Those who have attempted to wear artificial dentures but failed and are thoroughly discouraged. They are of a hysterical and nervous, temperament and will demand efficiency and appearance from the artificial dentures equal to that of the most perfect natural teeth.

Class IV - Indifferent

Those who are unconcerned about their appearance and feel very little or no necessity for teeth for mastication. They are therefore non-persevering and will inconvenience themselves very little, to become accustomed to dentures.

Patients may also be classified as follows:

A. Cooperative: These patients represent the optimum group. Stated in the most concise terms they may or may not recognize the need for dentures but they are open minded and are amenable to suggestion. Procedures can be explained with very little effort and they become fully cooperative.

B. Apprehensive: Even though these patients realize the need for dentures they have some irrational problem which cannot be overcome by ordinary explanation. They vary from the mildly apprehensive to definitely abnormal mental states and are hard to catalogue. The approach to all of these patients is to talk to them and to explore the anxiety.

A large group of prospective denture patients fear the outcome which may be quite well concealed from them and the dentist or which may be obvious. The more obvious expressions of anxiety are trembling, over-talkativeness; weeping, "touchiness" or the person may be sullen, withdrawn and uncooperative. There may be physical symptoms. Some of the most frequent types of apprehensive patients are the following:

i.Anxious: Those who are anxious and are upset about the uncertainties of wearing dentures often work themselves into a neurotic state. In extreme and rare cases they become psychotic. In most cases however, their apprehensions may be allayed if the dentist will probe for the cause. Some fear about the development of cancer; others fear that they will not be able to wear the denture; still others fear that the teeth will not look well.

ii. Obsessive or exacting: These persons are naturally of an exacting nature and give directions to others. They state their wants as to dentures and are inclined to tell the dentist how to proceed. In some instances the expectation esthetically, may amount to an obsession. Patients of this type must be handled firmly. They should be told tactfully at the outset that they will not be allowed to direct denture construction. If they cannot be made cooperative in this way, they will be a source of real trouble in the future.

iii. Chronic complainers: comprise a group who are habitually faultfinding and dissatisfied. They may be best handled by soliciting their cooperation and incorporating as many of their ideas as is compatible with good denture construction. It is best to have an understanding with such patients before work commences. In this way they are made to share responsibility for the outcome.

C. Uncooperative : These patients present themselves usually upon being urged by relatives or friends. They do not feel a need for dentures, though the need exists. Their general attitude is negative. They constitute an extremely difficult group of potential denture wearers and tax the dentist's patience to the limit.

Simon Gamer's Classification:

Gamer has classified patients into five types : ideal, submitter, reluctant, indifferent, and resistant. Each type is characterized by a rating on engagement and willingness to submit and by the stance the patient types are likely to take in reaction to being a dental patient.

a. Ideal patient, which corresponds to House's philosophical mind, is reasonably engaged and reasonably willing to submit to the dentist. These patients are considered mature with a healthy life balance. They are not vulnerable to regression or excessive dependence on authority figures. Therefore they are not prone to fixate on and be overly absorbed with their particular dental treatment. The ideal patient tends to be neither overly suspicious nor blindly accepting of the dentist's recommendations.

b. Submitter patient : lack discrimination and tend to idealize the dentist, which results in a high degree of engagement and utter surrender. This renders the submitter incapable of providing genuine informed consent because he/she has surrendered the use of critical faculties and therefore cannot be an active partner in the treatment.

c. Reluctant patient : is often leery of the dentist and skeptical of the treatment plan.

d. Indifferent patient : who corresponds to House's indifferent mind is usually coerced into seeing the dentist by a concerned family member or friend, the indifferent patient is minimally engaged and indifferent to the dentist to the extent that willingness to submit is not an issue.

e. Resistant patient : This patient corresponds to House's exacting mind and Boucher's critical patient. Resistant patients are skeptical of the dentist as a person and of being helped by anyone under any circumstance. The resistant patient is, paradoxically, very engaged with the dentist but in an adversarial way. Rather than being dependent, they challenge the dentist. And, like the indifferent patient, there is no trust.

VII. Extraoral observation

i. Facial form (Fig 2.7)

It is generally believed that form and arrangement of the teeth should harmonize with face form. Although a pure type is rarely found, face forms may be classified as follows:

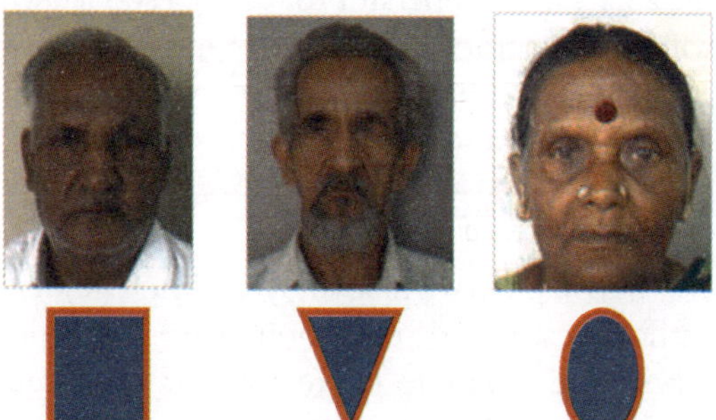

Fig. 2.7 Face-form–square, tapering, ovoid

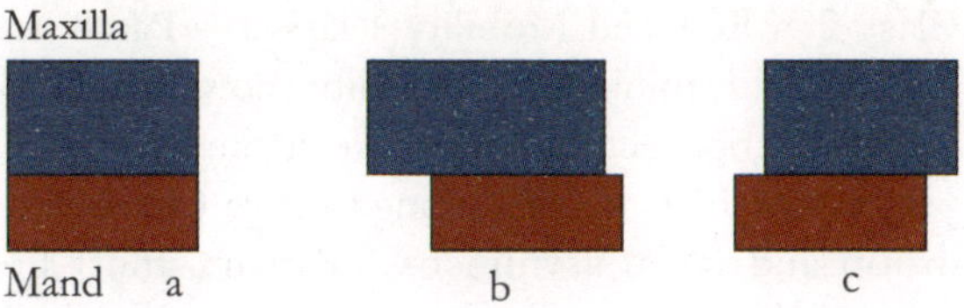

Fig. 2.8 Profile- a. straight b. Retrognathic c.Prognathic

A. Square: in this case the face is about equally wide in the temporalis region, the area of the zygomatic arch and the angles of the jaw.

B. Tapering: A decrease in width is generally found in these types as one progresses from forehead to chin.

C. Ovoid: the area of the zygomatic arch is widest in this case.

ii. Profile (Fig 2.8)

A patient's profile can be an early indicator of the patient's jaw classification. Examination of the facial profile is very important because it determine the jaw relation and occlusion and also helps in esthetics eg. In a convex profile a very prominent labial flange will make patients mouth look odd. Angle classified the facial profile as class:

Class I : Normal or straight or orthognathic profile.

Class II: Retrognathic profile

Class III: Prognathic profile

A patient's occluding vertical face height can easily be seen in profile and a judgment made whether the occlusal vertical dimension causes the patient's face to appear collapsed with excessive wrinkling around the mouth. A false prognathic relationship can be observed if the over closure is severe enough. An opened vertical dimension can mask the true relationship of the jaws as well as cause the facial tissues to appear strained and taut.

iii. Muscular tone

Muscular tone will be normal when no degenerative change occurs in the muscles of facial expression and mastication, or in the tactile sense of the jaw and mucosa. A marked loss of tone occurs in the absence of natural teeth, artificial substitutes or from wearing grossly inefficient dentures. Neurological deficiencies must also be considered. Classification according to House

Class 1 – The patient exhibits normal tension, tone, and placement of the muscles of mastication and facial expression. No degenerative changes are apparent. The majority of edentulous patients have experienced some degree of degeneration. Usually, only immediate denture patients have normal musculature.

Class 2 – The patient displays approximately normal function, but slightly impaired muscle tone. Maximum muscle function cannot be used following the loss of all natural teeth.

Class 3 – The patient exhibits greatly impaired muscle tone and function. This impairment usually is coupled with poor health, inefficient dentures, loss vertical dimension, wrinkles, decreased biting force, and drooping commissures.

iv. Lips

The lips should be examined for cracking ,fissuring at the corners, and ulceration. These changes could be caused by a Vitam,in B- Complex deficiency, infection from organisms as such as Candida albicans, an excessive over closure of an existing denture, or could be neoplastic in origin. The cause of this situation must be determined before proceeding with the denture construction. The lips are then examined for support, fullness, thickness, length and mobility.

a.Length : Classify the lip lengths as Long, Normal or Medium and Short. The length of the upper lip varies from 10 mm to 36 mm. When the maxillary lip length is 10-15 mm it is classified as short lip, 16-25 mm is medium lip and 26- 36 mm is long lip. Lip length plays an important role in esthetics. A long lip reveals very little of anterior teeth, where as a very short lip allows the display of the denture base. Mould selection and denture characterization can be critical factors in these cases.

b. Thickness : The thickness of the lip should also be noted. Any change in the labio lingual position of tooth can after fullness, support, or drape of a thin lip. A thick lips gives the dentist more freedom in setting the teeth before changes manifest themselves in lip contour. Thick lips need lesser support from the artificial teeth and the labial flange on the other hand thin lips relay on the appropriate labio lingual position of the teeth for their fullness and support.

c. Support (Fig 2.9): The contour and appearance of the vermillion border usually are altered by tooth loss. Restoration of lip support and vermillion border width must be considered during placement of anterior teeth. Classify the lip support as "adequately supported or un supported". Also comment on the amount of the vermillion border visible.

d. Mobility : Classify lip mobility as Class 1 – Normal, Class 2 – Reduced Mobility, Class 3 – Paralysis. Patients with minimal lip mobility show very little of the anterior teeth. Some stroke victims may have paralysis of half the lip, leading to unilateral mouth droop and facial asymmetry. Patients must be counseled regarding the treatment limitations when dealing with such physical challenges. Others wise patients may have unrealistic expectations regarding functional and esthetic results. Comment on the unilateral reduction of mobility.

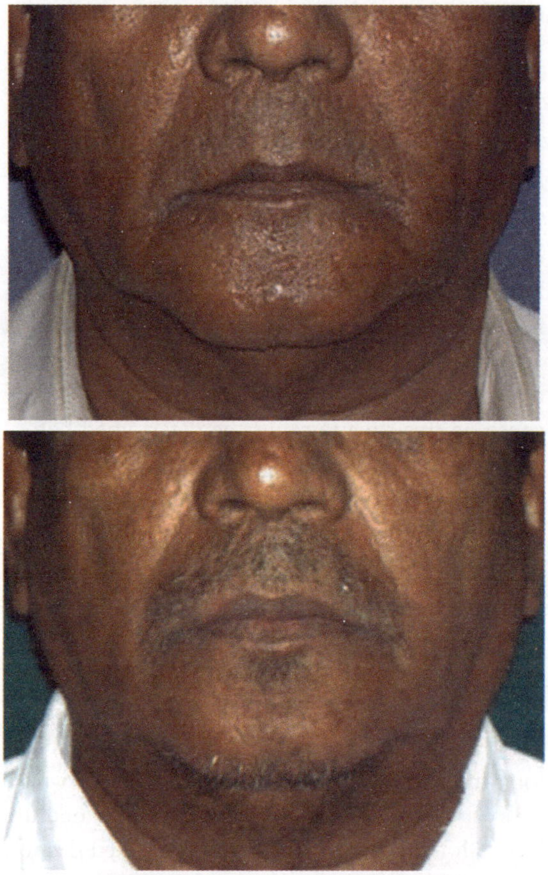

Fig. 2.9 Lip and the tooth support

v. Complexion

Hair, Eye and Skin color provide useful guides in shade selection. Skin color also can reveal underlined disease and pathology. Pale anemic looking patients may underlying systemic diseases and may require longer adjustment periods. Heavy wrinkles at the commissures and nafobial fold usually suggest decreased vertical dimension of occlusion or poor support of facial musculature by the denture.

vi. Temporo mandibular joint

Presence of pain in and around the TMJ and ear, difficulty in opening, clicking and crackling sound in the joint or any other problem in that area must be explored in detail. TMJ area is palpated for tenderness. Look for midline deviations when the patient opens and closes and evaluate any limitation of movements which may complicate the recording of centric relation and the other positions.

Mouth opening - A large opening is ideal for impression making and other procedures.A small opening, makes it difficult to remove the impression especially if the ridges have large arch form.

vii. Neuromuscular Evaluation

a.Speech: Patients who are capable of articulate speech with existing dentures (or natural teeth) usually have no problem producing articulate speech with new dentures. Patients with speech impediments or those who cannot articulate optimally with their existing dentures require special attention when the dentist places the anterior teeth and forms the palatal portions of the denture base. If normal muscle activity is altered by significantly changes in tooth placement and denture-base contour, a longer and more difficult period of adjustment may be anticipated. Classify speech as "normal" or "affected".

b. Coordination: Patients with good neuromuscular coordination can be expected to learn to manipulate dentures relatively quickly and likewise adapt readily to new dentures. Patients with poor coordination or a neurologic deficit (such as from a stroke) may never adapt to a denture completely. Classify neuromuscular coordination as follows: Class 1: Excellent, Class 2: Fair, Class 3: Poor

VIII. Intraoral examination

An overview of the oral mucosa should be obtained before a specific examination of the denture bearing area and the contiguous structures is conducted. The dentist should be looking for abnormalities or pathological lesions. The inside surface of the cheeks and lips, residual ridge, floor of the mouth, hard and soft palate and the tongue are closely examined. The tongue is pulled forward to expose the lateral borders. At the same time the anterior and posterior tonsillar pillars are viewed. This can be done effectively by wrapping an open 2 X 2 gauze pad around the anterior aspect of the tongue to aid in forcefully pulling it forward.

i. Arch form (Fig 2.10)

There are generally three forms of arches.This classification is based on the outline form of the ridges as observed in the horizontal plane.(Fig 2.10)

A. The Square type has a relatively flat curve of the anterior segment with the right and left posterior segments running backward parallel to each other.

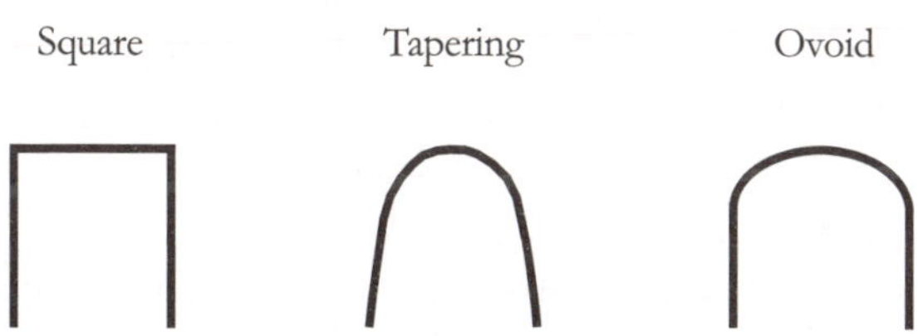

Fig. 2.10 Arch Forms

B. The Tapering type consists of flaring and diverging segments suggesting a triangle. The anterior segment may be decidedly triangular in form with its base at the cuspid line or it may be a continuation of the posterior flare. The apex of the anterior segment may be pointed, or it may be slightly round with less pronounced triangulation of the remainder of the segment. The posterior segment has a flare outward antero posteriorly.

C. The Ovoid type is rounded in the anterior and posterior segments. The curve of the anterior segment is greater than that of the square form. The posterior segment begins to swing outward at the cuspid region. The degree of outward curvature of the posterior segment varies considerably as does the size of the jaw and the alveolar process. Resorption influences the degree of observable curvature.

The square arch is more favorable for retention and stability. The ovoid is slightly less favorable and the tapering arch is the least favorable. Pure forms are seen only occasionally. It is not uncommon for the right side to differ from the left side. These variations between the anterior and posterior segments and between the right and left sides give the crossbite relation, and the variation between the upper and lower forms may result in prognathism or retrognathism. Thus a combination of arch forms may exist in one or both arches. Arch form may with more certainty be classified after casts have been obtained. This factor has an influence on the tooth set-up and alignment.

ii. Residual Ridge Form

Maxillary ridge and vault form should be classified as follows:

Class 1: Square to gently rounded,

Class 2: Tapering or "V" shaped,

Class 3: Flat

Mandibular Ridge Form: Mandibular ridge form is

classified as follows:

Class 1: Inverted "U" shaped (Parallel walls from medium to tall with broad crest),

Class 2: Inverted "U" shaped (Short with flat crest),

Class 3: Unfavorable, Inverted "W", Short inverted "V", Tall, thin inverted "V"

Undercut (results from all teeth in labial or lingual version)

iii. Inter arch space

While the patient maintains rest position part the lips and check for the space for dentures. If the space is limited, remember to use very thin base plates over the ridges and use acrylic resin teeth. A large intermaxillary space is also unfavorable because the teeth are to be placed well above the ridge, where undesirale leverage forces may be created on the ridges. 15mm inter arch space is adequate and it can be ascertained after the jaw relation stage.

Classify space as follows:

Class 1: Ideal Interarch space to accommodate the artificial teeth:

Class 2: Excessive Interarch space

Class 3: Insufficient Interarch space to accommodate the artificial teeth

iv. Ridge Parallelism

Classify ridge parallelism as follows

Class 1: Both ridges are parallel to the occlusal plane:

Class 2: The mandibular ridge is divergent from the occlusal plane anteriorly

Class 3: The maxillary ridge is divergent from the occlusal plane anteriorly or both ridges are divergent anteriorly.

v. Maxillo mandibular ridge relation

Class 1 – Normal : The lower ridge crest is slightly inside the upper ridge crest, except at the molar region where it runs outside the upper. No difficulty is expected in the positioning of teeth for proper leverage, for proper direction of stress and for obtaining maximum esthetic qualities

Class 2 – Retruded: The lower arch is smaller than the upper and the lower ridge crest is inside the upper ridge crest, more than in the normal. In retruded ridges(orthognathous) it is difficult to arrange teeth. Such patients often hold the mandible forward to improve appearance. They usually make a great range of jaw movements during function, and often require a large interocclusal distance.

Class 3 – Protruded: The lower arch is larger all around than the upper and hence the upper ridge crest is positioned inside of the lower ridge crest. When this ridge relationship is restricted to one or both posterior regions or to the anterior region, it is termed as crossbite relationship. The positioning of teeth may follow an atypical arrangement. In protruded ridges (prognathous) it is easier to arrange teeth. They usually function on a hinge (little or no protrusive component) and require a minimum of interocclusal distance. In any case, it should not be attempted to change a retrusive or protrusive position to a normal relationship.

vi. Throat form

A. Upper throat form

Throat form takes into consideration the posterior palatal seal area which is that area between the vibrating line and the posterior area of the hard palate. By virtue of variations in this region, ease or difficulty is encountered in denture adaptation. A wider post dam area is favorable for retention and is based on the throat form.

Class I - Large and normal in form with immovable tissue extending posteriorly from the hard palate for 5-12 mm. at which point the curtain of the soft palate makes an obtuse angle with the hard palate and becomes movable. It is usually present in cases with a low palatal vault and small tuberosities. It is the most favorable post dam configuration.

Class II - Medium and normal in form having immovable tissue approximately 3-5 mm. posterior to the hard palate. It is usually present in cases of moderate length and sweep of the soft palate. The junction between the hard and soft palate is more acute than in Class I.

Class III - Small with little or no immovable tissue posterior to the hard palate Such cases usually present a small short tense soft palate forming the most acute angle at the junction with the hard palate of all classes. The angle approaches a right angle. This is the least favorable post dam configuration.

Large tuberosities frequently are accompanied by a forward attachment of the tensor palatini muscle. Under these circumstances the posterior palatal periphery of the denture assumes a scalloped appearance.

One should test for displacement/compressibility of tissue by palpating the post dam area with a blunt instrument such as a T-ball burnisher. Marked displacement/compression is more favorable for good retention because a deeper posterior palatal seal can be used. Slight displacement/compression (especially with a flat ridge) can present severe retention problems.

B. Lateral throat form (Fig 2.11, 2.12a,b,c,d)

The retromylohyoid area which constitutes the lower throat form governs the distal and inferior extension of the lingual denture flange. It may be diagnosed by palpating the area while the tongue is alternately relaxed and extended. By this method, the relation of the tissue attachment to the ridge crest can be ascertained and described as:

Class I - Low - half inch or more from the mylohyoid ridge to the bottom of the retro-mylohyoid fold, visible when the tongue is in a slightly protruded position. It is the most favorable.

Class II - Medium - Less than half inch under the same conditions as above.

Class III - High - Retro-mylohyoid fold at same level as mylohyoid ridge. It is the least favorable.

The mucolingual tissues can not be displaced or compressed in the same sense as the mucobuccal tissues. Close apposition to the bone is neither desirable nor possible. The principal governing factor is the tongue in its protrusive action. Tongue position is described else where in this chapter.

At this point it may be desirable to note the patient's general muscle tone. This is in large measure controlled by the autonomic or involuntary nervous system. The ease with which impressions may be border molded depends in part on this factor as well as the patient's voluntary muscle action which may be sluggish, average or vigorous. Clinical experience will

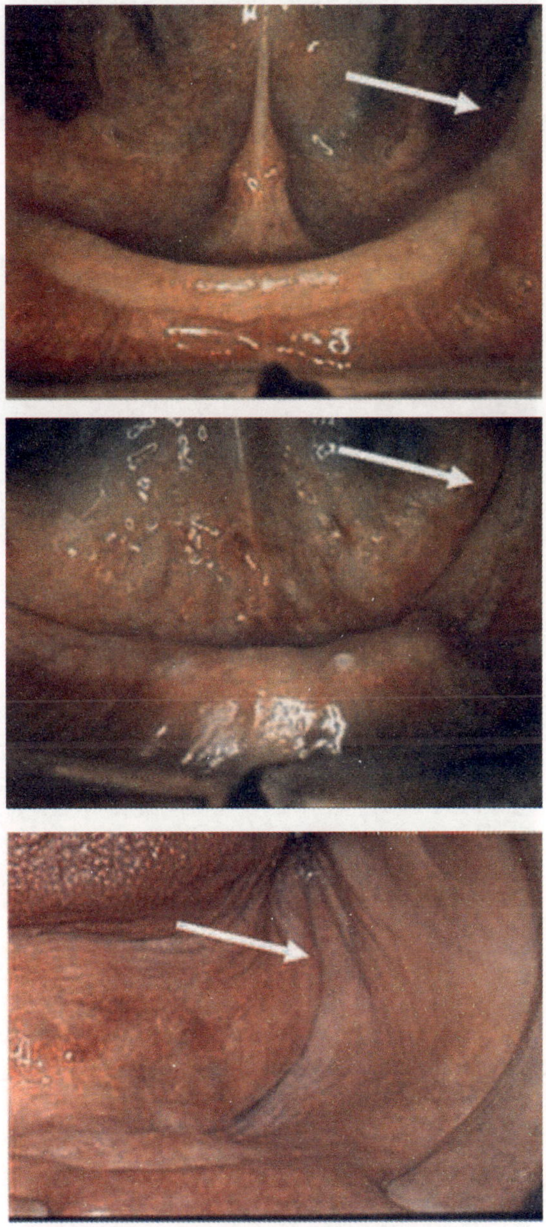

Fig. 2.11 Lateral throat form Cl. I II III

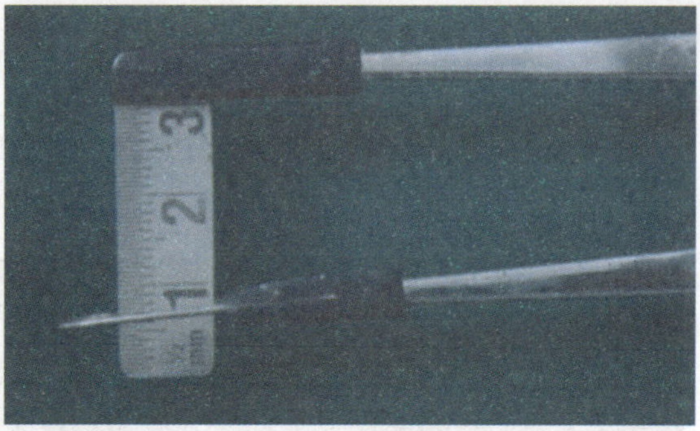

Fig. 2.12a Maaruti Chandra Sadhvi gauge to measure throat form

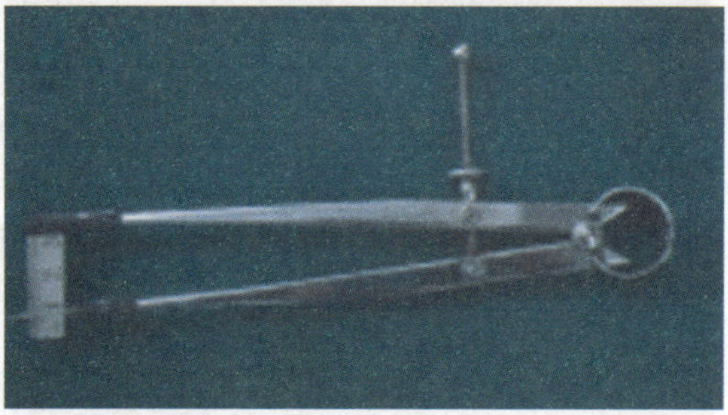

Fig. 2.12b Measuring tip consisting of (MCS Gauge) scale and the stop

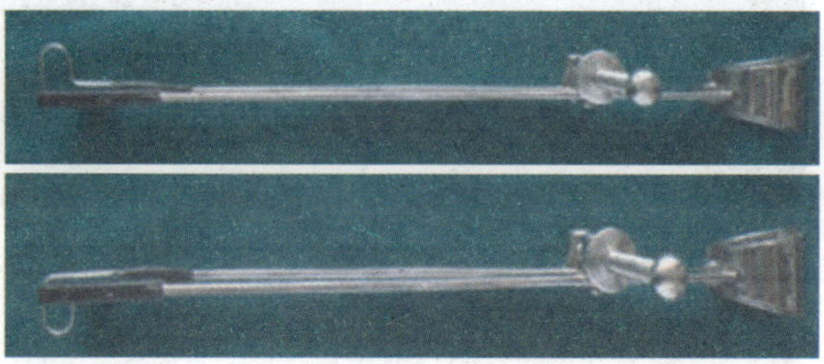

Fig. 2.12c Measuring tip repositioned for left and right side

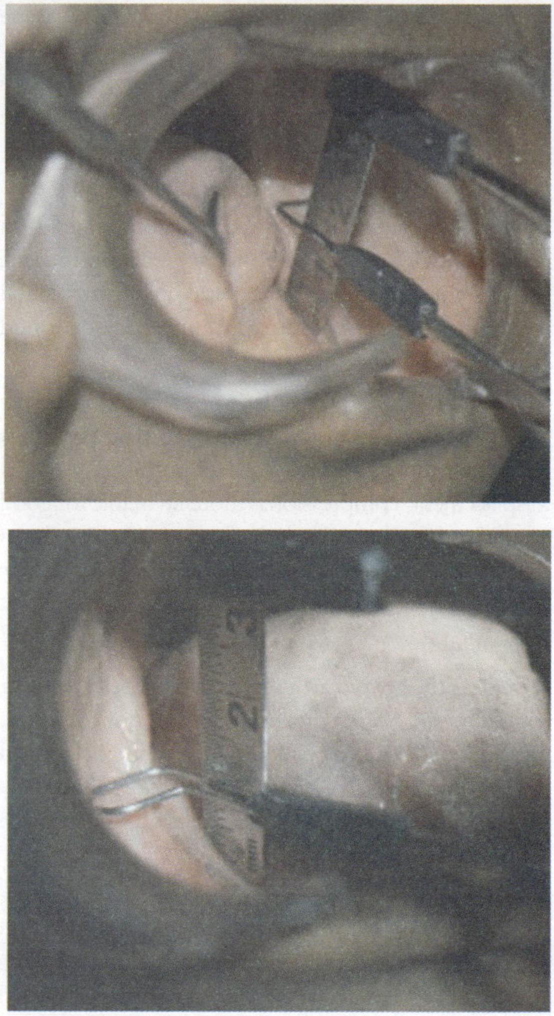

Fig. 2.12d Measuring throat form in the patient (right and left side)

determine the degree to which the operator may have to assist the patient in molding the denture borders.

vii. Soft palate : (Fig 2.13)

There are three classifications of soft palate configurations which are based on the degree of flexure the soft palate makes with the hard palate and the width of the palatal seal area.

Class I : Soft palate is rather horizontal and demonstrates little muscular movement. It is the most favorable condition because it allows for more tissue coverage for the palate seal.

Class II : Soft palate turns downward at about a 45 degree angle to the hard palate and the amount of potential tissue coverage for the palatal seal.

Class III: Soft palate turns downward sharply at about a 70 degree angle just Posteriorly to the hard palate. Since this is the most acute relation the

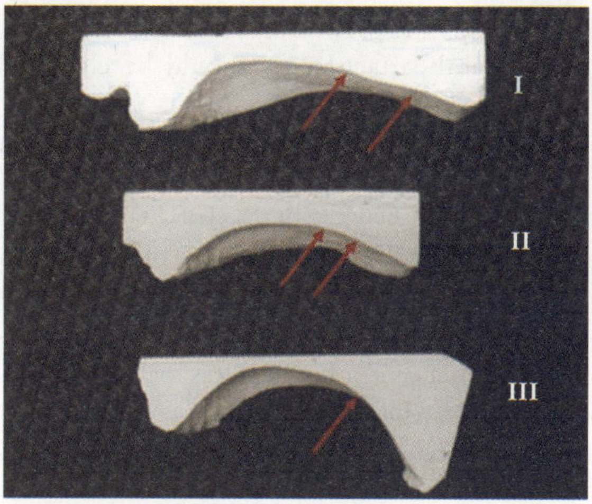

Fig. 2.13 Soft palate form Class I, II and III

Soft palate makes with the hard palate seal is at a minimum. Therefore ,This is the least favorable soft palate form. A V-shaped palate vault is usually associated with a class III soft palate. In such cases placement of the seal and its depth is most critical for maximum retention.

viii. Palatal sensitivity

Classify sensitivity according to House

Class 1: Normal

Class 2: Subnormal (Hyposensitive)

Class 3: Supernormal (Hypersensitive)

Patients tolerance to posterior extension of maxillary denture is checked. This is evaluated by lightly running the tip of the index finger over the soft palate. A slight or no response is favorable. Moderate gagging can be controlled by careful denture procedures, counseling and even medication.

Severe gaggers offer a poor prognosis and should be evaluated very carefully. Counseling and/or medication may also be indicated for the severe gaggers.

ix. Mucosa Condition

Classified according to House:

Class 1: Healthy

Class 2: Irritated

Class 3: Pathologic

Normal

Healthy mucosa is of light pink in color exhibiting no sign of injury or irritation, 1-1.5 mm. in thickness with an adequate keratin layer and evenly distributed over the ridge.

Atrophic

The mucosal covering of the bone is thin, the corium contains a reduced amount of connective tissue, the epithelial covering is also thin and the keratin is deficient or absent. Such tissue is usually seen in geriatric patients and presents problems with retention and soreness.

Hypertrophic

Here the mucosa is thickened. Usually all layers are well developed but frequently the thickening is due to an absence of connective tissue. When the keratin layer is thickened, it usually will appear white or grayish (leukoplakia) and is abnormal.

Fibrous and hyperplastic

This is most often seen in the maxillary anterior area, especially when the patient wears an upper denture against natural lower anterior teeth for a long period. If pendulous, this tissue requires careful consideration as it may be due to ill-fitting dentures, excessive vertical dimension, bruxism, allergy, or systemic conditions. Corrective surgical measures must be instituted before impression procedures are started.

More than one type of mucosa may be present in the same mouth. Tissue condition is important in providing retention, stability and support and consequently have a direct bearing on the comfort and efficiency of the denture. Atrophic mucosa lacks desired tissue resiliency and adequate seal at the periphery (especially posterior palatal seal area) is not obtained. Moreover, the tissues easily cause pain. Normal tissues are more advantageous to successful denture construction because of the optimal resiliency. However, when there is an excessive amount of tissue in a localized ridge area, it should be reduced. If surgical measures cannot be undertaken, proper placement of such tissue tends to minimize undesirable effects

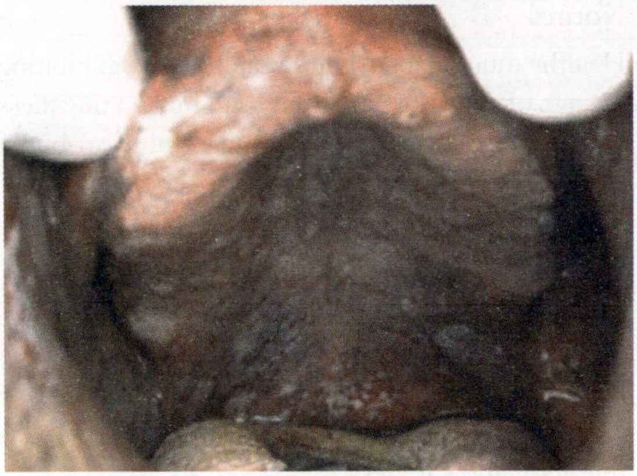

Fig. 2.14 Leukoplakia

on retention, stability and support. When a combination of tissue conditions exist in an arch, careful consideration must be given to the proper placement of the hypertrophied tissue with adequate relief over the thin tissue.

Other mucosal changes are of pathological nature and require special consideration.

Leukoplakia (Fig 2.14)

Leukoplakia is a premalignant condition which manifests as white patches on the mucous membrane of lips, tongue, and cheeks. Biopsy is the method of diagnosis. If the histologic examination indicates a premalignant lesion, the affected area should be removed. If reports state that the patch on the membrane is not premalignant and only heaped-up keratin, surgical intervention is not necessary and in that event it may be covered with a denture.

Irradiated mucosa is dark red in color, exhibiting an abraded or raw appearance, stretched and swollen. It is usually the result of ill fitting, poorly finished dentures. Impression should not be taken if signs of chronic irritation are present. Denture wearing should be avoided as far as possible and if not the denture should be modified with a tissue conditioner. Tissues previously subjected to radiation therapy are more apt to break down under the denture and special care must be exercised.

x. Attachments

a. Mucosal attachments should be classified according to House

Class 1: Attachments are high in maxilla or low in mandible with relation to ridge crest (0.5 inches/ 11mm or more between the level of attachment and crest of ridge)

Class 2: Attachment height in relation to the crest of ridge is between 0.25 and 0.5 inches or 6-11mm.

Class 3: Attachment height is less than 0.25 inches or 6mm from the ridge crest.

b.Frenal attachments should be classified according to the House (classified in similar manner as border attachments)

Class 1: High in maxilla or low in mandible with respect to crest of ridge.

Class 2: Medium

Class 3: Freni encroach on the crest of the ridge and may interfere with the denture seal. Surgical correction may be required.

xi. Saliva

Classify Saliva as follows

Class 1: Normal quality and quantity of saliva. Cohesive and adhesive properties of saliva are ideal.

Class 2: Excessive saliva contains mucus.

Class 3: Xerostomia, remaining saliva is mucinous.

The quantity of saliva is not easily discernible because all foreign bodies in the mouth excite the salivary secretions. Normal amount and viscosity is the most favorable. Thin watery saliva may affect retention. Abundant saliva is common when the denture is first inserted but usually gets adjusted with time. Thick ropy saliva complicates impression-making and is annoying to the patient as it clings to the denture. Deficient saliva is usually seen in the geriatric patient and in certain systemic disorders and poses a poor prognosis for retention and comfort.

xii. Tongue

a. Size : Classify Tongue according to House

Class 1: Normal size, development and function.

Sufficient teeth are present to maintain normal form and function.

Class 2: Teeth have been absent long enough to permit a change in the form and function of the tongue.

Class 3: Excessively large tongue. All teeth have been absent for an extended period of time, allowing for abnormal development of the size of the tongue. Inefficient dentures sometimes can lead to the development of a class 3 tongue.

b. Tongue Position: Classify according to Wright:

Normal: The tongue fills the floor of the mouth and is confined by the mandibular teeth. The lateral borders rest on the occlusal surfaces of the posterior teeth and the apex rests on the Incisal edges of the anterior teeth. There is no aberration in tongue size or activity.

Class 1: Retracted: The tongue is retracted. The floor of the mouth pulled downward is exposed back to the molar area. The lateral borders are raised above the occlusal plane and the apex is pulled down into the floor of the mouth.

Class 2: Retracted: The tongue is very tense and pulled backward and upward. The apex is pulled back into the body of the tongue and almost disappears. The lateral borders rest above the mandibular occlusal plane. The floor of the mouth is raised and tense.

Tongue position influences the establishment of the lingual contour of the denture and its retention. It helps the patient to get accustomed accustomed to use of the denture. To evaluate the position of tongue instruct the patient to open the mouth just enough to accomodate a small portion of food and observe the tongue carefully. In dentulous state, the tongue in relaxed position, completely fills the lower arch, and the apex lightly contacts the lingual surfaces of the lower teeth. This position is because of the long standing existence of teeth and is most favorable for maintaining the lingual border seal and retention in the edentulous state also. When teeth are missing for an extended period and denture replacement is delayed, the tongue becomes flattened and broadened creating a less favorable condition for denture construction particularly impression making.

Retracted position of the tongue is present in one third of the patients and has four forms:

1. Apex curls downward while the radix is elevated.
2. Apex curls up.
3. Apex seems to disappear into the body of the tongue giving it a square appearance
4. Body of the tongue is depressed.

The patient with a retracted tongue has poor lower denture prognosis unless the tongue position is improved with counseling and tongue exercises. It is easier to make an impression when the tongue is small but a seal for lower denture is often inadequate. The broad thick tongue is always in the way during the making of an impression but it provides an excellent seal for the lower denture.

IX. Investigations

Radiographs : Radiographs are usually taken to find out the presence of hidden abnormalities, to note the structure of cortical bone and trabeculae, sharp projections, thickness of soft tissue, etc. Retained roots with no apparent pathology can often be left alone provided the patient is informed of their presence and x-rayed periodically.

A. Based on Prosthodontic Diagnostic Index criteria classify bone height on oral panthogram as follows

Type I : A residual mandibular bone height of atleast 21mm, measured at the area of the least vertical bone height.

Type II : A residual mandibular bone height of 16-20mm, measured at the area of the least vertical bone height.

Type III : A residual mandibular bone height of 11-15mm, measured at the area of the least vertical bone height.

Type IV: A residual mandibular bone height of 10 mm or less, measured at the area of the least vertical bone height.

B. Lateral Cephalogram :is useful in finding out the skeletal relationship of maxilla and mandible viz. Angle Class I, Class II, Class III.

X. Diagnosis

Prosthodontic Diagnostic Index (PDI) for complete edentulism. The American college of Prosthodontics develops the official classification system for edentulisam. The system classifies, edentulous patient treatment complexity using 4 diagnostic criteria:

1. Mandibular bone height
2. Maxillomandibular relationship
3. Maxillary residual ridge morphology
4. Muscle attachments

These 4 criteria identify patients as

1. Class 1 (ideal or minimally compromised)
2. Class 2 (moderately compromised)
3. Class 3 (substantially compromised)
4. Class 4 (severely compromised)

The PDI for the Edentulous Class 1 Patient (Fig 2.15)

A patient who presents with ideal or minimally compromised complete edentulism that can be treated successfully by conventional prosthodontic techniques. The class 1 patient exhibits

- A residual mandibular bone height of at least 21mm measured at the area of least vertical bone height
- A maxillomandibular relationship permitting normal tooth articulation and an ideal ridge relationship
- A maxillary ridge morphology that resist the horizontal and vertical movement of the denture base
- Muscle attachment location conductive to denture base stability and retention

The PDI for the Edentulous Class 2 Patient (Fig 2.16)

The patient who presents with moderately compromised complete edentulism and continued physical degradation of the dentures supporting anatomy. The class 2 patient exhibits

- A residual mandibular bone height of 16-20mm, measured at the area of the least vertical bone height.
- A maxillomandibular relationship permitting normal tooth articulation and an appropriate ridge relationship.

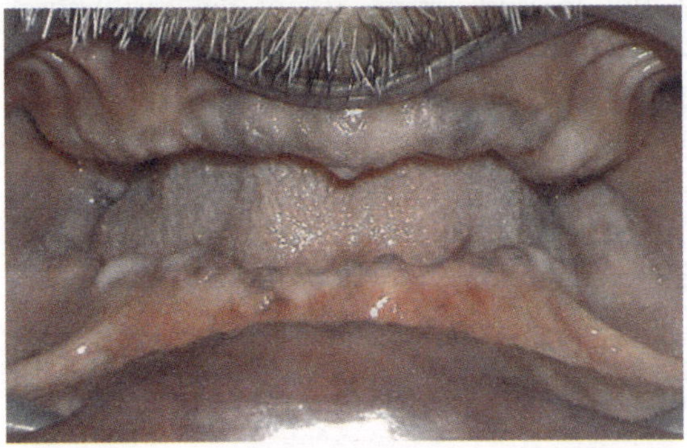

Fig. 2.15 Class I

- residual mandibular height 21mm
- maxillomandibular relation permits normal tooth articulation
- maxillary ridge resists horizontal and vertical movement of denture
- muscle attachment conducive to stability and retention

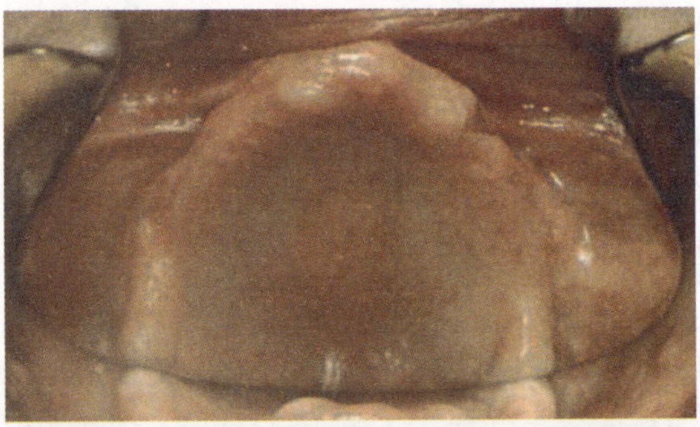

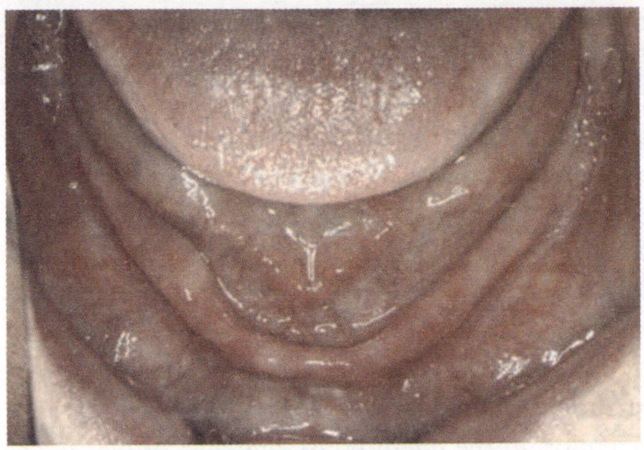

Fig. 2.16 Class II

- residual mandibular height at least 16-20mm
- maxillomandibular relation permits normal tooth articulation
- maxillary ridge resists horizontal and vertical movement of denture
- muscle attachment exerts limited compromise on stability and retention

- A maxillary residual ridge morphology that resist horizontal and vertical movement of the denture base.
- Muscle attachments that exert limited compromise on denture base stability and retention.

The PDI for the Edentulous Class 3 Patient (Fig 2.17)

A patient who presents with substantially compromised complete edentulism and exhibits

- A limited interarch space of 18-20 mm and / or temporomandibular disorders
- A residual mandibular bone height of 11-15mm measured at the area of least vertical bone height
- An angle class I, II, III maxillomandibular relationship
- Muscle attachments that exert a moderate compromise on denture base stability and retention.
- A maxillary residual ridge morphology providing minimal resistance movement of the denture base.

The PDI for the Edentulous Class 4 Patient (Fig 2.18)

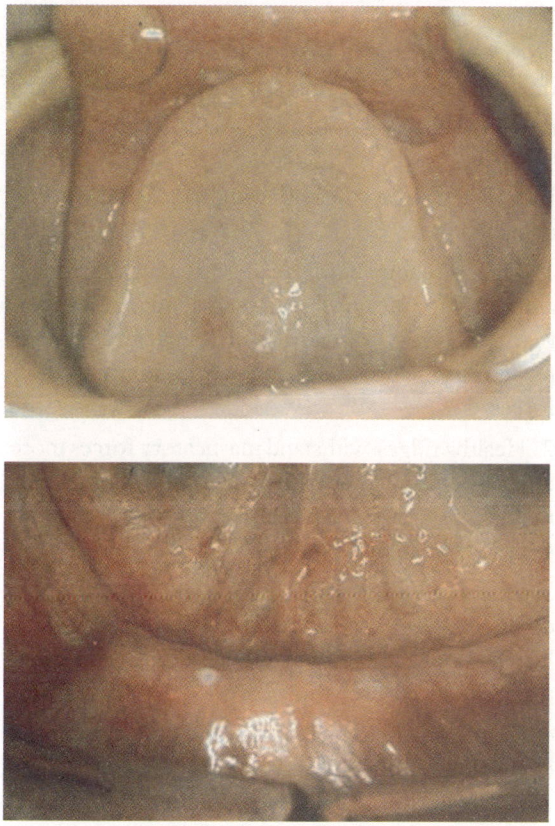

Fig. 2.17 Class III

- residual mandibular height at least 11-15mm
- maxillomandibular relation Angle Cl I, II, III
- limited inter arch space 18-20mm
- maxillary ridge offers minimum resistance to horizontal and vertical movement of denture
- muscle attachment exerts moderate compromise on stability and retention

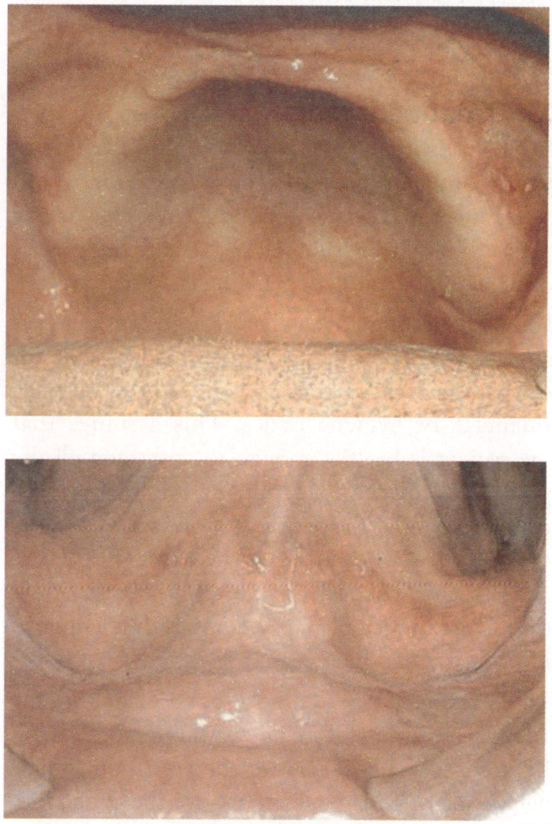

Fig. 2.18 Class IV

- residual mandibular height at least 10 mm or less
- maxillomandibular relation Angle Cl I, II, III
- limited inter arch space 18-20mm
- maxillary ridge offers no resistance to horizontal and vertical movement of denture
- muscle attachment exerts significant compromise stability and retention

A patient who presents with the most debilitated form of complete edentulism, where surgical reconstruction is usually indicated and specialized prosthodontic techniques are required to achieve an acceptable outcome.

The class 4 patient exhibits

- A residual mandibular bone height of 10mm or less
- An angle class I, II, or III maxillomandibular relationship
- A maxillary residual ridge morphology providing no resistance to movement of the denture base
- Muscle attachments that exhibit a significant compromise on denture base stability and retention.

XI. Treatment plan

While considering the prosthodontic treatment, every clinician aims for the most refined and scientific plan. Always it may not be possible to give the most ideal treatment. Hence the different levels of achievable treatment planning is discussed.

Ultimate Treatment Plan- This may be considered as absolutely the best that dentistry could provide for the patient if there were no confounding medical, financial, or hygiene issues. This assumes that the patient is healthy enough to withstand all the procedures you will do for him/her without financial restriction, and if the patient demonstrates excellent oral hygiene. For example, if the dentists expertise and patients financial condition is not a restriction, the ideal treatment plan for a completely edentulous individual would be implant supported prosthesis.

Ideal Treatment Plan- This may be very similar to the Ultimate Treatment Plan, but may need modification because of medical, or hygiene constraints. This will be the best plan tailored to give the patient the finest that dentistry can offer and one that is likely to succeed in that person's mouth. Financial restrictions are not considered.

Realistic Treatment Plan- This plan considers the entirety of the patient's problem list when developing a treatment plan. This plan is one the patient can AFFORD. The Realistic Treatment Plan may represent compromises from the ideal plan, for example conventional removable complete dentures of implants

Stabilizing Treatment Plan- This is a minimalist plan, generally driven by patient finances, but one that recognizes that the patient's future financial status, health, attitude about the importance of his/her dentition may improve. This is a plan which ensures that urgent dental needs will be resolved until such time as the patient has the desire to proceed toward establishing the best 'form, function, and esthetics.

XII. Prognosis

Prognosis provides an indicator to the course of disease or treatment. In complete denture treatment the prognosis should indicate the number of years, patient can successfully use the prosthesis with satisfaction.

In order to do so the following factors need to be considered:

1. The present mandibular bone height, after giving allowance for the inevitable residual ridge resorption that may occur, should be sufficient after 5 years to support the prosthesis and withstand masticatory forces.
2. Healthy ridges withstand masticatory forces more efficiently than flabby tissues. The flabby tissues may reduce the time of efficient denture service if not surgically treated.
3. Limited mouth opening – In substantially compromised patients - ACP class III, the vertical height is reduced. The patient's masticatory efficiency may be reduced, even though a good denture is made.
4. Nutritional status of patient – As the completely edentulous individual cannot chew well, lack of adequate nutrition will be experienced. The rate of formation of new cells may be less and new bone may not form which will affect the dynamics of remodeling of bone.
5. Medical condition of the patient – Diabetes may increase rate of residual ridge resorption, may affect healing of tissues, decreased stress tolerance. Hypertensive patients may have xerostomia, reduced

stress tolerance etc. which may reduce the expected duration of trouble free service of prosthesis

Based on these factors, the clinician can predict the prognosis of the prosthesis and rate it as good/ fair/poor.

SOAP Summary

Chart entries for initial visits, periodic evaluations, and emergency visits are well understood and legally complete if done in the form of a SOAP note. Subsequent treatment visits do not need such detail.

S=Subjective--- what the patient tells you viz. patients chief complaint, history of present illness (this complaint), past medical history, past dental history, patient expectation.

Example: Patient complains of missing teeth. States that the teeth were extracted as they were mobile or were decayed. Past medical history is non-contributory, however patient admits to smoking 1/2 pack per day of cigarettes. Past dental history – Patient's past experiences with dentist, treatments received including restorations and prosthesis if any.

O=Objective--- what you see on extraoral examination viz face – form, symmetry, profile, muscle tone development, lip, TMJ and intraoral examination, including radiographic findings if any.

Example: Extaroral examination findings including Intra-oral exam reveals displaceable fibrous tissue in the maxillary anterior region, knife edge mandibular ridge, Class III palate throat form, pigmentation in buccal mucosa,white patches on buccal mucosa, inflamed papillae on dorsal surface of tongue. Radiographic exam mandibular bone height of less than 12 mm in premolar region,impacted third molar.

A=Assessment-- problem list, or diagnoses.

Based on ACP classification criteria.

1) Bone height – mandibular
2) Residual ridge morphology – maxillary
3) Muscle attachments – mandibular
4) Maxillomandibular relationship
5) Interarch space

P=Plan—includes treatment options, materials used, stages of fabrication, financial considerations.

Example: Mention the type of treatment plan that is finalized after discussing with the patient whether removable complete dentures or removable implant retained or fixed implant supported prosthesis. Then the sequence of the treatment planning is also mentioned. Example: Primary and final impressions with elastomers, face bow transfer use of semiadjustable articulator, type of teeth selected, type of occlusal scheme planned viz lingualised, balanced etc.

Suggested reading

1. House, M. M. *Relationship of oral examination to dental diagnosis.* J Prosthet Dent l958;8:208-219.
2. Collet, B. A. *Background for psychological conditioning of the denture patient.* J Prosthet Dent 1961;11:608-616.
3. Barone J.V.*Diagnosis and prognosis in complete denture prosthesis.* J Prosthet Dent 1964;14:207-213
4. Brewer, A. A. *Treating complete denture patients.* J Prosthet Dent 1964.;14:1015-1030
5. Koper, A. *Why dentures fail.* Dent Cli N Am 1964; 8:721-734.
6. Collet, H. A. *Motivation: A factor in denture treatment.* J Prosthet Dent 1967;17:5-14.
7. Koper, A. *Difficult denture birds.* J Prosthet Dent 1967;17:532-539
8. Bolender, C. L., Swoope, C. C., and Smith, D. E. *The Cornell Medical Index as a prognostic aid for complete denturepatients.* J Prosthet Dent 1969;22:20-29.
9. Koper, A. *The initial interview with complete denture patients:Its structure and strategy.* J Prosthet Dent 1970 23:590-597.
10. Koper, A. *Human factors in prosthodontic treatment.*J Prosthet Dent 1973;30:678-679.
11. Swoope, C. C. *Predicting denture success.* J Prosthet Dent 1973;30:860-865.
12. Winkler, S. *The geriatric complete denture patient.* Dent Cli N Am 1977;21:403-425.
13. The Academy of Denture Prosthetics. *Principles,concepts, and practices in prosthodontics* - 1982. J Prosthet Dent 1982;48:467-484.
14. Alvi, H. A., Agrawal, N. K., Chandra, S., and Rastogi, M. *A psychological study of self-concept of patients in relation to artificial and natural teeth.* J Prosthet Dent 1984;51:470-475
15. Bergman, B, and Carlsson, G. E. *Clinical long-term study of complete denture wearers.* J Prosthet Dent 1985 ;53:56-61,
16. Pitts, W. C. *Difficult denture patients: Observations and hypothesis.* J Prosthet Dent 1985;53:532-534
17. Gamer.S, *M.M House classification revisited,* J Prosthet dent 2003;89:297-300
18. Perezous F Letecia, *Colonisation of candida species in denture wearers with emphasis on HIV infection : A literature review.* J Prosthet dent 2005; 93: 288-93
19. Huang Pei - Sheng et al, *The proportion of 3 classes of lateral throat form.* Int J Prosthodont 2007; 20:640-42.
20. Friedman, N, Landesman, H.M. & Wexler, M. *The influence of fear, anxiety and depression on the patient's adaptive response to complete dentures. Part I.* J Prosthet dent 1987;58: 687-693.
21. Friedman, N., Landesman, H.M. & Wexler, M. *The influence of fear, anxiety and depression on the patient's adaptive response to complete dentures. Part II.* J Prosthet dent 1988;59: 45-8.
22. Friedman, N., Landesman, H.M. & Wexler, M. *The influence of fear, anxiety and depression on the patient's adaptive response to complete dentures. Part III.* J Prosthet dent 1988;59: 169-73.

3

Case sheet – completely edentulous patients

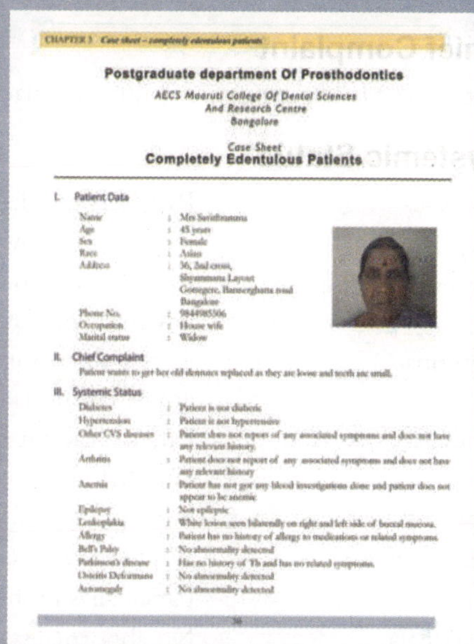

CHAPTER 3 Case sheet – completely edentulous patients

Postgraduate department Of Prosthodontics

AECS Maaruti College Of Dental Sciences
And Research Centre
Bangalore

Case Sheet
Completely Edentulous Patients

I. Patient Data

Name	:	Mrs Savithramma
Age	:	45 years
Sex	:	Female
Race	:	Asian
Address	:	36, 2nd cross, Shyammana Layout Gottegere, Bannerghatta road Bangalore
Phone No.	:	9844985506
Occupation	:	House wife
Marital status	:	Widow

II. Chief Complaint

Patient wants to get her old dentures replaced as they are loose and teeth are small.

III. Systemic Status

Diabetes	:	Patient is not diabetic
Hypertension	:	Patient is not hypertensive
Other CVS diseases	:	Patient does not report of any associated symptoms and does not have any relevant history.
Arthritis	:	Patient does not report of any associated symptoms and does not have any relevant history
Anemia	:	Patient has not got any blood investigations done and patient does not appear to be anemic
Epilepsy	:	Not epileptic
Leukoplakia	:	White lesion seen bilaterally on right and left side of buccal mucosa.
Allergy	:	Patient has no history of allergy to medications or related symptoms.
Bell's Palsy	:	No abnormality detected
Parkinson's disease	:	Has no history of Th and has no related symptoms.
Osteitis Deformans	:	No abnormality detected
Acromegaly	:	No abnormality detected

36

Patient data must be recorded in a systematic manner so that no important factor is missed

Case Sheet

Completely Edentulous Patients

I. Patient Data

Name	:	Mrs xxxxxxxxxxxxxxxxx
Age	:	xx years
Sex	:	Female
Race	:	Asian
Address	:	xx, xxxxxxxxxxxxx, xxxxxxxxxxxxxxxxxxxxxxxx xxxxxxxxxxxxxxxxxxxxxxxxx Bangalore
Phone No.	:	xxxxxxxxxx
Occupation	:	House wife
Marital status	:	Widow

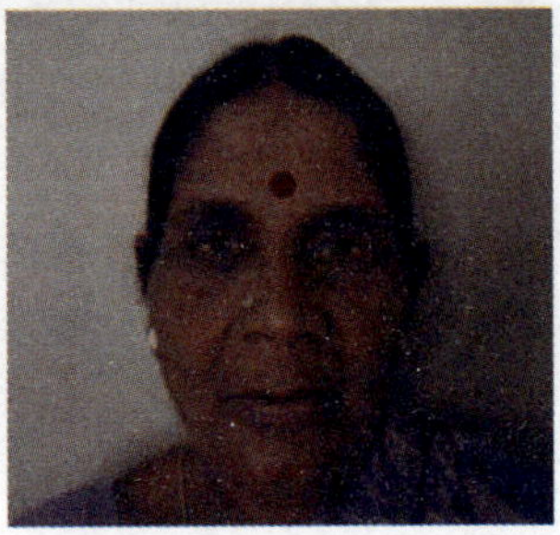

II. Chief Complaint

Patient wants to get her old dentures replaced as they are loose and teeth are small.

III. Systemic Status

Diabetes	:	Patient is not diabetic
Hypertension	:	Patient is not hypertensive
Other CVS diseases	:	Patient does not report of any associated symptoms and does not have any relevant history.
Arthritis	:	Patient does not report of any associated symptoms and does not have any relevant history
Anemia	:	Patient has not got any blood investigations done and patient does not appear to be anemic
Epilepsy	:	Not epileptic
Leukoplakia	:	White lesion seen bilaterally on right and left side of buccal mucosa.
Allergy	:	Patient has no history of allergy to medications or related symptoms.
Bell's Palsy	:	No abnormality detected
Parkinson's disease	:	Has no history of Tb and has no related symptoms.
Osteitis Deformans	:	No abnormality detected
Acromegaly	:	No abnormality detected

IV. Personal History

Diet : Mixed

Habits :

1. Smoking : Non smoker
2. Pan chewing : Chews paan since 30 years and has a habit of keeping the quid in the buccal mucosa for longer durations.
3. Alcohol : Non alcoholic
4. Clenching : Has no history of clenching teeth when teeth were present
5. Bruxism : Is not a bruxer

V. Dental History

i. History of dental extraction

Maxillary:

Reason for extraction - Pulpal

Duration of edentulism - 7 years

Mandibular:

Reason for extraction - Pulpal

Duration of edentulism - 7 years

ii. Number and type of previous denture

a) RPD: Nil

b) CD: one pair for seven years

iii. Examination of existing denture

(Subjective : what the patient feels, Objective : what the operator finds)

a. Tooth shade: A1

Tooth Material - acrylic

b. Esthetics : Subjective: Fair, Objective - Fair

c. Phonetics : Subjective / Objective - good

d. Retention : Subjective: Upper - Good, Lower - Poor

Objective : Upper - Good, Lower - Poor

e. Stability : Objective - Fair

f. Extensions : Objective - Fair

g. Contours : Objective - Fair

h. Centric relation : Objective - acceptable

i. Vertical dimension at occlusion: Inadequate

j. Occlusal plane orientation : Acceptable

k. Palate form : acceptable

l. Post palatal seal : Acceptable

m. Base adaptation : Acceptable - upper, Unacceptable - lowr

n. Midline : Acceptable

o. Buccal vesituble : Acceptable

p. Characteriuzation : Uncharacterized

q. Comfort : Acceptable - upper, Unacceptable - lower

r. Hygiene : Poor

s. Wear : Moderate wear.

* Subjective : Patient's opinion, Objective : Operator evaluation

iv. Pre extraction Records : None available
Photographs: Not available
Diagnostic casts : Not available

VI. Mental Attitude: Ideal

VII. Extra Oral Examination

i.	Facial form	:	Ovoid
ii.	Profile	:	Straight
iii.	Muscle tone	:	Class II
iv.	Lips (Static Position)		
	a) Length	:	The length of the upper lip when measured from the depth of buccal vestibule to the dry wet junction is 22 mm.
	b) Thickness	:	6mm
	c) Support	:	Unsupported
	d) Mobility	:	Normal – no pathology found during function
	e) Inter commissural width	:	Passive – 59 mm, Active – 81 mm
v.	Complexion	:	Dark
vi.	Temporomandibular joint		
	a) Tenderness	:	No tenderness on palpation
	b) Mouth opening	:	Normal, has no pain during opening or closing the mouth, the distance between the upper and lower vermilion border at maximum opening – 56 mm
	c) Deviation	:	No deviation of the mandible observed on closing the mouth
	d) Clicking	:	No clicking sounds detected on auscultation of the TMJ area
vii.	Neuro muscular evaluation:		
	a) Speech	:	Normal
	b) Co-ordination	:	Excellent on asking the patient to touch the right shoulder with left hand and vice- versa

VIII. Intra oral Examination

i.	Arch form	:	Square tapering
ii.	Residual Ridge Form	:	
	Maxillary	:	Class II
	Mandibular	:	Class II – short with flat crest
iii.	Inter arch space	:	23mm when measured in the premolar region at rest position.
iv.	Ridge Parallelism	:	Class I – As the ridges are parallel to each other
v.	Ridge Relationship	:	Angle's Class I
vi.	Throat form	:	
	a. Upper throat form	:	Class I
	b. Lateral Throat form	:	Class I – functional height -5 mm when measured from the floor of the mouth to height of lower ridge in region of retro mylohyoid fossa.

vii. Soft Palate : Class I
viii. Palatal Sensitivity : Absence of gagging on normal stimulation
ix. Mucosa Condition : Class II – Inflamed
x. Attachment
Mucosal :
Maxilla : Class I – 11 mm
Mandible : Class III – 5 mm
Frenal :
Maxilla : Class II – 8 mm
Mandible : Class III – 5 mm
xi. Saliva : Class I
Quality : Serous
Quantity : Adequate
xii. Tongue:
Size : Normal
Position : Normal

IX. Investigations

Radiographs :

1. O.P.G - Mandibular height - Type I – 20mm
2. Lateral ceph. - Angle's Class I

Routine blood investigations: Adv. RBS, Blood pressure.

X. Diagnosis

According to PDI patient belongs to Class I Ideally or minimally compromised because

a. Residual mandibular bone height is greater than 21mm when measured at the area of least vertical bone height.
b. The maxillomandibular relationship allows normal tooth articulation and ideal ridge relationship is present
c. The maxillary ridge morphology resists horizontal and vertical movement of the denture base
d. Muscle attachment location is conducive to denture base stability and retention.

XI. Treatment Plan

Tissue conditioning : Tobacco induced mucositis on buccal mucosa, advised to apply Retino A ointment locally thrice daily for a month. Patient has been infomed of ill effects of tobacco on oral health and is advised to refrain from the same.

Preprosthetic surgery : Not indicated

Impression procedure :

Primary impression : Putty and light body impression for - upper and lower.

Final impression : Border molding with putty and impression with light body – upper and lower

Jaw relations and Articulator:

Face bow transfer : Hanau Arbitrary Spring bow earpiece type

Articulator : Semi adjustable, Arcon type, Hanau wide view

Control settings
- 30^0 horizontal condylar guidance
- 30^0 lateral condylar guidance
- 0^0 incisal guide angle

Tooth selection :

Shade : A2

Mold : 45 mm -Total mesiodistal width of the upper anterior teeth

Material : Acrylic resin

No. of teeth : 24

Denture base material: Heat – cured PMMA resin

XII. Prognosis:

Fair

Doctors' Signature

SOAP Summary

A 45 year old female patient named xxxxxxxxxxxxxxx reported to the clinic with the chief complaint of replacement of existing dentures as they are loose and teeth have worn down. Patient has no significant medical history except that she has gastric ulcer and is on medication for the same. She has been completely edentulous in both maxilla and mandible since 7 years with history of extraction of teeth due to decay. Extraoral examination reveals ovoid facial form, with straight profile. Intra oral examination reveals sq. tapering arch form, Class II maxillary and Class II mandibular ridge form, Class I ridge relationship, ideal interarch space, Class I ridge parallelism, Class I palate, Class III frenal and mucosal attachments in the mandible, Class I mucosal and Class II frenal attachments in the maxilla, Cl. I Lateral throat form. Patient has been in the habit of chewing paan for the past 30 years and so has tobacco induced muocistis on right and left buccal mucosa. OPG reveals bone is of adequate quantity and is loosely packed trabaculae. Saliva is of adequate quantity and serous in nature. The Patient belongs to ACP Class I Ideal or minimally compromised. Informed consent is obtained after explaining the treatment procedure and is also informed about the various treatment options including implants. Treatment planning involves primary impression with putty for - upper and lower. For the final impression, border molding will be done with putty and impression with light body. Face bow transfer will be done using Hanau Arbitrary Spring bow earpiece type face bow and will be transferred to a semi adjustable, Arcon type, Hanau wide view Articulator. The mold of artificial teeth that is selected is 45 mm mesiodistal width of upper anteriors and shade A2. Prognosis is fair.

4

Nutrition for complete denture wearers

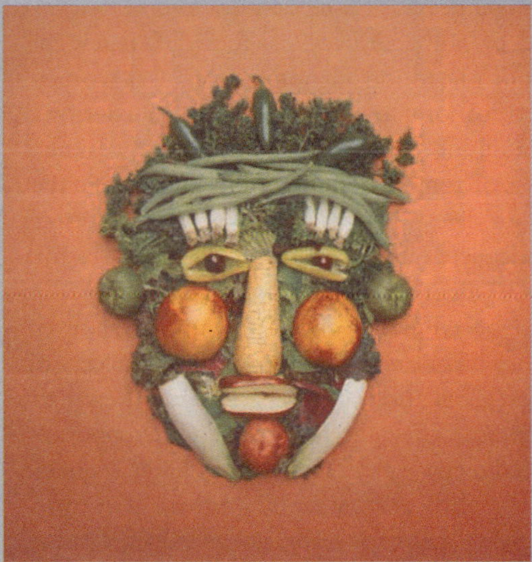

Edentulous individual and denture wearer are prone to nutritional dificiencies because of the handicap experienced in chewing.

Nutrition is the science that deals with composition of food, the role of food in the maintenance of good health and the various methods to bring about proper nourishment. The council on Food and Nutrition of the American Medical Association defines nutrition as, "the science of foods, the nutrients and the substances therein, their action, interaction and balance in relation to health and diseases". The average nutritional requirements of different groups of people are fixed and that will depend on various factors such as age, sex, height, weight, degree of activity and rate of growth. Nutrition is greatly depended on oral health status. One in five of the older people reported that oral condition prevented them from eating the food they would choose, 15% took longer time to complete their meal and their enjoyment of food was limited by oral condition, 5% avoided eating certain food because of chewing problems. In addition, a poor diet coupled with a sedentary lifestyle are known to be risk factors for life- threatening chronic diseases viz heart disease, stroke, hypertension, diabetes and some form of cancer and death. Tissue dehydration, xerostomia caused by polypharmacy, calcium deficiency and osteoporosis found in postmenopausal women, fragility of oral mucosa resulting in frictional trauma during denture wearing, muscle weakness and loss of tonicity resulting from low protein diet and poor digestion and absorption are the results of inadequate nutrition. Presence of these factors should be identified and the patients and caretakers should be educated about the importance of adequacy of nutrition and its role in the success of dental rehabilitation. Complete denture treatment may adversely affect the health of denture supporting tissues directly or indirectly. The direct sequelae include denture stomatitis, denture irritation, hyperplasia, traumatic ulcer, flabby ridges, residual ridge resorption, mucosal ulcerations, altered taste perception, burning mouth syndrome and gagging. Indirect sequelae are related to reduced chewing ability with an overall reduction in the functional capacity and general health. Inadequate diet can lead to reduced tolerance of the tissues to normal wear and tear and this reduced resistance, in turn, can result in poor adaptation to dentures. Loose denture, sore spots under denture, severely resorbed mandible, difficulty in chewing, eating less food, inability to arrange food for oneself, unexpected excessive weight gain or weight loss, alcohol or drug abuse, and undergoing chemotherapy or radiation therapy can be considered as risk factors related to nutritional deficiencies.

Nutritional guidelines

The recommended dietary requirement calls for an average caloric intake of 2400 Kcal/day for men and 2000 Kcal/day for women. Health problems arise when the intake is less than 1600 Kcal/day. Out of the total daily caloric intake, about 60 per cent should come from the carbohydrates, 25 per cent from the fats and 15 per cent from the proteins. One gram of carbohydrates gives about 4 calories and so is the case with proteins, while 1 gram of fat gives about 9 calories.

Carbohydrates: The richest source is plant starch present in wheat, rice, corn and potatoes. It should be not less than 100 gms per day.

Proteins: There are two sources in our diet. One is animal protein (its sources are meat, egg, milk, paneer, etc) and the other is plant protein. (sources: pulses, soyabean peas, mushrooms, etc) Adequate dietary protein intake is crucial for senior citizens. Four eggs a week can be safely included in the diet.

Fats: There are two types of fats in our daily diet. One is saturated fats — the sources are cream, butter, ghee, meat, yolk of egg, milk, coconut oil, etc. The second type is unsaturated fats which are mono-unsaturated and polyunsaturated fats. The sources of mono-unsaturated fats are mustard oil, olive oil, til oil, etc. while the sources of poly-unsaturated fats are refined oils, especially Saphola and Ricela (rice bran). Emphasis should be on reducing the intake of saturated fat and choosing unsaturated fat.

TransFats: Commonly known as vanaspati, are the most harmful of the dietary fats. They are more atherogenic than saturated fats and can raise total cholesterol and LDL-C ("bad cholesterol") and lower HDL-C ("good cholesterol"). Eliminating trans fats (Vanaspati) from the diet is very important to prevent chronic disease. Read food labels carefully and avoid foods which mentions trans fats (partially and hydrogenated vegetable oils). Trans fats are the commonly used in most restaurants, fast-food chains, road side stalls, commercial baked foods and Indian sweets and savouries. The food industry uses trans fats as they are cheaper and they are known to impart a longer shelf life to the food products. (Fig. 4.1)

Minerals and vitamins

An adequate intake is essential as the agents that enhance the health of the elderly. The important minerals are calcium, zinc, iron, copper, sodium, potassium, etc. and their sources are essentially from green leafy vegetables, fruits, carbohydrates and milk. Important vitamins are Vitamin-E, Vitamin-C, Vitamin-A, Vitamin-D, Riboflavin and Vitamin B12. The sources are green leafy vegetables, yellow fruits, cod liver oil, fish oil, carrots, sprouted grams/dals, milk, butter, citrous fruits, amla, chillies, etc. Seasonal cheap and easily affordable fruits and vegetables are rich in minerals, vitamins and fibres.

Calcium

It is very essential for an average elderly person. As people become older, the bones become demineralised. This is called osteoporosis. So calcium intake should be not less than 400 mg per day. Food rich in calcium are ragi, green leafy vegetables, milk, fenugreek leaves, drumstick leaves and sea food. Phosphorus, dietary fibre, drugs, alcohol, menopause, illness and exercise may all affect absorption of minerals in the body.

Iron

Deficiency of iron leads to anaemia. So the diet of the elderly should contain sufficient amount of iron. Greens are rich in iron, cheaper than other vegetables and are available easily most of the time. Elders should include some variety of greens in their diet everyday. Other foods rich in iron are wheat flour, ragi, jaggery, dates and liver. The recommended daily allowance is 30 mg. per day.

Water

Though water has no caloric value, it should be taken in sufficient quantity along with food or otherwise. The elderly do not recognise the need to maintain the volume of water excreted. The fluid intake should be atleast 1.5 - 2 lts per day in a normal elderly person.

Fibre

The elderly require sufficient fibre or roughage in their diet to avoid constipation. Fibre is the undigestible carbohydrate present in the food. Rough fibre is not well-tolerated by the intestine in old people. But, the tender fibre of vegetables, fruits and whole-grain cereals will encourage normal bowel movements. The elderly tend to use harmful laxatives and mineral oils. This should be substituted by a fibre-rich diet and adequate fluid intake. Fibres help in lowering blood cholesterol (fat circulating in blood) levels which are risk factor for coronary artery disease. Some good sources of dietary fibre are ragi, wheat, Italian millet, horsegram, green leafy vegetables, plantain stem, drumstick, bittergourd, fruits like dates, figs, guava, wood apple and sweet lime

Vegetables

Habitual consumption of a variety of fresh vegetables everyday reduces the risk of hypertension, stroke, coronary heart disease, cancer, diabetes and other chronic diseases. Vegetables have unique combinations of nutrients like folate, vitamins, minerals, fiber, anti-oxidants and are relatively low in calories. All these work together to protect the body from disease. They have a high water content and low energy density which also assist in weight control. It is recommended that all age groups should consume a minimum of 300-400 gms of vegetables everyday (along with a minimum of 200- 250 gms fruits everyday). A variety of seasonal, locally available and cheap vegetables can be opted for. Locally available berries and greens are desirable.

Fruits

Fruits contain unique combinations of micro and macronutrients and anti-oxidants. Daily regular consumption of fruits leads to lower the risk of high blood pressure, stroke (paralysis), coronary artery disease, cancer, diabetes and other chronic diseases. It also enhances the body's immune system, prevents acute diseases and delays ageing. It lowers blood pressure in persons already having high blood pressure. It is recommended that all age groups should consume a minimum of 200-300 gm of fruits daily (along with a minimum of 250 gm or more of vegetables).

Grains

Grains form the integral part of Indian diet providing proteins, iron, fiber and many micronutrients. Whole grains are more nutritious and disease preventing than refined grains. Freshly made refined grain products like boiled rice, idli, upma, dosa etc are better then packed refined grain products (pasta, noodles). Rotis are better than buns. Wheat ground from a chakki is better rather than buying readymade flours. Partially polished rice is better than polished rice. In India, foods labeled with "stone ground", "100% wheat", "bran" are usually not whole grain products. Draining the excess of water while cooking rice depletes them of valuable vitamins and it should be avoided. Idlis and dosas made with brown rice are preferable to those made from white rice.

Pulses (dals)

Pulses in the Indian diet are the primary source of protein. It is important to eat dal every day more so in vegetarians. Each dal has a unique combination of amino acids . Dal needs to be combined with

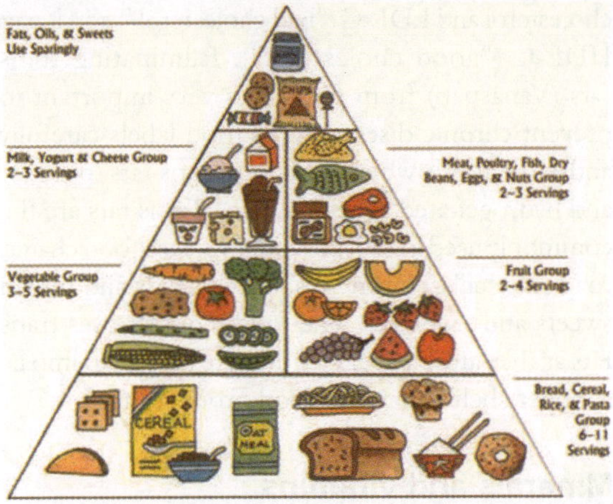

Fig. 4.1 Food Pyramid

grains or another dal to provide total protein to the body. In non vegetarians pulses can be substituted with fish, chicken and meat. Pulses provide vegetable protein, complex carbohydrate, dietary fiber, vitamins, minerals and isoflavones. All pulses have low glycemic index and are rich in soluble fibre. A variety of dals can be included in daily diets that. All freshly made dals are healthy and nutritious. Dehusking or milling of dals decreases their nutritive value and fiber content.

Table 4.1 Recommended Daily Allowances for Indian Elderly (ICMR)

Nutrients	Male	Female
Calories (Kcal)	1800	1400
Protein (gms)	60	50
Fat (gms)	50	40
Calcium (mg)	400	400
Iron (mg)	28	30
Vitamin A (microgram)	2400	2400
Thiamine (mg)	1.2	0.9
Niacin (mg)	16	12
Riboflavin (mg)	1.4	1.1
Vitamin C (mg)	40	40

Ideal diet for Edentulous Indian

Early morning : 1 cup coffee/tea

Breakfast : Idly – 3 or Pongal- 1½ cup or Upma 1½ cup or Bread – 4 slices or Apple- 1

Mid morning : Milk – 3/4th cup or Buttermilk – 1 cup or Soup – 1 cup or Fruit juice – 1 glass

Lunch : Cooked rice 1½ cups or Chappatis 3 medium, Dhal ½ cup or sambhar ¾ cup or or minced chicken or well cooked fish, rasam, curd 1/2 cup or butter milk 1 cup or Greens – ¾ cup

Tea : 1 cup coffee/tea, Biscuits 2

Dinner : Cooked rice- 1 ½ cup, soft raw fruits like banana, papaya, cooked apples, paneer or egg white or greens ¾ cup

Bedtime: 1 cup of milk (Table 4.1)

Excessive intake of Zinc

Zinc is used in denture adhesives to improve the bond between dentures and residual ridge. Zinc concentrations ranging from about 17,000 to 34,000 g/g were identified in denture adhesives. Chronic, excess zinc intake can result in copper deficiency and profound neurologic disease. Many people have claimed that they've suffered neurological damage leading to numbness, partial paralysis. Dietary zinc prime sources include meat, poultry, beans, nuts and oysters is good for people, to a point. It bolsters the immune system and promotes wound healing, among other benefits. But too much zinc has long been known to cause neurological problems. Many manufacturers have started producing zinc free denture adhesives. Recommended dietary intake of Zinc is 8-11 mg per day.

Suggested reading

1. Maury Massler, *Geriatric nutrition: The role of taste and smell in appetite,* J Prosthet Dent, 1980;43(3):247 -50
2. Maury Massler, *Geriatric nutrition II: Dehydration in the elderly,* J Prosthet Dent, 1979;42(5):489-91
3. James V. Barone, *Nutrition-Phase one of the edentulous patient,* J Prosthet Dent, 1978;40(2):122-26
4. Robert E. Schifferle, *Nutrition and Periodontal Disease,* Dent Clin N Am 2005; 49 595–610
5. Hutton Brian, Feine Jocelyne, Morais José, *Is There an Association Between Edentulism and Nutritional State?* J Can Dent Assoc 2002; 68(3):182-7
6. Boyd D Linda, *Importance of Nutrition for Optimum Health of the Periodontium,* The Journal of Contemporary Dental Practice, 2001; 2(2): 1-14

5

The face and the mouth

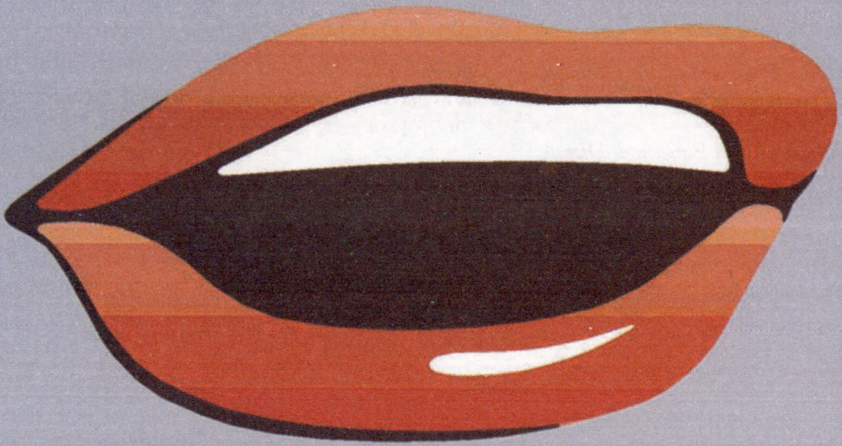

Facial features and oral conditions will influence the design of the denture

A person requiring complete dentures must first be examined for the facial features. The overall shape of the face can be rectangular, ovoid, tapering or a combination of these three. For this assessment the angle of the mandible, the zygomatic arch and the sides of the forehead will provide valid information. If a person is observed from the front, an operator will get an impression of the general outline of the face. Understanding the outline form of the face will provide a basic frame work on which the outline of the incisors can be worked out. A similarity in the outlines will make the teeth harmonize with the facial features and hence artificiality of the dentures can be masked to a greater extent. Then the face must be observed from the side to get a profile view. In the profile, the position of the chin is to be observed first. If the observer feels that the chin is positioned much anterior to the nose tip, a discrepancy in the arch size can be expected. Similarly if the chin is positioned far back, again a discrepancy in the arch size can be observed. In the former condition the mandibular arch will be bigger where as in the latter the mandibular arch will be smaller.

The soft tissue contour of the upper lip should then be observed. In an edentulous individual, the angle formed by the columella of the nose and the upper lip will be more than 90 degrees. If the angle is 90 degrees or less than that in an edentulous individual, it can be presumed that the residual ridge is so prominent and adequate space for the labial flange may not be available. The philtrum may be ill developed in an edentulous individual because of lack of support. On providing adequate support, philtrum will appear slightly concave in the profile view. Convex contour of the philtrum is unnatural. Face should then be examined for symmetry. If there is an asymmetry in the over all outline, further investigation must be done to find out the reasons for the asymmetry. Mid sagittal plane is to be identified in determining the symmetric features of the face. The tubercle of the philtrum and the centre of the eye brows if connected by a straight line will provide valid information in determining the mid sagittal plane. Nose cannot always be relied upon because it gets tilted in many individuals. Mid sagittal plane is identified to develop the smile symmetrically. If midline of the dental arch and midline of the face are coincided, aesthetics is easily achieved.

Complete dentures are placed on residual ridges. Residual ridges are formed by the loss of teeth and the subsequent remodeling of alveolar bone. Maxillary residual ridges become smaller in dimensions when compared to that of the dental arches where as the mandibular ridges become bigger. This is because of the direction of the resorption which eventually makes the maxillary arch smaller than the mandibular arch especially in width. Maxillary denture bearing area including the ridges and the palate will be around 20 sq cm and the mandibular 12 sq cm. The masticatory load is to be transmitted to these limited areas. The masticatory load in the dentulous state was transmitted to an area of 40 sq.cm. provided by the specialized tissue of periodontium. The reduction in the area makes the residual ridges more vulnerable and hence in the course of the use of complete dentures residual ridges undergo resorptive changes. In the dentate condition, the bones were subjected to tensile loading applied through the periodontal ligament which is well tolerated. However, dentures provide compressive loading, which is not well tolerated by the bone and hence it can set in resorption. Size of the residual ridges becomes important in this context.

Broader ridges will support the dentures well. Both the maxillary and mandibular ridges have a mucosal covering which by its viscoelastic nature dampens the load applied on to the ridges when an individual masticates with the dentures. In the maxilla, the ridges and the palate are covered by masticatory mucosa which is well adhered to the underlying bone. In the midpalatine region, the mucosal cover has got very limited compressibility where as on the ridges and on the slopes, the compressibility goes up to 1or 2 mm. On the outer periphery of the ridge, the mucosa appears glossy and it lines the muscles attached to the bone forming a sulcus which when copied in an impression will have a width of 3 to 6mm. Posteriorly the hard palate continues as the soft palate which moves during swallowing, speech, breathing and related functions. The movement of the soft palate is to be identified so that the posterior border of the denture can be limited to the soft palate tissue which will not move in a pronounced fashion. The line on which the curling movement visibly occurs is known as vibrating line.

The border tissues of the maxillary ridges have a profound influence in shaping the borders of the denture. In the midline, the labial frenum has to function freely so that the dentures are provided a

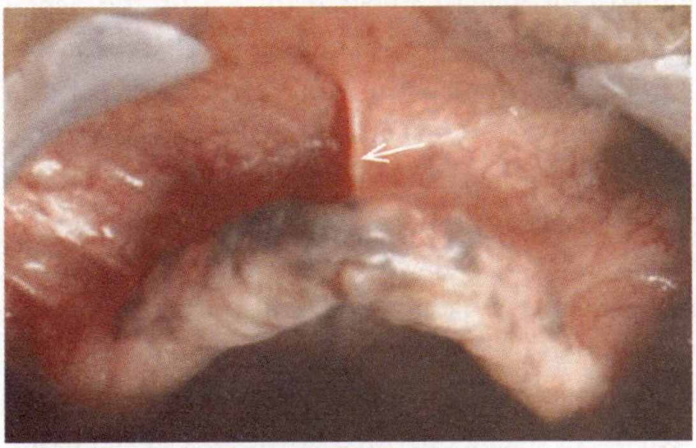

Fig. 5.1 Labial frenum

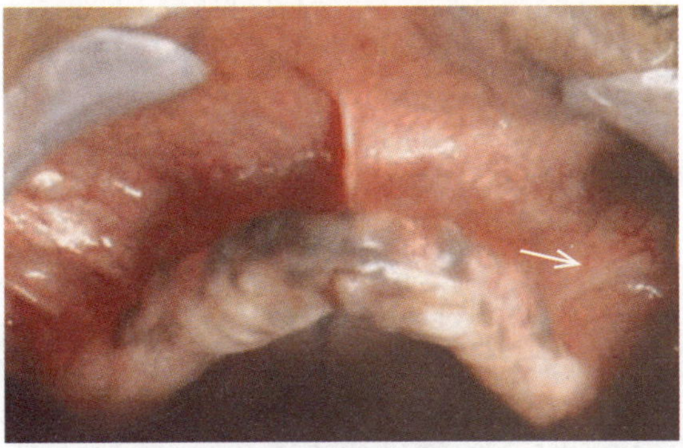

Fig. 5.2 Buccal frenum

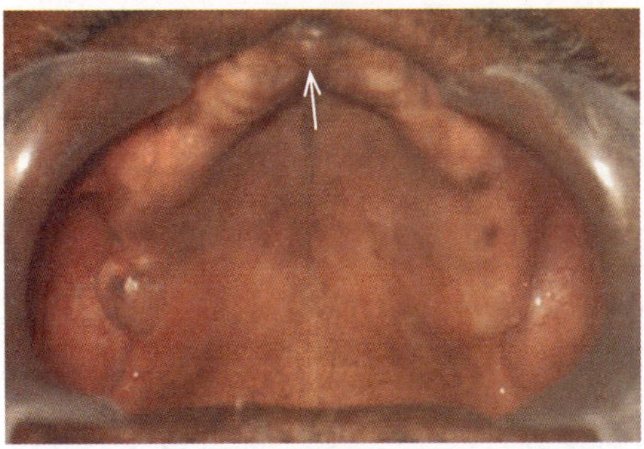

Fig. 5.3 Incisive papilla

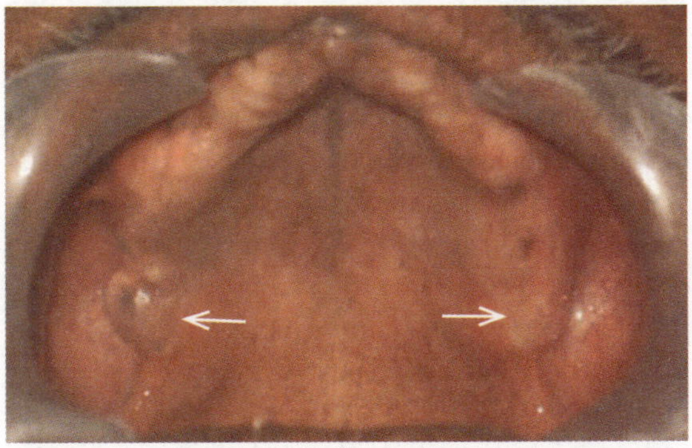

Fig. 5.4 Maxillary tuberosity

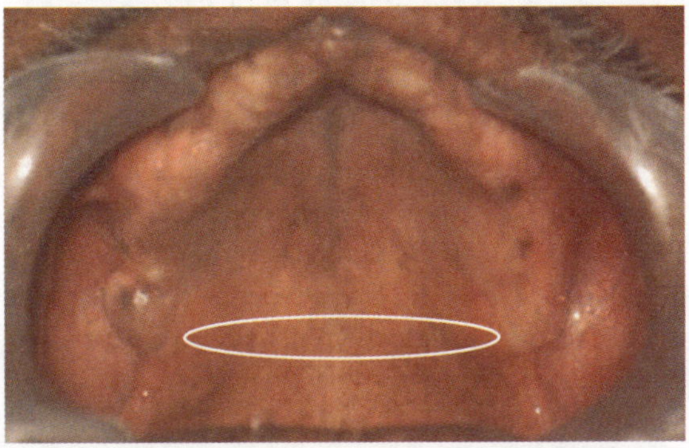

Fig. 5.5 Posterior palatal seal area

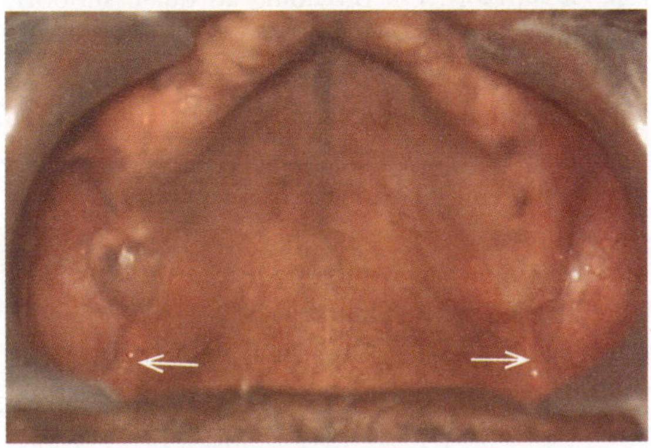

Fig. 5.6 Hamular notch

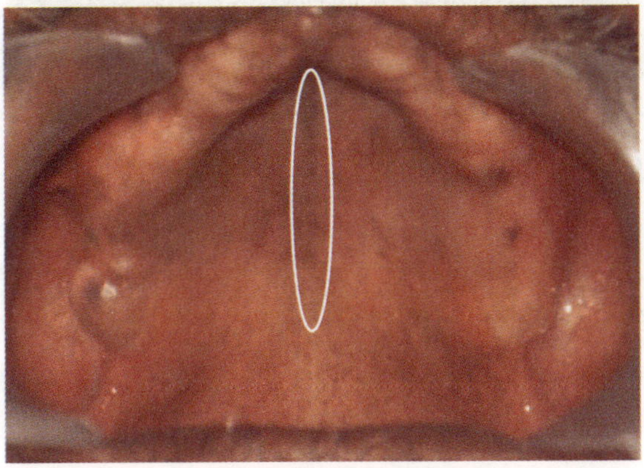

Fig. 5.7 Mid-palatine raphae

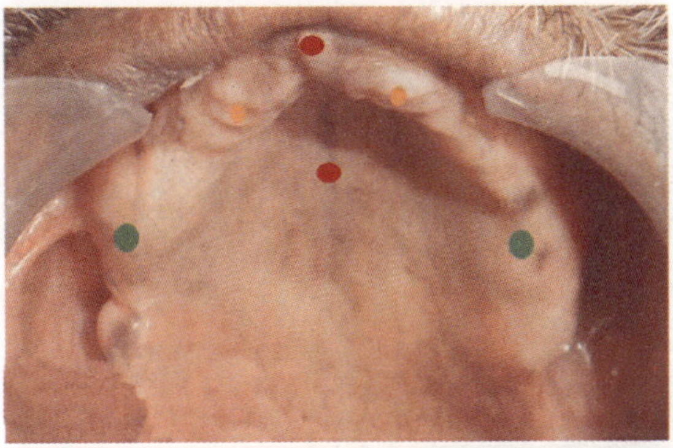

Fig. 5.8 Green: Primary stress bearing area Residual alv. ridge, Yellow: Secondary stress bearing area: Rugae, Relief Areas: incisive papilla, mid palatine raphae

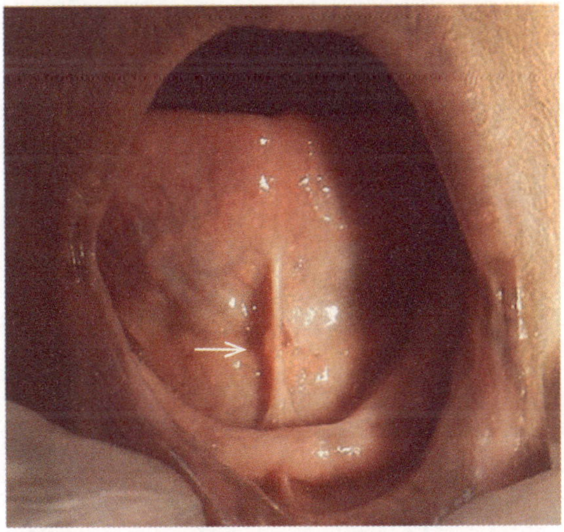

Fig. 5.9 Lingual frenum

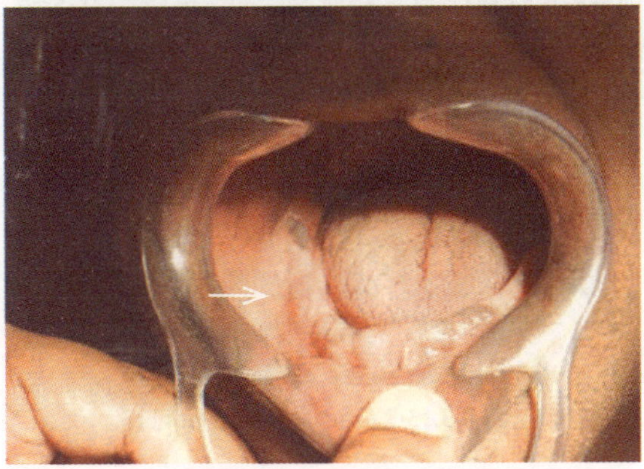

Fig. 5.10 Buccal sulcus

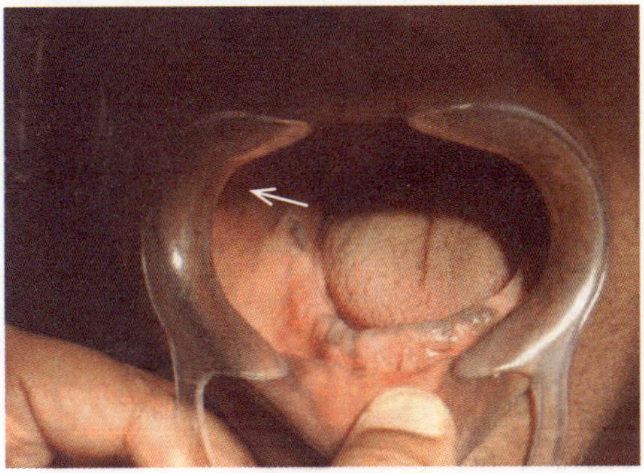

Fig. 5.11 Massetric notch

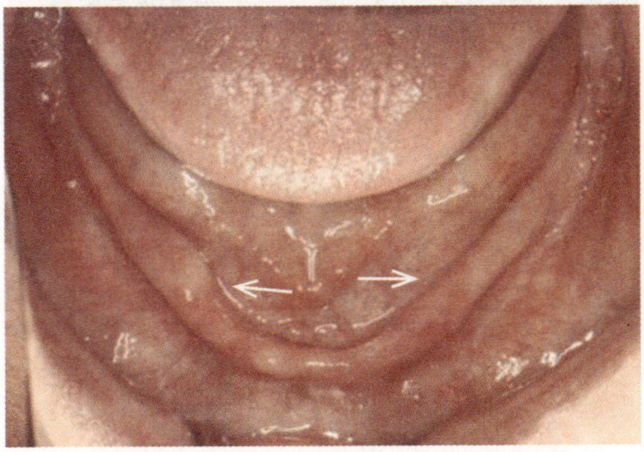

Fig. 5.12 Lingual sulcus

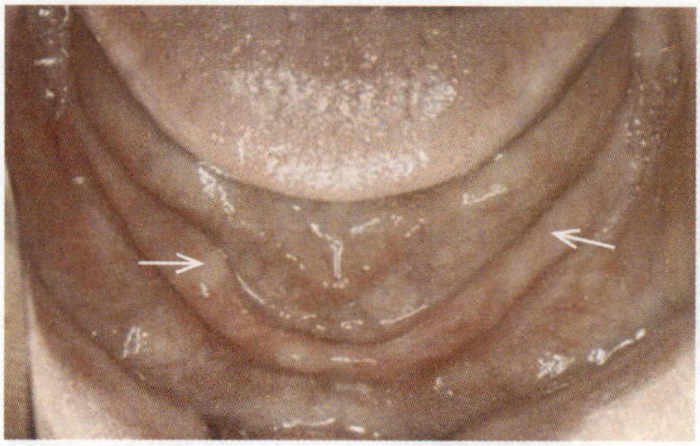

Fig. 5.13 Resdiual alveolar ridge

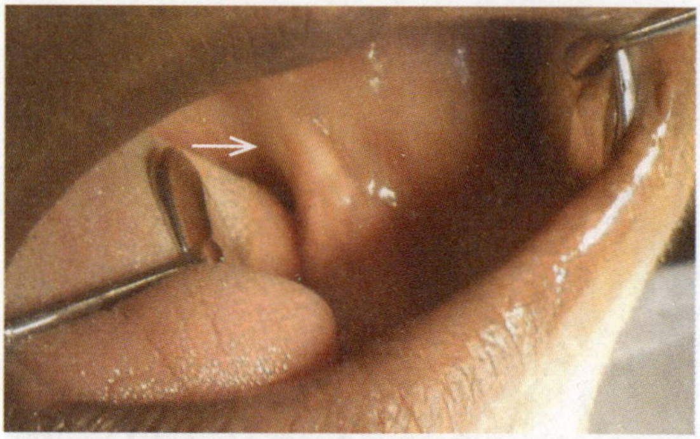

Fig. 5.16 Retromylohyoid curtain

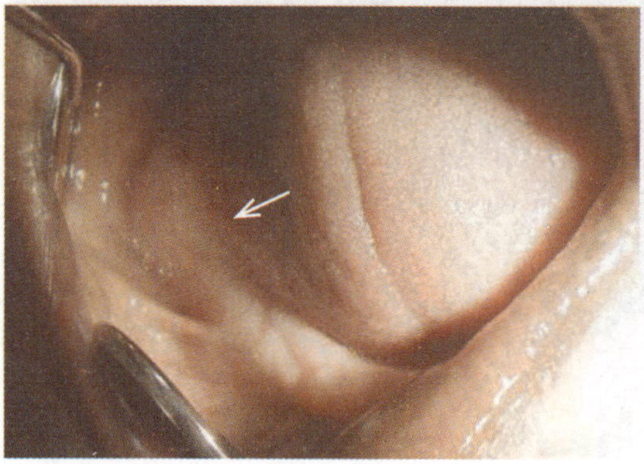

Fig. 5.14 Mylohyoid ridge

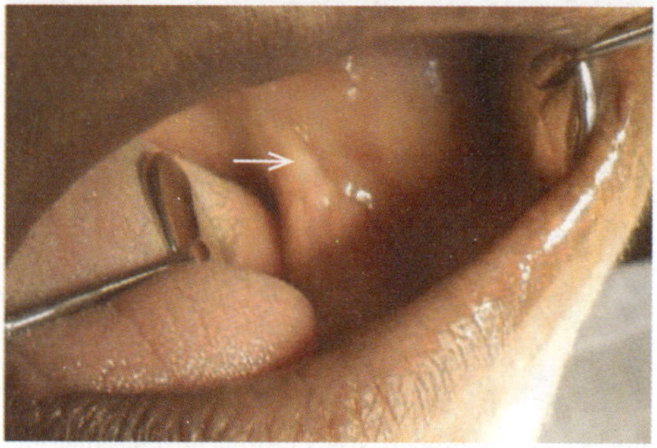

Fig. 5.17 Retromolar pad

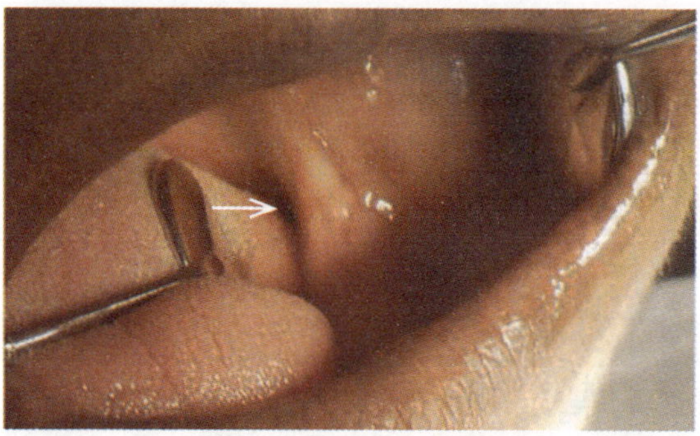

Fig. 5.15 Retromylohyoid fossa

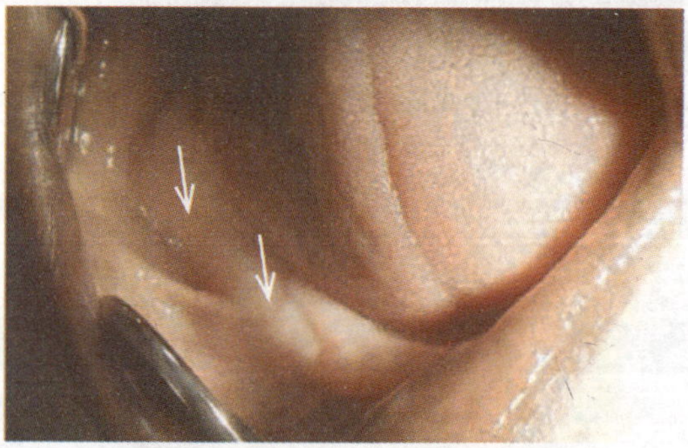

Fig. 5.18 Primary stress bearing area

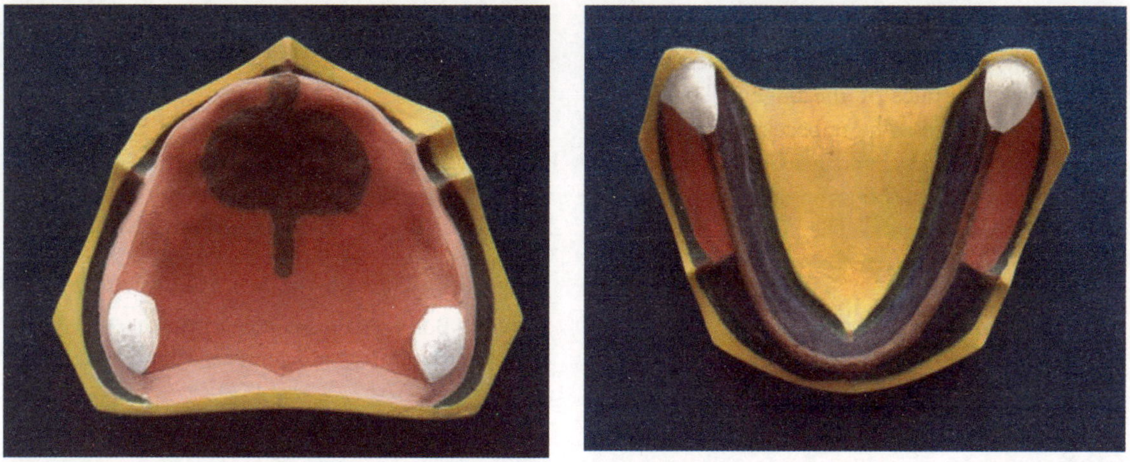

Fig. 5.19 Anatomic landmarks

notch like relief area, to accommodate the frenum. From midline to the angle of the mouth orbicularis oris and the elevator muscles of lip influence the shape of labial sulcus. The buccal frenii come next to the labial sulcus which should also be provided with adequate relief in the denture. Behind that the buccinator muscle determines the shape of the buccal sulcus. The width of the sulcus in the tuberosity region will be influenced by the position of the coronoid process of the mandible. At the posterior end of the tuberosity the influencing structures are the pterygomandibular raphe, a delicate tendinous band that runs between the hamulus of the pterygoid bone, mandible and the hamular notch. The hamular notch can be identified by palpation and this will limit the posterior border of the denture that covers the tuberosity. The soft tissue present over the hamular notch provides seal for the denture. (Fig. 5.1-5.8)

Mandibular ridge which is limited both by lingual and labial buccal sulci is covered by the masticatory mucosa. Lingual frenum that is present anteriorly reduces the effective width of the ridge and a relief given to accommodate this frenum weakens the denture. On the labial sulcus the frenii are not very prominent but the buccal freni are comparatively thick. The mandibular ridge is surrounded by labial and buccal sulcii externally and the lingual sulcus internally. The width of the sulcii usually measures between 3 to 6mm. Labially the limiting structures are the frenii and the muscles of lip viz. the orbicularis oris and the depressor muscles of the lip. Posterior to that, the buccinator muscle is the major influence. At the posterior termination of the mandibular ridge the retromolar pad is seen, the posterior half of which moves with the movement of the cheek. When denture is made usually the anterior half is covered. The lingual surface of the mandibular denture will be limited by the pterygomandibular raphe, the superior constrictor muscle and the palatoglossus muscle. In this region the muscles are vertically directed and hence the denture borders can be given a shape mainly by the movement of the tongue. Majority of the lingual borders especially in the anterior region are influenced by the floor of the mouth which is formed by the mylohyoid muscle, the genioglossus muscle, the geniohyoid muscle and the sublingual salivary gland. By appropriately directing the movements of the mandible and tongue the lingual borders of the denture can be shaped. The sulcus depth has to be ascertained to find out the dimensions of the denture bearing area. (Fig. 5.9-5.19)

The next anatomical feature to be identified is the bone and its structure. A well mineralized bone, if present on the surface of the ridge will adequately support the dentures. The trabecular pattern should also be checked for its abundance because it supports the outer contour of the bone through a well connected mesh of interior structure. The bone assessment can be done through an X - ray.

Residual ridge and its anatomy should be subjected to periodic evaluation because ridges undergo resorptive changes altering its shape and making it poorly supportive. Age and harmonal changes can also aggravate the reduction in the contours of the ridge. Many a time the ridges become flabby or fibrous. The former is seen in the anterior region and the latter in the posterior region.

Suggested reading

1. Sheldon Winkler, *Essentials of complete Denture Prosthodontics,* 2nd edition,1996, AITBS Publishers, India, Pp 88-105
2. Zarb- Bolender, Prosthodontic treatment for edentulous areas, Complete dentures and implant supported prosthesis, *Developing analogue/ Substitute for the maxillary denture bearing area, Developing analogue/ Substitute for the mandibular denture bearing area,* 12th edition, Mosby 211-31

6

Saliva

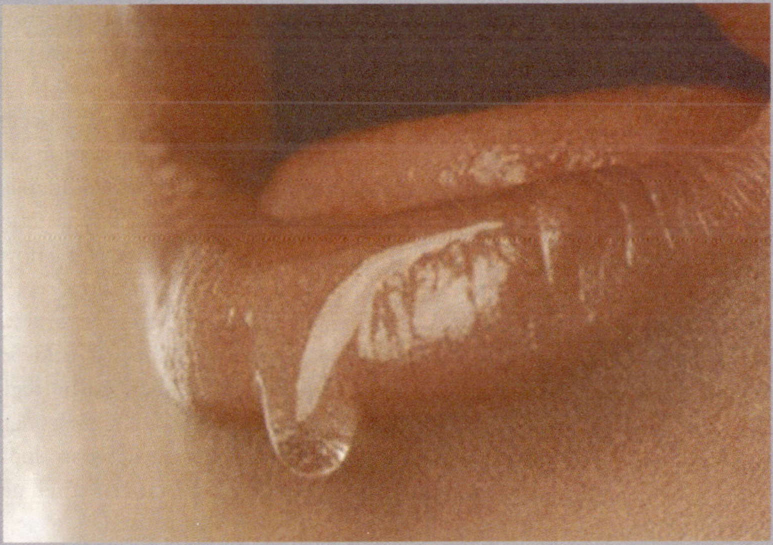

A vital biologic medium assisting complete dentures both biologically and mechanically

Saliva is the most valuable oral fluid, which is important for the preservation and maintenance of oral health.

Saliva is a clear, slightly acidic mucoserous, exocrine secretion. Whole saliva is a complex mix of fluids from the major and minor salivary glands and from the gingival crevicular fluid which contains oral bacteria and food debris.

Composition of saliva

Saliva is composed of:-

1. 99% of water and variety of electrolytes such as
   - Sodium
   - Potassium
   - Calcium
   - Magnesium
2. Bicarbonates, Phosphates, urea - These components act to modulate pH and the buffering capacity of saliva. The normal pH of the saliva is 6 to 7 that is slightly acidic. The pH in salivary flow ranges from 5.3 (low flow) to 7.8 (peak flow).
3. Macromolecular proteins and mucins - These components of saliva serve to cleanse aggregate and / or attach oral micro-organism and contribute to dental plaque metabolism.
4. Calcium- works together with phosphates and protein as an antisolubility factor and modulate demineralization and remineralisation.
5. Immunoglobulins and enzymes - Saliva consists of IgA, IgG and IgM. Saliva also participates in digestion by providing fluid environment for solubilisation of food and through the action of certain digestive enzymes, principally amylase. Several isoenzymes of amylase have been identified in humans; two of these representing 25% to 30% of the total amylase protein have small amounts of bound carbohydrate.
6. Other organic molecules present in saliva are cyclic AMP and cyclic AMP binding proteins, aminoacids, uric acid, various lipids and corticosteroids.

Saliva is not considered as an ultrafiltrate of plasma. Initially saliva is isotonic as it is formed in the acini, but it becomes hypotonic as it travels through the duct network.

The hypotonicity of saliva allows the taste buds to perceive different tastes without being masked by normal plasma sodium levels. Hypotonicity specially during low flow periods also allows expansion and hydration of mucus glycoproteins which protectively blankets tissues of the mouth. Lower levels of glucose, bicarbonate and urea in unstimulated saliva augment the hypotonic environment to enhance taste.

Flow

The average daily flow of whole saliva varies in health between 1 to 1.5 L. Percentage contribution of the different salivary glands during unstimulated flow are as follows:

Gland	Percentage Contribution
Parotid	20%
Submandibular	65%
Sublingual	7 - 8%
Minor salivary glands	<10%

Stimulated high flow rates drastically change the percentage contribution from each gland with the parotid contributing more than 50% of total salivary secretions.

Salivary flow does not occur evenly throughout the mouth. Regional variation intraorally is site specific with the mandibular lingual being a site of high volume and maxillary anteriors and interproximals being sites of low volume flow. These areas of higher and lower volume flow regions have been referred to as Salivary Highways and Biways respectively. The regional clearance of acid produced from bacteria is directly influenced by regional variation in flow within the mouth. Consequently salivary biways are areas in which acid by products may remain in longer contact with oral structures, unless mechanical means of cleansing is used.

Functions of saliva

Salivary functions can be organized into 5 major categories that serve to maintain oral health and create on appropriate ecologic balance:

1. Lubrication and protection
2. Buffering action and clearance
3. Maintenance of tooth integrity
4. Antibacterial activity.
5. Taste and digestion.

1. Lubrication and Protection - As a seromucous coating, saliva lubricates and protects oral tissues acting as a barrier against irritants. These irritants include:

a. Proteolytic and hydrolytic enzymes produced in plaque.
b. Potential carcinogens from smoking and exogenous chemicals
c. Dessication from mouth breathing.

The best lubricating components of saliva are mucins that are excreted from minor salivary glands. These mucins have low solubility, high viscosity, high elasticity and strong adhesiveness. Any intraoral contact between the soft tissues and teeth or between the soft tissue and prosthesis benefits from lubricating capability of saliva supplied largely by mucins. Mastication, speech and swallowing are aided by lubricating effects of mucins.

Mucins also perform an antibacterial function by selectively modulating the adhesion of micro-organism to oral tissue surfaces which contributes to the control of bacterial and fungal colonization.

2. Buffering action and clearance - This function of saliva is through the following components

a. Bicarbonate
b. Phosphate
c. Urea
d. Amphoteric Proteins
e. Enzymes

Bicarbonate diffuses into the plaque and act as a buffer by neutralizing acids. Urea, that is the another buffer present in saliva releases ammonia after being metabolized by plaque and thus increases plaque pH.

Phosphate is likely to be important as a buffer only during unstimulated flow.

3. Maintaining tooth integrity - This function facilitates the demineralisation and remineralisation process.

Demineralisation occurs when acids diffuse through plaque and the pellicle into the liquid phase of enamel between the enamel crystals. Resulting crystalline dissolution occurs at the pH of 5 to 5.5 which is the critical pH range for the development of caries. Dissolved minerals subsequently diffuse out of the tooth structure into the saliva surrounding the tooth. The buffering capacity of saliva greatly influence the pH of plaque surrounding the enamel thereby inhibiting caries progression. Supersaturation of minerals in saliva is critical to this process. The high salivary concentration of calcium and phosphate account for maturation and remineralisation of enamel.

More importantly the presence of flouride in saliva speeds up crystal precipitation forming a flourapatite like coating more resistant to caries than the original tooth structure. In that sense small amounts of demineralization is advantageous for tooth because enamel components of magnesium and carbonate are replaced by stronger, more caries resistant flourapatite crystals.

4. Antibacterial Action - Salivary glands are exocrine glands and as such secrete fluid containing immunologic & non-immunologic agents for the protection of teeth and mucosal surfaces.

Immunologic contents of saliva include secretory IgA, IgG and IgM.

Non immunologic salivary contents are proteins, mucins, peptides and enzymes.

Secretory IgA, the largest *immunologic component* of saliva is an immunoglobulin produced by plasma cells in connective tissue and translocated through the duct cells of major and minor salivary glands. IgA acts to neutralize viruses, it serves as an antibody to bacterial antigens and works to aggregate or dump bacteria, thus inhibiting bacterial attachment to host tissues.

The *non immunologic* antibacterial salivary contents are the products of acinar gland cells. They help protect teeth against physical, chemical and microbial insult.

5. Taste and Digestion - The hypotonicity of saliva enhances the tasting capacity of salty foods and nutrient sources. The enhanced tasting capability depends upon the presence of protein and gustin which bind zinc. Saliva has an early but limited role in total digestion by beginning the breakdown of starch with amylase, a major component of parotid saliva that initially dissolves sugar. More importantly saliva serves to lubricate the food bolus which aids in swallowing.

Factors controlling the secretion of saliva

The secretion of saliva is controlled by a salivary center composed of nuclei in the medulla but there are specific triggers for this secretion.

There are three types of triggers or stimuli for secretion or production of saliva which are as follows:

1. Mechanical: the act of chewing
2. Gustatory: Acid which is the most stimulating trigger.
3. Olfactory.

Other factors affecting secretion are psychic in nature:

1. Pain
2. Certain types of medication
3. Various local & systemic diseases affecting glands.

Salivary glands are innervated by both sympathetic and parasympathetic nerve fibres. Various neurotransmitters and hormones stimulate different receptors, different salivary glands and different responses.

When sympathetic innervations dominate, the secretions contain more protein from acinar cells; where as when parasympathetic innervations predominate, they produce more watery secretion.

Dysfunction of salivary secretion

Xerostomia or impaired salivary secretion or oligosialia

Causes

It has long been noted that xerostomia is likely to occur in diseases with fever and in diabetes mellitus, cholera and chronic nephritis. A reliable correlation probably exists between Sjogren Kerato conjunctivitis sicca (KCS) and decreased salivary secretion because according to Sjogren 10% of KCS patients also suffer from xerostomia.

In some cases a relatively satisfactory explaination is available of local disturbances of the activity of the salivary glands. These include salivary concrements and swellings which some times cause mechanical obstruction of salivary ducts.

Effects of radiation

Irradiation of the oral cavity can also result in the destruction of glandular tissue. The glandular architecture is replaced by ductal remanants and loose fibrous connective tissue which is moderately infiltrated with lymphocytes and plasma cells.

The acinar cells of parotid glands being the most radiosensitive, 2.25Gy causes 50% reduction in resting flow rate.

If all the major salivary glands are included in the treatment field a thick, ropy, viscous saliva results.

Radiation dose exceeding 40 Gy causes permanent hyposalivation.

Effects of aging

As a result of regressive changes in the salivary glands particularly atrophy of the cells lining the intermediate ducts, there is decrease in salivary flow in aged. The diminished function of glands also results in a change in the saliva itself which shows a decrease in ptyalin content and an increase in mucin content and becomes more viscous and ropy. The change in the character of saliva contributes to plaque formation and creates a favourable environment for the growth of cariogenic bacteria.

Drugs causing xerostomia

1. Antihistamines e.g., diphenhydramine
2. Glycopyrolate, propanthelene decrease gastrointestinal secretions and motility to control conditions of stress and tension
3. Many antihypertensives
4. Nitroglycerin for angina pectoris

5. Most antipsychotic drugs
6. Antiparkinsonian agents especially those with anticholinergic effects e.g., procyclidine
7. Antiarrythmic agents e.g., procaineamide; guanidine.
8. Tricyclic antidepressants eg:imipramine
9. Antianxiety agents e.g., diazepam and alprazolam
10. Amphetamines used in the control of obesity and as a central nervous system stimulant
11. Antisialogogue drugs purposely used to dry up the mouth. e.g., atropine
12. Decongestants e.g., phenylpropanolamine

Prosthodontic causes of xerostomia

1. Extended lingual flanges - cases have been described in which extended lingual flanges have obstructed the salivary secretion from the submandibular gland because of compressing on to the long salivary duct from the gland to its opening in curuncula sublingualis.
2. Denture plate - denture plate can obstruct the majority of the opening of palatine glands. These obstructions first result in the dilation of salivary glands due to retention of saliva which in turn causes the degeneration of glandular tissue.

The resulting dryness of the oral cavity due to the above mentioned factors will lead to other symptoms such as abnormal taste sensation, burning of the oral tissues and tongue, cracking of the lips and fissuring of the tongue. The oral mucosa will become dry, smooth and translucent and the tongue can assume an abnormal coating. Pain in the oral cavity is not uncommon.

Treatment of xerostomia

The treatment of Xerostomia is generally unsuccessful but various treatment options are there which may be helpful. These are:

1. Use of Salivary substitutes
2. Frequent use of mouth rinses, particularly during meals.
3. Use of sialogogues, drugs that stimulate the flow of saliva without affecting ptyalin content.

Salivary substitutes

1. Carboxymethyl cellulose based substitute, (MAS 84) which contains:
   i) carboxymethylcellulose - 500 mg.
   ii) Sodium flouride - 20 mg.
   iii) Xylito1- 3.0 mg
   iv) Potassium phosphate - 35 mg.
   v) Sodium chloride - 90 mg.
   vi) Potassium chloride - 120 mg.
   In 100 m1 of water solution.
2. Porcine mucin based substitute (Saliva Orthana) which contains.
   i) Porcinmucin - 3.5 mg
   ii) Xylitol- 2.0 gms
   iii) Methyl paraben - 100 mg
   iv) EDTA - 50 mg
   v) Benzalkonium chloride - 2 mg
   vi) Sodium flouride - 0.42 mg
   In 100 m1 of water solution.
3. Salinum, based on a linseed extract which contains:
   i) water soluble polysacchrides
   ii) metagin 0.1 %
   iii) potassium phosphate

Clinical studies on the effectiveness of saliva substitutes frequently report results claiming that xerostomia patients prefer mucin containing substitutes.

Sialogogues

Drugs which are used are:

1. Pilocarpine hydrochloride in 5 mg doses before meals which cause a pronounced flow for two to five hours. This drug also causes excessive sweating and discomfort so it is seldom prescribed.
2. Nicotinamide (250 - 400 mg three times daily) This drug is given if the decrease in salivary flow is due to nutritional deficiencies and it is usually given for a period of two weeks.

Sialorrhoea (profuse secretion)

Although occasionally it is of endogenous origin as in pregnancy or due to local irritation such as that caused by carious teeth, sharp edged restoration or ill fitting removable prosthesis, psychic tensions associated with the adaptation to new prosthesis can also cause sialorrhea.

Drugs causing sialorrhea

a. Cholinesterase inhibitors e.g., neostigmine.
b. Adrenergic stimulating drugs e.g., epinephrine.
c. Sailogogues e.g., pilocarpine.

Treatment

Drugs advised are parasympatholytics such as atropine or methyl scopolamine nitrate.

Role of saliva in the retention of complete dentures

1. Interfacial force

It is the resistance to separation of two parallel surfaces that is imparted by a film of liquid between them. It is provided by interfacial surface tension, interfacial vioscous tension

Interfacial surface tension - results from a thin layer of fluid that is present between the two parallel planes of rigid material. It is dependent on the ability of the fluid to wet the rigid surrounding material. If the surrounding material has low surface tension as oral mucosa does, fluid will maximize its contact with the material thereby wetting it readily and spreading out in a thin film. If the material has high surface tension, fluid will minimize its contact with the material, with the result that it will form beads on the material's surface.

Most denture base materials have higher surface tension than oral mucosa, but once coated by salivary pellicle, they display low surface tension that promotes maximizing the surface area between liquid and base.

Interfacial surface tension may not play an important role in retaining the mandibular denture as it does for the maxillary one. In many patients there is sufficient saliva to keep the external borders of the mandibular denture a wash in saliva, there by eliminating the effect of interfacial surface tension. This is not so in maxilla.

Interfacial viscous tension - It refers to the force holding two parallel plates together that is due to the viscosity of the interposed liquid. Viscous tension is described by Stefan's law.

For two parallel, circular plates of *radius (r,)* that are separated by a Newtonian liquid of *viscosity (k)* and *thickness (h)* this principle states that the *force (f)* necessary to pull the plates apart at a *velocity (v)* in a direction perpendicular to the radius will be:

$$F = \frac{(3/2)\,\Pi\, kr^4}{h^3} V$$

The relationship expressed by Stefen's law makes it clear that the viscous force increases proportionally to increases in the viscosity of the interposed fluid. The viscous force drops off readily as the distance between the plates increases. The force increases proportionally to the square of the area of the opposing surfaces.

When applied to denture retention the equation demonstrates the essential importance of an optimal adaptation between denture and basal seat, the advantage of maximizing the surface area covered by the denture and the theoretical improvement in retention made possible in increasing the viscosity of medium between the denture and its seat.

2. Adhesion

Adhesion is a physical attraction of unlike molecules for each other. The adhesive action of a thin film of saliva between the denture base and the underlying soft tissues is considered to be one of the principal factors in denture retention. Adhesion of saliva to mucous membrane and denture base is achieved through ionic forces between charged salivary glycoproteins and surface epithelium or acrylic resin.

Another version of adhesion is observed between denture bases and the mucous membranes themselves, which is the situation in patients with xerostomia. The denture base materials seem to stick to the dry mucous membrane of the basal seat, and other surfaces. Such adhesion is not very effective for retaining dentures and predisposes to mucosal abrasions and ulceration due to lack of salivary lubrication.

An ethanol free rinse containing aloe or lanolin or water soluble lubricating jelly can be helpful in this situation.

It is important to note that the amount of retention provided by adhesion is proportionate to the area covered by the dentures. Mandibular dentures cover less surface area than the maxillary prosthesis and therefore are subject to lower magnitude of adhesive retentive forces. Similarly patients with small jaws or very flat alveolar ridges cannot expect retention to be as great as, patients with large jaws of prominent alveoli.

3. Cohesion

Cohesion is the physical attraction of the like molecules for each other. It is a retentive force because it occurs with the layer of saliva that is present between denture base and the mucosa and works to maintain the integrity of the interposed fluid. Normal saliva is not very cohesive, so that most of the retentive force of the denture mucosa interface comes from adhesive and interfacial factors unless the interposed saliva is modified.

Suggested reading

1. Gray H., Gray's *Anatomy*, 37th Ed, 1989 London, Pg. 1290–1297.
2. Chaurasia B.D., *Human Anatomy*, Vol III, 2nd Ed., India Pg. 108–112, 131–134.
3. Grant J.C.B., *Grant's Atlas of Anatomy*, 10th Ed.,U.S.A., Pg. 725.
4. Singh I, *Textbook of Anatomy with colour Atlas*, 2nd Ed., 1998, India. Pg. 922.
5. Heidegger W., *Atlas of Human Anatomy* 4th Ed., 1990, Barcelona, Pg. 139–140.
6. Winkler S., *Essentials of Complete Denture Prosthodontics* 1996, U.S.A., Pg. 400–402.
7. Boucher, *Prosthodontic Tratment for Edentulous Patient*, 11th Ed., 1999, India, Pg 400–402.
8. Sharry, J., *Complete Denture Prosthodontics*, 3rd Ed., 1974, South Carolina, Pg. 29–32.
9. Heartwell C.M., *Textbook of Complete Dentures,* 5th Ed., 1992, Pg. 156.
10. Orban, B.J., *Oral Histology and Embroylogy*, 10th Ed.,1990, Canada, Pg. 328–329, 335, 341.
11. Humphery Sue P., Russel T. Williamson, A *Review of Saliva: Normal Composition, flow and function*, J Prosthet Dent 2001; 85:162–166.
12. Christianson Cecillia E, *Film forming Properties and Viscosities of Salivary substitutes and human whole saliva*, European J oral science, 2000; 108 :419–420.
13. Edgar W.M. O'Mullane D.M., *Saliva and oral health* second edition 1996 BDJ. Pub. British Dental Association.

7

Preprosthetic surgery

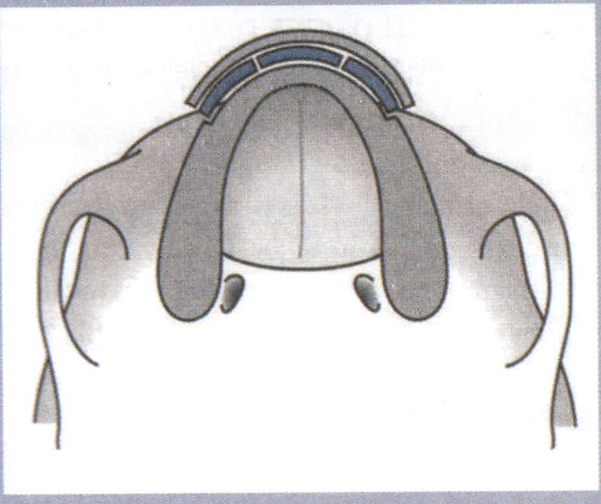

A paradigm shift has happened in complete denture therapy. Denture is not made according to existing conditions rather conditions are altered to suit a stable, retentive denture

A complete denture wearer will get satisfaction for a longer duration if the edentulous ridge has the following qualifications:

- adequate quality and quantity of bone to support the denture during rest and function
- ridge should have healthy attached soft tissue
- ridge should have a well rounded cross sectional configuration
- ridge should not have sharp crest, protuberances and undercuts
- buccal and lingual sulcii should be well defined and adequate
- attached muscle fibres, frena or scar bands which are capable of unseating the denture should not be present
- ridge and sulcii should not contain tissue folds, redundant tissues and hypertrophic tissues
- ridges should not have pathologic tissue

Ideal characteristics of the residual ridge can be partly planned before the dental extraction but on most of the occasions preprosthetic surgeries have to be planned when the patient report for denture fabrication. Common minor surgical procedures are described below.

Alveoloplasty

This is a common surgical procedure performed on patients who require complete dentures. Undercuts of the residual ridges are eliminated through alveoloplasty. If bone is removed from the buccal surface, it may lead to considerable resorption. Instead intraseptal alveoloplasty may be adopted which avoids reflection of buccal muco periosteum and which retains attached mucosa. The undercut is reduced by infracturing of the buccal alveolus. Advantages of this procedure is the maintenance of periosteal attachment to the labial plate of bone which decreases postoperative bone resorption and remodeling. By this method buccal undercut is reduced without reducing the height of the alveolar ridge. Intraseptal alveoloplasty results in less overall alveolar bone resorption than when the buccal reduction technique is used. Regardless of the alveoloplasty technique, when a mucoperiosteal flap is reflected, primary closure is preferred; but care must be exercised not to distort the adjacent soft tissues or to decrease the depth of the buccal vestibule. (fig. 7.1)

Reduction of maxillary tuberosity and removal of exostoses

Excess tissue in the region of the maxillary tuberosity that interferes with denture insertion is not uncommon. The tissue may present clinically as mobile or redundant soft tissue, vertical bony or soft tissue hyperplasia, or excessive bony undercuts in the lateral maxilla. Radiographs help to determine the relative tissue content of the enlarged tuberosity and the amount of pneumatization of the maxillary sinus. Articulated models help to plan the quantity and location of tissue removal.

If the excess tissue is fibrous, an elliptical incision is made, the mucosa is undermined, and the fibrous tissue is removed. The excess mucosal tissue then is trimmed and primary closure is obtained. If the excess tissue primarily is bone, then an elliptical incision is made, the mucoperiosteum is reflected,

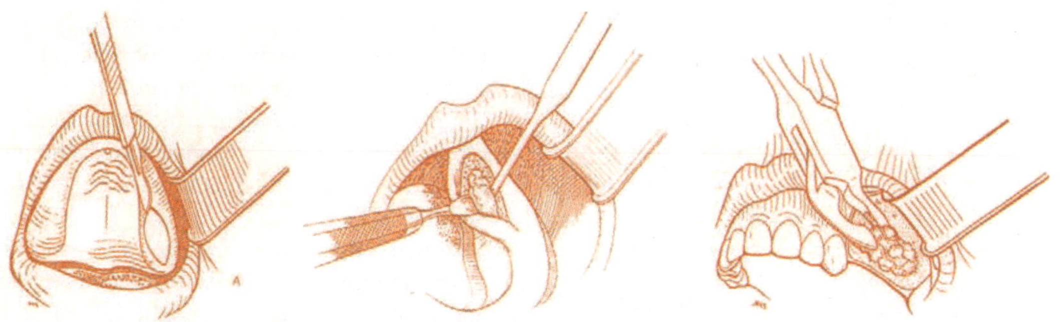

(a) (b) (c)

Fig. 7.1 a,b,c Alveoloplasty

a rongeur or rotary bur is used to remove adequate bone (being careful to avoid sinus perforation), and excess mucosal tissue is removed. Care must be taken to smooth the area with a bone file and to irrigate with saline copiously prior to primary closure. If sinus perforation should occur, postoperative antibiotics and a decongestant are prescribed for 7 days. In addition, the patient is cautioned to avoid vigorous nose blowing for 14 days.

Buccal exostoses are common in the maxilla and create undercuts which necessitate surgical removal. Adequate exposure is obtained with a mucoperiosteal flap and the bone can be reduced with a rongeur or rotary bur. Before primary closure, the area should be irrigated with saline copiously, and if necessary the excess soft tissue should be trimmed.

Removal of the redundant soft tissue present on crest of the ridge

Excess non-inflammatory tissue is formed due to long-term wear of dentures with poor fit or a single denture functioning against natural dentition. This is found commonly in the anterior mandible and maxilla. The possibility of bony augmentation should be considered prior to the excision of any soft tissue and in every case an attempt should be made to preserve attached mucosa.

When soft tissue excision is necessary it should be performed with minimal trauma to the remaining tissues. In general the excess tissue can be excised as a simple procedure. When subperiosteal dissection is necessary, the extent of the periosteal reflection should be limited, in order to minimize resorption of the underlying bone. Care must be taken not to excise too much tissue. Excessive tissue excision may obliterate the vestibule, committing the patient to a secondary ridge extension procedure. (fig. 7.2)

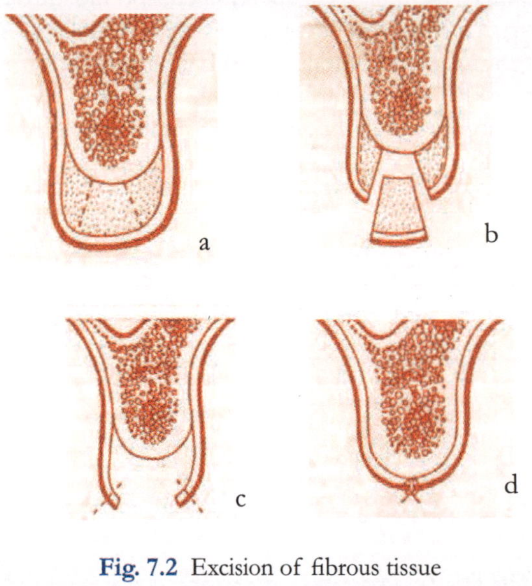

Fig. 7.2 Excision of fibrous tissue

Frenectomy

When extension of the denture base is impeded by a band of fibrous tissue that attaches near the crest of the residual ridge, or a frenum is present that displaces the denture prosthesis continually during function, a frenotomy or frenectomy is indicated. The maxillary midline frenum most commonly is a problem, followed by the lingual frenum and the maxillary frena in the bicuspid molar region. Different surgical techniques have been described to treat various clinical situations. The diamond excision

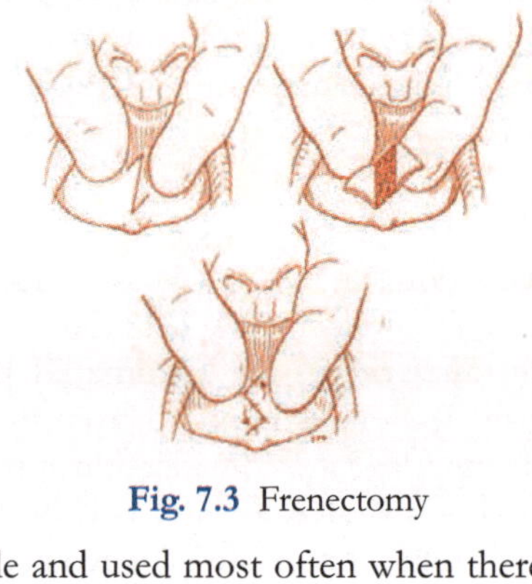

Fig. 7.3 Frenectomy

is simple and used most often when there is not a lack of soft tissue. It is used commonly to release the lingual and maxillary midline frena. (Fig. 7.3) The technique is somewhat more difficult to perform but useful when the frenum is broad and short. Its use simultaneously can eliminate the frenum and deepen the vestibule. A V-Y advancement technique can be used when a concomitant decrease in nasal base width is desired.

When a mandibular frenectomy is performed a tongue traction suture is helpful to improve visibility, and control of the tongue. The incision is made close to the tongue and the fibrous tissue is excised. Care must be taken to avoid the submandibular duct orifice. Good closure must be obtained and tongue movement should be encouraged postoperatively to prevent scar adhesions.

Broad frena in the bicuspid-molar regions of the maxilla are treated best with a localized vestibuloplasty. A semilunar incision is made at the mucogingival junction, a supraperiosteal dissection is performed, and the flap edge is sutured apically to the periosteum. The area either is grafted with soft tissue or allowed to heal by secondary epithelialization.

Epulis fissuratum and palatal papillary hyperplasia

Epulis fissuratum is a lesion of benign redundant tissue frequently associated with dentures having overextended borders. Different techniques have been described for the removal of epuli including sharp excision, electrocautery, cryosurgery and laser excision. All the methods are effective. Cryosurgery may require repeated attempts. Laser excision offers the advantage of good hemostasis and decreased postoperative pain. Again, the soft tissues must be managed carefully and an attempt must be made to prevent any decrease in the depth of the labial vestibule.

Palatal papillary hyperplasia is secondary to chronic denture irritation, usually under a poorly fitting prosthesis, and often involves varying degrees of candidal infection. Approximately ten percent of maxillary denture wearers exhibit this phenomenon. Relief of the denture in this area or a tissue conditioner and oral antifungal agents can be used preoperatively to reduce the size of the lesion and the extent of inflammation. While doing supraperiosteal removal of this tissue with a circular electrosurgery loop, care must be taken not to cauterize periosteum or bone because this causes bone necrosis and significantly delays healing. Soft tissue removal techniques using a large rotary bur, curettage, cryosurgery, or laser ablation are also acceptable. Regardless of the technique used, a splint or denture with soft tissue liner can be helpful in decreasing postoperative patient discomfort.

Palatal Torus

Palatal tori are bony protuberances composed mainly of cortical bone. Some may have a cancellous component. The cause of these bony protuberances is unknown. Fortunately, most tori do not require removal prior to prosthesis fabrication. The indications, for their removal include:

- large torus filling the palatal vault
- torus that extends beyond the posterior palatal seal area
- traumatized mucosa over the torus
- undercuts
- interference with speech and deglutition
- malignancy phobia

To remove tori an anteroposterior incision is made over the middle of the torus with a Y-shaped releasing incision at each end. A full-thickness mucoperiosteal flap is raised carefully, and the bone is sectioned with a bur and removed in pieces with a chisel. A large rotary bur also can be used to grind the torus away. In either case care must be exercised to prevent perforation into the nasal cavity or maxillary antrum. The mucosal tissue is replaced following torus removal, the excess tissue is trimmed away, and primary closure is obtained using horizontal mattress sutures. A stent or denture should be placed to support the palatal tissue and to prevent hematoma formation under the wound closure. Possible complications of torus removal include nasal perforation, oronasal or antral fistula formation, palatal tissue necrosis, and hematoma.

Mandibular Torus

Mandibular tori may be single, multiple, or lobulated. Removal is indicated when tori produce lingual undercuts or interfere with lingual flange extension of the prosthesis. If teeth are to be extracted, they should be removed prior to addressing the torus. A mucoperiosteal envelope flap is raised only on the lingual aspect of the mandible, so that the flap may later be sutured back to a fixed base. Care is taken not to tear or perforate the lingual flap when dissecting over the torus. Releasing incisions are not recommended because they may compromise blood supply to the flap or damage the lingual nerve. After adequate exposure, the tori are reduced with a large rotary bur or removed initially by making a groove adjacent to the lingual cortex with a fissure bur followed by sectioning with an osteotome. The bone should be smoothened carefully with a bone file, the wound irrigated copiously to remove debris, and primary closure obtained. Possible complications of mandibular tori removal include floor of the mouth hemorrhage and infection. The former can be a life threatening sequela and must be managed accurately to prevent possible airway compromise.

Reduction of mylohyoid ridge

The mylohyoid ridge of the mandible is a common area of painful denture irritation. Vertical bone resorption in the posterior mandible causes this ridge to become prominent, thereby limiting extension of the lingual flange of the prosthesis. If this occurs, relocation of the mylohyoid muscle and osseous reduction of the mylohyoid ridge are indicated.

An incision is made in the posterior aspect of the mandible on the crest of the alveolar ridge. Care must be taken not to incise too far lingually because the lingual nerve may traverse the retromolar pad region in some patients. Exposure of the mylohyoid ridge is obtained by raising a mucoperiosteal flap and sharply dissecting the muscle fibers from their bony insertion. A rotary bur or bone file may be used to decrease the prominence of the ridge. Copious wound irrigation, primary closure with sutures, and immediate placement of a stent or modified denture to position the muscle inferiorly are required. After a week the stent is removed and a new prosthesis is fabricated. As with mandibular tori removal, possible complications include infection and hemorrhage into the floor of the mouth.

Pre prosthetic surgery includes many other procedures listed below description of which can be had from concerned speciality text books.

- Transpositional flap vestibuloplasty is useful for the patient with inadequate vestibular depth caused due to mandibular atrophy and high soft tissue attachments.
- Mandibular vestibuloplasty with split thickness skin or palatal mucosal grafting is useful if adequate tissue is not available for vestibuloplasty.
- Bony augmentation procedures like visor osteotomy, onlay border grafting, interpositional bone grafts, inferior bone grafts
- Dental implant surgery to obtain additional support.

Suggested reading

1. Warneke SC. *The pre prosthetic management of the edentulous patient.* Aust Dent J. 1978 Apr;23(2):167-70
2. Hopkins R, Stafford GD, Gregory MC. *Pre-prosthetic surgery of the edentulous mandible.* Br Dent J. 1980 Apr 1;148(7):183-8.
3. Benington IC. *Post-surgical prosthodontics: clinical notes.* J Oral Rehabil. 1983 Jan;10(1):31-40.
4. Peterson, L. J. *Principles of Oral and Maxillofacial Surgery.* Vol. II. J. B. Lippincott Co., Philadelphia, 1992.
5. Zarb, G. *Prosthodontic View of Traditional and Contemporary Preprosthetic Surgery.* Chapter 42, pp. 1091-1102.
6. Tucker, R.M. *Ambulatory Preprosthetic Reconstructive Surgery.* Chapter 43, pp. 1103-1132.
7. Stoelinga, P.J.W. *Preprosthetic Reconstructive Surgery.* Ch. 43, pp. 1169-1207.
8. Chase, D.C. and Laskin, D.M. *Procedure to Improve the Alveolar Soft Tissue. Basic Preprosthetic Surgery,* Vol. II, Oral Surgery.
9. Chase, D.C. and Laskin, D.M. *Procedure to Improve the Alveolar Soft Tissue.* Basic Preprosthetic Surgery. Chapter 9, pp. 293–347.
10. Chase, D.C. and Laskin, D.M. *Procedure to Improve the Alveolar Soft Tissue.* Basic Preprosthetic Surgery. Chapter 10, p.349-361.
11. Peterson, L.J., *Contemporary Oral and Maxillofacial Surgery,* 2nd ed., Mosby Year-book Inc., St. Louis, 1993.
12. Tucker, M.R. *Basic Preprosthetic Surgery.* Chapter 13, pp. 395-334.
13. Tucker, M.R. *Advanced Preprosthetic Surgery.* Chapter 14, pp. 335-368.
14. Fonseca, R.J. and Davis, W.H. *Reconstructive Preprosthetic Oral and Maxillofacial Surgery.* W.B. Saunders Co., Philadelphia, 1986.
15. Scott, R.F. and Olson, R.A. *Minor Preprosthetic Procedures.* Ch 4, pp. 61-68.
16. Davis, W.H. *Surgical Management of Soft Tissue Problems.* Ch 5, pp 69-116.
17. Fonseca, R.J. *Osseous Reconstruction of Edentulous Bone Loss.* Chapter 6, pp 117-165.

8

Resorption of residual ridges

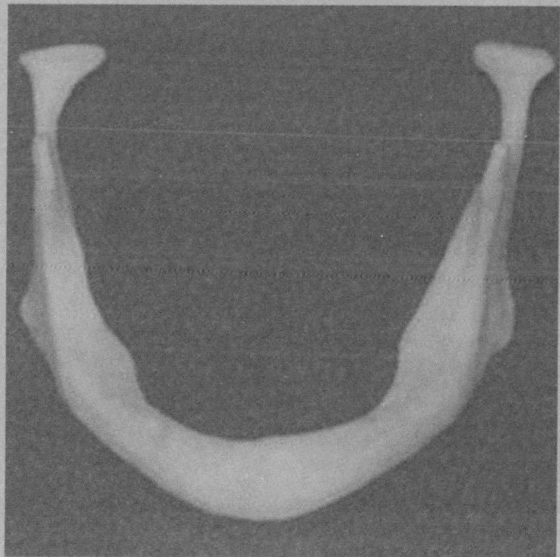

Resorption of residual ridges is the greatest obstacle in the long term prognosis of complete dentures

The present day world shows a contrasting picture of edentulism. In countries like Sweden, individuals requiring complete dentures are seldom found in dental clinics where as in India patients queue up for longer duration to get a complete denture. This picture is brought in to highlight the importance of the health of residual ridge in the context of our country. The story of residual ridges begins soon after dental extraction. The natural physiologic processes remodel the alveolar bone to form a well shaped ridge that serves as a foundation to the complete denture. It was well identified that the ridge changes its shape in the course of denture wearing. The well rounded ridge progressively narrows down and finally attains a flat or concave surface topography towards the terminal stages of complete denture wearing. The terminal phase is now extended because of the increasing life expectancy. (fig. 8.1, 8.2)

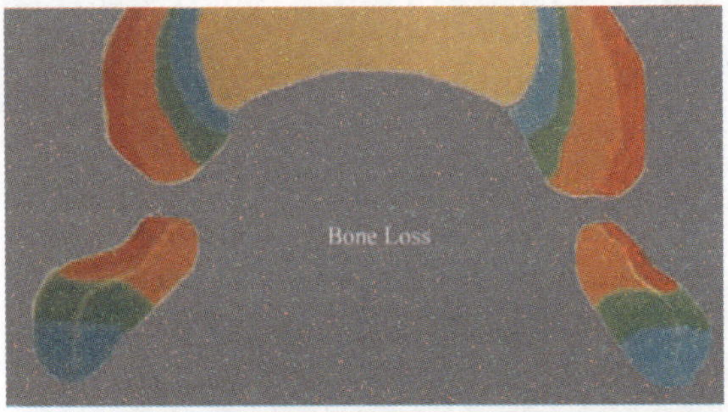

Fig. 8.1 Pattern of bone loss in maxilla and mandible

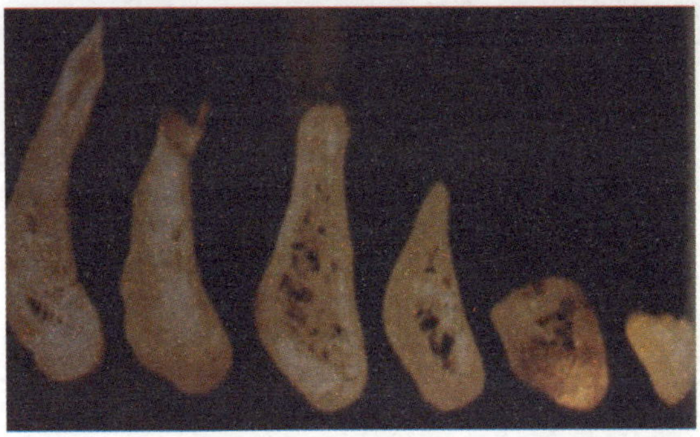

Fig. 8.2 Stages of bone resorption-mandible

Changes in the residual ridges of complete denture wearers was considered to be a normal physiologic phenomenon, the validity of which was first questioned by Atwood through the renowned article published in 1971 on reduction of residual ridges (RRR). This has brought in the thinking that reduction of residual ridge is a pathologic process. RRR can be considered as a pathologic process because it was not inevitably seen in all the denture wearers. While some easily succumb to this phenomenon, others do resist without any marked change. There is no uniformity in the process between sites, between individuals, between sexes and between age groups. In severe cases, RRR has proceeded beyond the alveolar bone indicating the

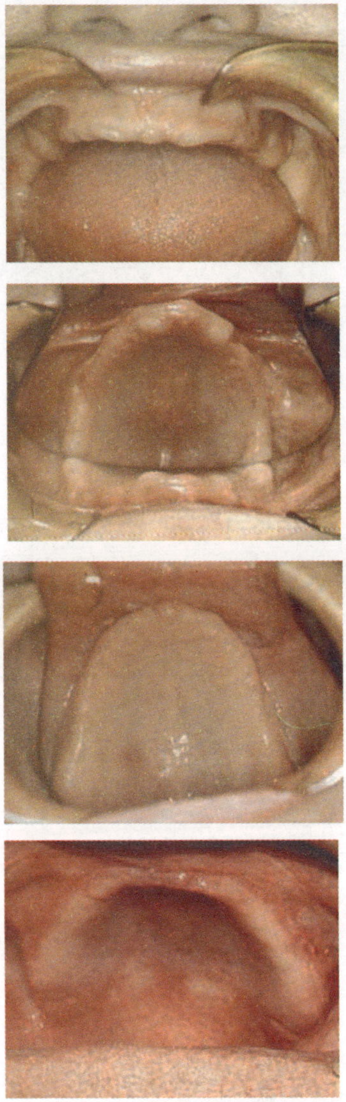

Fig. 8.3 Different stages of resorption-maxilla(clinical)

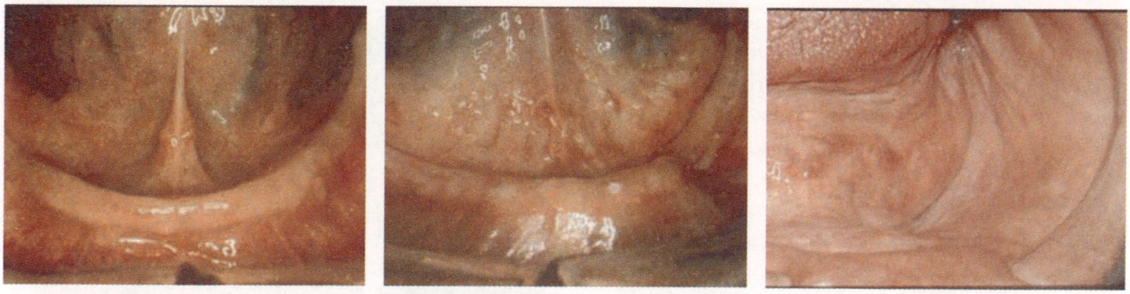

Fig. 8.4 Different stages of resorption-mandible(clinical)

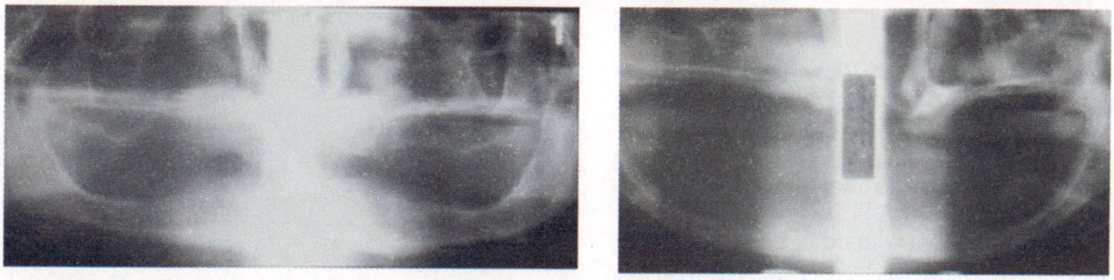

Fig. 8.5 Different stages of resorption-mandible(Radiographic)

fact that the resorption superceded bone formation. These arguments cast the shadow of pathology on the process of RRR. (fig. 8.3-8.5)

While recognizing the fact that great individual variations do exist in the causation of RRR, Woelfel et al listed nearly 63 factors that could possibly be related to bone resorption under removable dentures. Even today we are at a loss to find out the important causative factors of RRR. The commonly related factors include gender, age, facial structure, duration of edentulousness, habits, oral hygiene, parafunctions, masticatory load, nutritional status, medications, systemic diseases, hormones and osteoporosis.

It is generally believed that old age and womanhood are related to residual ridge resorption. Human skeleton accumulates bone up to the age of approximately 30 years and then gradually starts to lose bone. Post menopausal osteoporosis in which trabecular bone is predominantly lost is mainly associated with inadequacy in estrogen and progesterone. The senile osteoporosis is characterized by the loss of both cortical and cancellous hone. RRR in women and in old age can be viewed as an oral manifestation of osteoporosis but statistically significant associations cannot always be found out. The force by which bone in subjected to can be a possible reason for RRR. More light was thrown on this by implant studies. (fig. 8.6)

Asthmatics have been associated with RRR because most of them undergo corticosteroid therapy. Interestingly alcohol intake is not correlated to RRR greatly. Fluoridated water supply has a positive effect on the residual ridges if an individual is exposed for more than ten years. Smoking seems to cause implant failures due to peri-implant bone loss. This might probably emerge as a causative factor for RRR, if multivariate

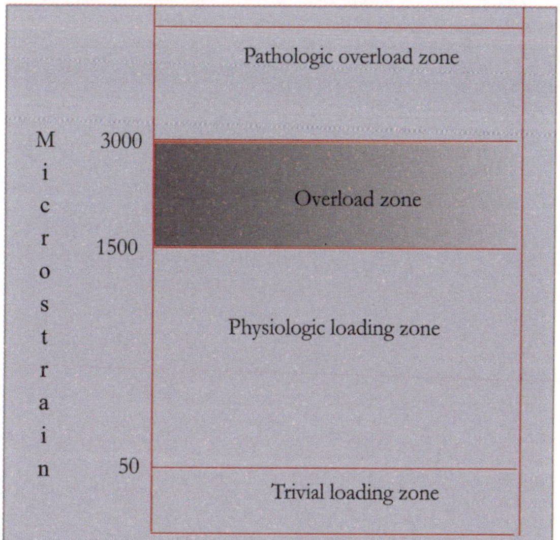

Fig 8.6 Chart showing different types of loading and the corresponding microstrain.

analyses are applied to the presently available research data. The conventional etiologic factors like more the ridge more the RRR, the bone resorptive factors, the negative bone formative factors, endotoxins from dental plaque, prostaglandins, heparin, ill-fitting dentures, do seem relevant but do not seem to be useful in the prevention of RRR. Hence the clinician is at a loss to help the edentulous individual in sustaining the health of ridges. A recent reference on the use of Indomethacin in the control of RRR is worth studying. Indomethacin controls the production of prostaglandins and thereby bone resorption. (Table 8.1)

A silver lining of hope for the edentulous individuals is present in the use of dental implants. Implants are capable of providing an altered functional stimulus to the bone tissue and in individuals wearing implant supported prosthesis, bone loss was substantially reduced. The stark reality is that only one in thousand of the edentulous individuals is benefited by the implant. In a vast country like India which is nursing a huge geriatric population, implant is not going to offer a feasible solution. Even ridge augmentation procedures do not seem to brighten the picture. The treatment option to prevent RRR would be retention of healthy roots, fabrication of overdentures and careful use of dental implants.

Table 8.1 Etiologic factors related to reduction of residual ridges (RRR)

Etiologic factor	Correlation with RRR
Anatomic factor	
Mandible	RRR in mandible is nearly four times greater than in maxilla. This finding is inconclusive.
Short and square face	RRR is more evident in short and square faces -may be due to direct effect of masticatory force.
Large alveolar process	Increased RRR. No correlation with the jaw size.
Density of alveolar bone	No correlation with bone density.
Labial alveoloplasty	Increased RRR.
Prosthodontic factor	
Immediate denture	Decreased RRR.
Zero degree teeth	Increased RRR.
Metabolic and systemic factor	
Age and Sex	No correlation with the rate of RRR.
Osteoporosis	No correlation with the ridge height.
Smaller maxillary ridge.	Knife edge type mandible.
Calcium and Vitamin D supplement	Decreased RRR.
Zinc sulfate supplement	Better healing in hamsters.
Dichloromethane diphosphonate supplement.	Decreased RRR in rats.
Sodium fluoride supplement	Better clacification.
Indomethacin supplement	Decreased RRR in rats.
Functional factor	
Intensive denture wearing	Increased RRR
Regular denture wearing	Combination syndrome No correlation with the rate of RRR
Bioelectric potential	Decreased RRR by exogenous pulsed electromagnetic fields in dogs.

Suggested Reading

1. Douglas Allen Atwood. *Reduction of residual ridges A major oral disease.* J. Prosthet Dent 1971; 26: 266-277.
2. Woelfel JB, Winteer CM. Igarashi T. *Five year cephalometric study of mandibular ridge resorption with different posterior occlusal forms. Part I . Denture construction and initial comparison.* JProsthet Dent 1976; 36: 602-23.
3. Leila Jahangiri. *Current perspectives in residual ridge remodelling and its clinical implication. A review*, JProsthet Dent 1998; 80(2): 224-237.
4. John N.M. Heerche. *The decrease in bone mass associated with aging and menopause.* J Prosthet Dent 1998; 79: 14-16.
5. Gunnar.E.Carlsson. *Clinical morbidity and sequelae of treatment with complete dentures.* J Prosthet Dent I998;79: 17-22.
6. Tallgren. A. *The continuing reduction of the residual alveolar ridges in complete denture wearers: a mixed longitudinal study covering 25 years* J Prosthet Dent 2003; May 89(5): 427–35.

9

Informed consent for dentures

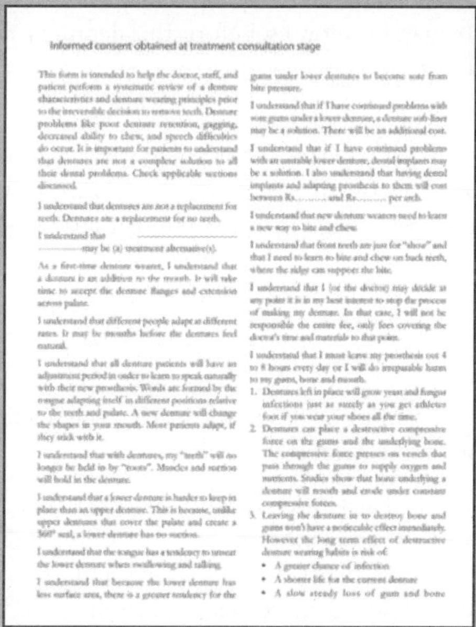

Informed consent obtained at treatment consultation stage

This form is intended to help the doctor, staff, and patient perform a systematic review of a denture characteristics and denture wearing principles prior to the irreversible decision to remove teeth. Denture problems like poor denture retention, gagging, decreased ability to chew, and speech difficulties do occur. It is important for patients to understand that dentures are not a complete solution to all their dental problems. Check applicable sections discussed.

I understand that dentures are not a replacement for teeth. Dentures are a replacement for no teeth.

I understand that ______________ may be (a) treatment alternative(s).

As a first-time denture wearer, I understand that a denture is an addition to the mouth. It will take time to accept the denture flanges and extension across palate.

I understand that different people adapt at different rates. It may be months before the dentures feel natural.

I understand that all denture patients will have an adjustment period in order to learn to speak naturally with their new prosthesis. Words are formed by the tongue adapting itself in different positions relative to the teeth and palate. A new denture will change the shapes in your mouth. Most patients adapt, if they stick with it.

I understand that with dentures, my "teeth" will no longer be held in by "roots". Muscles and suction will hold in the denture.

I understand that a lower denture is harder to keep in place than an upper denture. This is because, unlike upper dentures that cover the palate and create a 360° seal, a lower denture has no suction.

I understand that the tongue has a tendency to unseat the lower denture when swallowing and talking.

I understand that because the lower denture has less surface area, there is a greater tendency for the gums under lower dentures to become sore from bite pressure.

I understand that if I have continued problems with sore gums under a lower denture, a denture soft-liner may be a solution. There will be an additional cost.

I understand that if I have continued problems with an unstable lower denture, dental implants may be a solution. I also understand that having dental implants and adapting prosthesis to them will cost between Rs.......... and Rs.......... per arch.

I understand that new denture wearers need to learn a new way to bite and chew.

I understand that front teeth are just for "show" and that I need to learn to bite and chew on back teeth, where the ridge can support the bite.

I understand that I (or the doctor) may decide at any point it is in my best interest to stop the process of making my denture. In that case, I will not be responsible the entire fee, only fees covering the doctor's time and materials to that point.

I understand that I must leave my prosthesis out 4 to 8 hours every day or I will do irreparable harm to my gums, bone and mouth.

1. Dentures left in place will grow yeast and fungus infections just as surely as you get athletes foot if you wear your shoes all the time.
2. Dentures can place a destructive compressive force on the gums and the underlying bone. The compressive force presses on vessels that pass through the gums to supply oxygen and nutrients. Studies show that bone underlying a denture will smooth and erode under constant compressive forces.
3. Leaving the denture in to destroy bone and gums won't have a noticeable effect immediately. However the long term effect of destructive denture wearing habits is risk of:
   - A greater chance of infection
   - A shorter life for the current denture
   - A slow steady loss of gum and bone

No treatment can be undertaken without the consent of the patient

A. Informed consent obtained at treatment consultation stage

This form is intended to help the doctor, staff, and patient perform a systematic review of a denture characteristics and denture wearing principles prior to the irreversible decision to remove teeth. Denture problems like poor denture retention, gagging, decreased ability to chew, and speech difficulties do occur. It is important for patients to understand that dentures are not a complete solution to all their dental problems. Check applicable sections discussed.

I understand that dentures are not a replacement for teeth. Dentures are a replacement for no teeth.

I understand that ------------------------------- -------------may be (a) treatment alternative(s).

As a first-time denture wearer, I understand that a denture is an addition to the mouth. It will take time to accept the denture flanges and extension across palate.

I understand that different people adapt at different rates. It may be months before the dentures feel natural.

I understand that all denture patients will have an adjustment period in order to learn to speak naturally with their new prosthesis. Words are formed by the tongue adapting itself in different positions relative to the teeth and palate. A new denture will change the shapes in your mouth. Most patients adapt, if they stick with it.

I understand that with dentures, my "teeth" will no longer be held in by "roots". Muscles and suction will hold in the denture.

I understand that a lower denture is harder to keep in place than an upper denture. This is because, unlike upper dentures that cover the palate and create a 360° seal, a lower denture has no suction.

I understand that the tongue has a tendency to unseat the lower denture when swallowing and talking.

I understand that because the lower denture has less surface area, there is a greater tendency for the gums under lower dentures to become sore from bite pressure.

I understand that if I have continued problems with sore gums under a lower denture, a denture soft-liner may be a solution. There will be an additional cost.

I understand that if I have continued problems with an unstable lower denture, dental implants may be a solution. I also understand that having dental implants and adapting prosthesis to them will cost between Rs.......... and Rs......... per arch.

I understand that new denture wearers need to learn a new way to bite and chew.

I understand that front teeth are just for "show" and that I need to learn to bite and chew on back teeth, where the ridge can support the bite.

I understand that I (or the doctor) may decide at any point it is in my best interest to stop the process of making my denture. In that case, I will not be responsible the entire fee, only fees covering the doctor's time and materials to that point.

I understand that I must leave my prosthesis out 4 to 8 hours every day or I will do irreparable harm to my gums, bone and mouth.

1. Dentures left in place will grow yeast and fungus infections just as surely as you get athletes foot if you wear your shoes all the time.
2. Dentures can place a destructive compressive force on the gums and the underlying bone. The compressive force presses on vessels that pass through the gums to supply oxygen and nutrients. Studies show that bone underlying a denture will resorb and erode under constant compressive forces.
3. Leaving the denture in to destroy bone and gums won't have a noticeable effect immediately. However the long term effect of destructive denture wearing habits is risk of:
    - A greater chance of infection
    - A shorter life for the current denture
    - A slow steady loss of gum and bone support

- Future possibility I may not be able to wear a denture at all.

I understand that gums and bone continually change under my denture and that dentures will need to be evaluated every 6 months to insure that a change in fit is not doing irreparable damage to the gums and bone.

I understand that regular dental exams are essential to staying healthy and functioning well with a denture. The most important reason for denture patients to have examinations is to screen for oral cancer. It is also important to determine the appropriate time to reline a denture before it fits so poorly that damage to tissues has occurred.

I understand that the time will come when my denture will have to be relined or remade. That time may be as short as 6 months or as long as 8 years.

I understand that the use of "do-it-yourself denture relining products is strongly discouraged. Denture relines using these products are more porous, harbor more bacteria, and the resulting fit can lead to severe bone and soft tissue damage.

I have been given an opportunity to have all my questions answered.

I give permission to have my teeth extracted and that the resulting condition will be that I have no teeth.

I give my permission to have a denture made to deal with the resulting condition of having no teeth.

I understand that dentures have their own challenges and are not a complete solution to all my dental problems.

________________________ ____________

Patient's Signature Date

B. Informed consent obtained at wax try in stage

This form is intended to help the doctor or expanded function dental assistant and patient perform a systematic review of a denture and denture wearing principles prior to final processing and delivery. While it is possible to correct problems after processing, it is easier and less expensive for the patient to correct problems at this stage. Correction of problems after processing will result in additional costs. Check each applicable section discussed.

Checklist for patient approval of denture prior to final processing

I have been afforded the opportunity to bring a friend or family member with me to give me a second opinion about the appearance of the denture.

When my lips are relaxed, I like the way the denture looks.

When I smile, I like the way the denture looks.

The teeth arch form seems to fit my mouth.

The placement of the edges of the upper front teeth seems natural when I smile.

The way that each tooth is set looks natural.

The shade of the front teeth seems acceptable.

The shade is too dark.

The shade is too light.

The size of the front teeth seems acceptable.

The size is too big / too tall / too wide.

The size is too small / too short / too narrow.

When I bite straight together, the bite seems fine.

The right side seems to hit first.

The left side seems to hit first.

When I grind side to side or forward and back, the bite still feels fine.

I wish to have the following changes made:

____

____

____

I wish to have an additional wax try-in to insure that I like the looks of the denture.

I do not want an additional wax try-in.

I understand that changes to the denture after processing will be at additional cost.

General Considerations Checklist

I understand that dentures are not a replacement for teeth. Dentures are a replacement for no teeth.

If I am a first-time denture wearer (immediate dentures), I understand that a denture is an addition to the mouth and it will take time to accept the denture flanges and extension across palate.

I understand that different people adapt at different rates. It may be months before the dentures feel natural.

I understand that all denture patients will have an adjustment period in order to learn to speak naturally with their new prosthesis. Words are formed by the tongue adapting itself in different positions relative to the teeth and palate. A new denture will change the shapes in your mouth. Fortunately most all patients adapt, if they stick with it.

I understand that new denture wearers need to learn a new way to bite and chew. My "teeth" will no longer be held in by "roots", muscles and suction hold in the denture.

I understand that front teeth are just for "show" and that I need to bite and chew on back teeth, where the ridge can support the bite.

I understand that I must leave my prosthesis out 4 to 8 hours every day or it will do *irreparable harm to my gums, bone and mouth.*

1. Dentures left in place will grow yeast and fungus infections just as surely as you get athletes foot if you wear your shoes all the time.
2. Dentures can place a destructive compressive force on the gums and the underlying bone. The compressive force presses on vessels that pass through the gums to supply oxygen and nutrients. Studies show that bone underlying a denture will resorb and erode under constant compressive forces.
3. Leaving the denture in to destroy bone and gums won't have a noticeable effect immediately. However the long term effect of destructive denture wearing habits is risk of:

- A greater chance of infection
- A shorter life for the current denture
- A slow steady loss of gum and bone support
- Future possibility I may not be able to wear a denture at all.

I understand that gums and bone continually change under my denture and that dentures will need to be evaluated every 6 months to insure that a change in fit is not doing irreparable damage to the gums and bone.

I understand that regular dental exams are essential to staying healthy and functioning well with a denture. The most important reason for denture patients to have examinations is to screen for oral cancer. It is also important to determine the appropriate time to reline a denture before it fits so poorly that damage to tissues has occurred.

I understand that the time will come when my denture will have to be relined or remade. That time may be as short as 6 months for immediate dentures or as long as 8 years.

I understand that the use of "do-it-yourself denture relining products is strongly discouraged. Denture relines using these products are more porous, harbor more bacteria; and the resulting fit can lead to severe bone and soft tissue damage.

I have been given an opportunity to have all my questions answered.

I give permission to have my denture processed. I understand that changes made after processing will be at an additional cost.

____________________ __________

Patient's Signature Date

10

Impression – the concept and technique

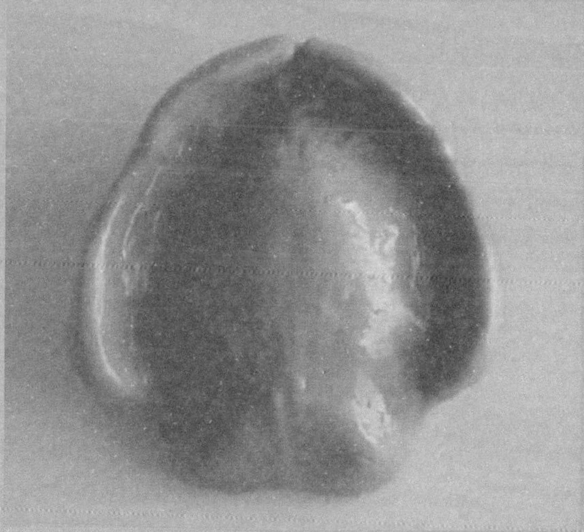

The foundation on which the dentures function must be duplicated because denture is fabricated mainly outside the mouth. Hence the impressions

Impressions are made to make a positive replica of the residual ridges which will serve as a foundation for the dentures. When an impression is made it should ensure faithful copying of the tissue surface so that the dentures made later can make a very close contact with the tissues. Most of the impression materials copy details measuring 50 microns and above. Details below that are not very relevant because those details might vanish during the laboratory phases of complete denture fabrication namely preparation of the cast, preparation of the transfer bases and preparation of the mould for packing acrylic. Dentures made on casts of edentulous ridges, copied in its anatomic form may not be successful during function. Edentulous ridges have a soft tissue cover the thickness of which varies from 0.5 to 3 mm in different areas. During mastication the soft tissue cover of the residual ridges will undergo compression which varies from place to place. If the denture is made on an anatomic replica, during mastication the denture will start rocking or in other words the denture becomes unstable. The area of minimum compression will act as a fulcrum. For example in a maxillary denture the mid palatine raphe region will act as a fulcrum causing a rocking movement of the denture. If an individual uses such an unstable denture, either the central region of palate will get injured or the denture will get fractured in the midpalatal region. To avoid instability, the minimally compressible areas are not compressed during the impression procedure where as all other areas are subjected to compression. By this selective application of compression instability and injury can be controlled. From this point of view the philosophy of selective pressure impression was evolved. The maxillary residual ridge has an area ranging from 25 to 35 sq.cms and selective pressure can optimally be applied. The mandibular residual ridge area is only 10 to 15 sq.cms and the distinction between the compressible and minimally compressible areas is not very evident. Hence in the mandibular ridge, selective pressure cannot be applied with great success. When this particular technique of selective pressure is applied, the cast obtained out of the selective pressure impressions will not be an anatomic duplication where as it will be a duplication with appropriate functional modification. A denture made out of such a cast will make faithful contact with the tissue in all the areas only when the denture is subjected to masticatory load. On other occasions at the minimally compressible regions, between the denture and the tissue there may be a gap filled by the salivary film. This situation will remain optimal for a limited period of time only because tissues can undergo morphologic changes in the course of wearing the denture. That is why periodic refabrication of dentures is recommended i.e., once in every 5 years.

In order to obtain a functionally modified cast of denture bearing area impressions are made in two stages. In the first stage, impression is made using a very viscous impression material which will compress the soft tissues of the denture bearing area uniformly. A cast is made out of it and on that cast the area which are to be compressed minimally are relieved using a spacer. Over this a tray is fabricated which when placed in the mouth will compress all the areas excepting that relieved by the spacer. In other words an impression made of this tray will compress the desired areas and spaced areas will not be subjected to compression.

Preliminary Impression

To obtain a preliminary impression, an impression tray that would cover the entire denture bearing area is

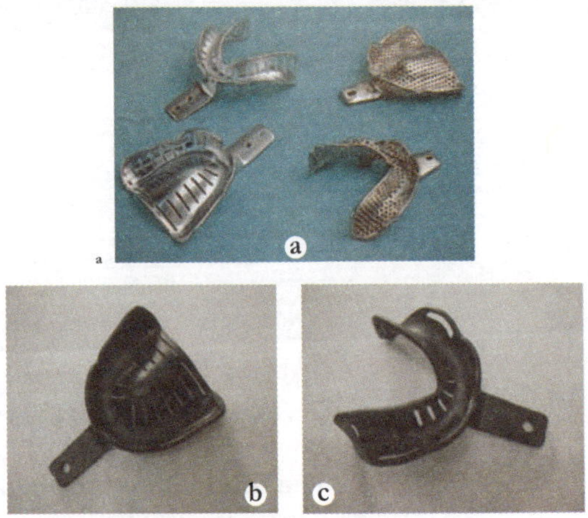

Fig. 10.1 a,b,c Stock trays used for completely edentulous ridges

necessary. At the same time there must be space of 5 mm between the tissue surface and the tray. Dimension of the tray can be selected by measuring the width of the denture bearing area using a caliper. For maxillary tray selection, the caliper should be placed between right and left buccal sulcii and for madibular arch it should be placed between the right and left lingual sulcii. However, final selection of the tray should be done only after placing the tray in the mouth and verifying the coverage and space. Minor modifications to the tray can be made by bending the tray to suit individual situations. Impression trays are available in different sizes denoted by numbers from 0 - 4 in an ascending order corresponding to the size of the arch. This will help the operator in selecting the tray with minimum attempts and if it is written in the patient's record it can be used as a reference on subsequent uses. (fig 10.1)The materials of choice for primary impression are Putty Silicones, Alginate, Impression Compound

Impression compound is a thermoplastic material which has to be softened using a water bath kept at a temperature of 70^{0}C. The compound should be softened and kneaded well inside the hot water so that it will become uniformly soft and flow will be improved by the hot water incorporated in it. Softened impression compound is made into a ball without making any crease on the surface and moulded on to the tray roughly simulating the final form of the impression.

The compound surface is again exposed to hot water and a thin layer of petrolatum jelly is smeared over it. It is then carried to the mouth and is pressed against the tissue. The compound will flow adequately if a load of 1500 gms is applied. While the maxillary impression is made, it is appropriate if the operator stands behind the patient. Once the material has flown through the borders, the lips and cheeks are pressed against the compound and later the lips and cheeks are pulled away from the respective sulcii and folded towards the inner aspect. In case of mandibular impression lingual borders are moulded by asking the patient to protrude the tongue horizontally to mould the lingual crescent area and to reach for the philtrum and the corners of the mouth in an open mouth posture to mould the mylohoyid and the retromylohyid regions. In the maxillary impression pressure should also be applied on the posterior most border so that a possible gap in the posterior border between the tissue and the compound can be avoided. With the impression in position and the compound in a softened state the patient can be encouraged to move the mandible gently in a side to side movement also. Once the compound is hardened impression can be removed and observed for the following.

The impression should cover the entire borders of the denture bearing area and the border need have a thickness of 5mm only in normal cases. However the lingual borders will be comparatively thicker because the moulding of which is done only by the tongue of the patient where as all other borders are moulded with operator assistance.

The border should accommodate labial, buccal and lingual frenii in clearly formed notches which are created by the tissue manipulation in a vertical as well as side to side movements of the respective frenii.

A faithful copying of the surface is essential for a good impression. Details up to 75 microns will be copied in impression compound. Areas of loss of

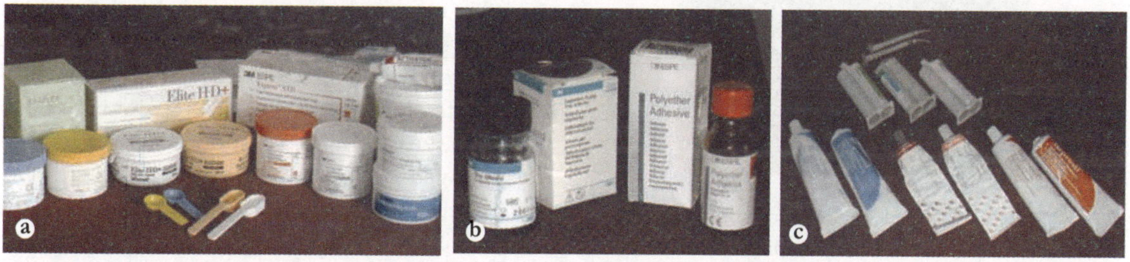

Fig. 10.2 a) Different brands of putty consistency elastomeric impression materials. b) Tray adhesives for both poly vinyl siloxane and polyether impression materials. c) Light and regular body polyvinylsiloxane impression materials

contact can be identified easily. Bigger folds of 100 microns and above in width and having more than 5 mm length have to be corrected. Minor defects can be eliminated by heating the impression surface using a dry flame, tempering it in hot water and reseating it in the mouth. If the defects cannot be corrected then that it is better to repeat the impression. Such an attempt more than once is not desirable for reasons of inaccuracy caused by warpage.

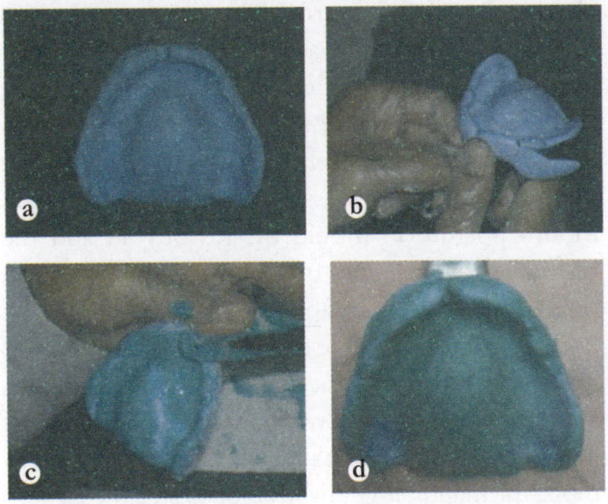

Fig. 10.3 a.) Maxillary preliminary impression obtained with putty elastomeric impression material. b.) Border thickness modified with scalpel. c.) Putty impression linned with light body polyvinyl siloxane material. d.) Completed impression

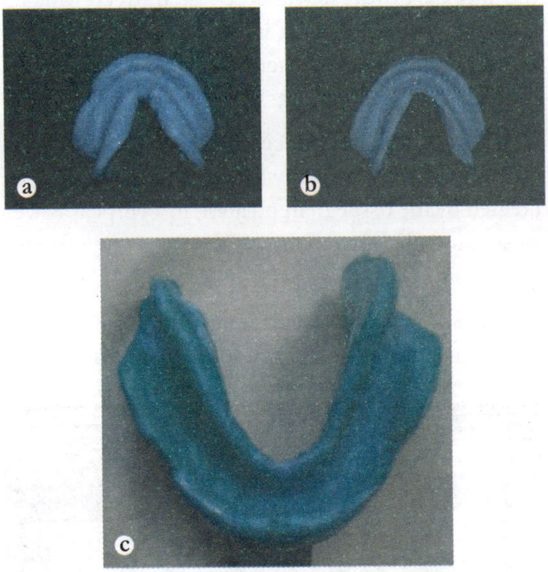

Fig. 10.4 a.) Mandibular preliminary impression obtained with putty elastomeric impression material. b.) Border thickness modified with scalpel. c) Putty impression linned with light body polyvinyl siloxane

Instead of impression compound, putty consistency silicone impression material can be used. It can be modified for extensions by the addition of newer increments. (fig 10.2a) It is supplied in two paste form and equal quantity of both the base and reactor pastes are mixed using hand with polyvinyl or nitryl gloves. It is moulded on to a tray the surface of which is previously coated with tray adhesive and dried with air. (fig 10.2b and 10.5d) Moulding is done as in the case of impression compound. Once the reaction is completed, the impression can be removed and checked for the quality. Mandibular impressions are easily under extended in the mylohyoid and the retromylohyoid regions which has to be extended by additional increments of the same material. Undercuts in the region of the mylohyoid are copied with ease when putty is used which may not be possible with impression compound where possibility of distortion cannot be ruled out. In order to check the rate of setting reaction of the material it is always desirable to keep a small portion of the mixed material outside the mouth and periodically testing it for the flow during the procedure. The impression can be lined with light body silicone to improve the copying of surface details. It is very comfortable to work with materials both for the clinician and for the patient. Results are also superior. (fig 10.2c, fig 10.3, fig 10.4)

On a satisfactory impression, cast can be made in dental plaster. It is desirable to observe 0.6 water powder ratio to ensure strength of the cast. If the impression is made in putty silicone, a cast of dental stone is preferred to facilitate easy removal without fracture because it is a comparatively tough material. Cast from the compound impression can be removed by softening it in warm water. The cast is then trimmed retaining the sulcular details all round. Maintenance of 3mm lateral wall of the sulcus is essential to decide upon the borders of the special tray.

A line is drawn at the fornix of the sulcii. 2mm above this line, another parallel line is drawn and which designates the borders of the special tray. Wherever there is a frenum, the line should dip to maintain relief. In the maxillary cast the extent of the rugae is outlined and it is extended along the median raphae for a width of 6mm. Posteriorly the out line should terminate short of the posterior palatal seal area. In the outlined area, one sheet of wax is adapted and the borders of which are merged to the surface of the cast. This is the design for relief to achieve minimum pressure in the non compressible area out lined while applying pressure on all other areas.

On the mandibular cast outlines are made as in the case of maxillary cast. Care should be taken to include retromolar pads within the outline in the posterior region. If the ridges have well formed parallel sided walls and 4mm wide crestal surface, it is considered to provide adequate support to the denture during function. In such a case incorporation of relief areas in non compressible areas may not be required. But if the ridge has low side walls and the width of the crest is narrow, it is desirable to direct the forces mainly to the buccal shelf areas. In such a case spacer wax is adapted on the entire surface of the residual ridge within the second line drawn to indicate the borders of the tray. Then the wax over the buccal shelf areas is removed. Care should be taken not to uncover the crest of the ridge. The buccal shelf area is demarcated from the anterior border of the retromolar pad to the distal border of the premolar area. This will ensure stability of the special tray during the process of impression making. During impression making pressure is applied exclusively on buccal shelf areas and not on the anterior region.

Alginate separating medium is then applied on to the casts with a brush using unidirectional strokes. Two coats of separating medium are desirable. Self cure acrylic is mixed and poured into a template kept over moistened cellophane sheet to make a sheet of

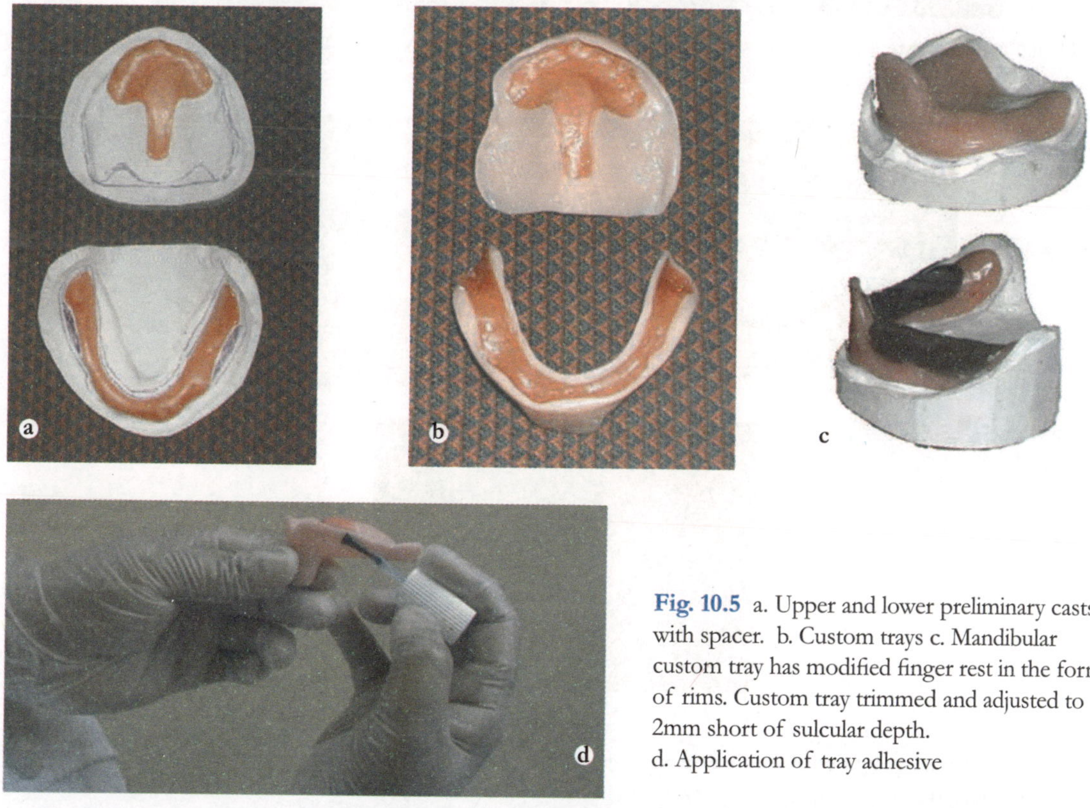

Fig. 10.5 a. Upper and lower preliminary casts with spacer. b. Custom trays c. Mandibular custom tray has modified finger rest in the form of rims. Custom tray trimmed and adjusted to 2mm short of sulcular depth.
d. Application of tray adhesive

acrylic. This is adapted to the already prepared cast. The thickness should be within 2-3mm. A handle can be made in the anterior region which should not be bulkier to interfere with the contour and movements of the lip. Over the buccal shelf area of the mandibular tray and over the posterior border of the maxillary tray additional strengthening can be done to withstand the pressure applied by the operator during impression making. If the width of the tray is smaller than the width of the operator's finger it is better to add a rim over the tray for finger rest. Once the acrylic resin is cured, the trays are removed and trimmed. (fig 10.5) The spacer wax can be retained till border moulding process is completed. However wax should not interfere with the border moulding material. The spacer wax can be removed sectionally from border.

Dentures should be designed to have borders which maintain contact with the border tissues during functional movements. During the opening and closing movements and during the movements of speech and mastication, tissues will stretch but

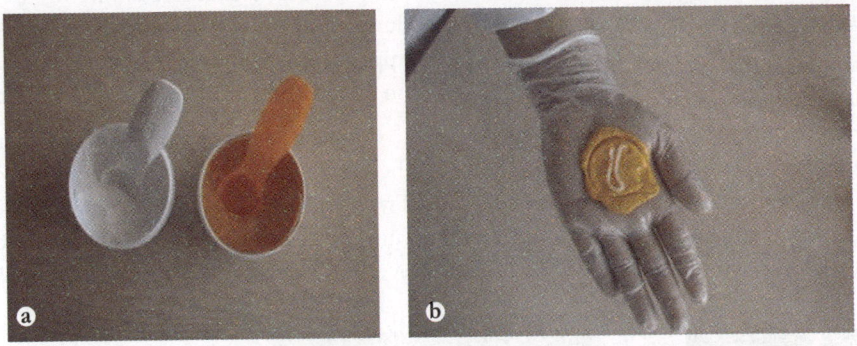

Fig. 10.6 a. Putty consistency polyvinyl siloxane with measuring spoon. b. Vaseline incorporated to each component

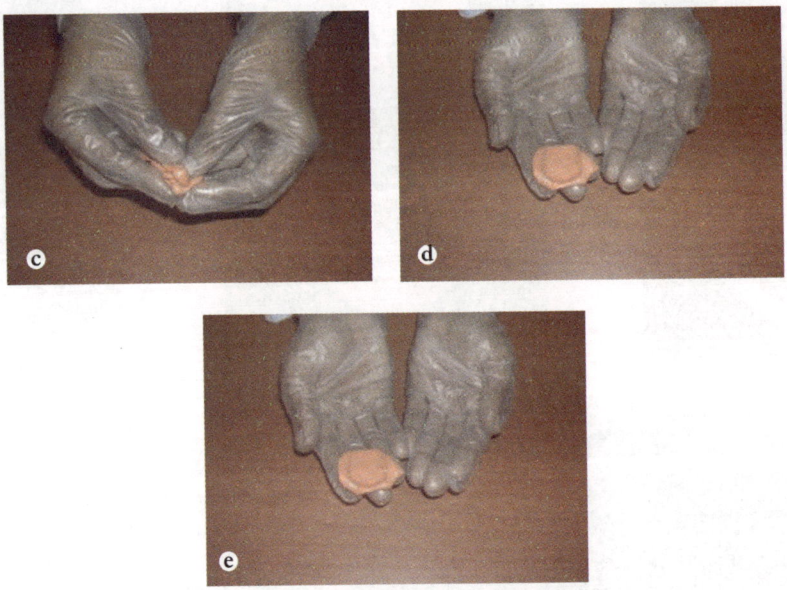

Fig. 10.7 c,d,e Equal quantities of both base and catalyst pastes mixed with finger tips till uniform color is obtained

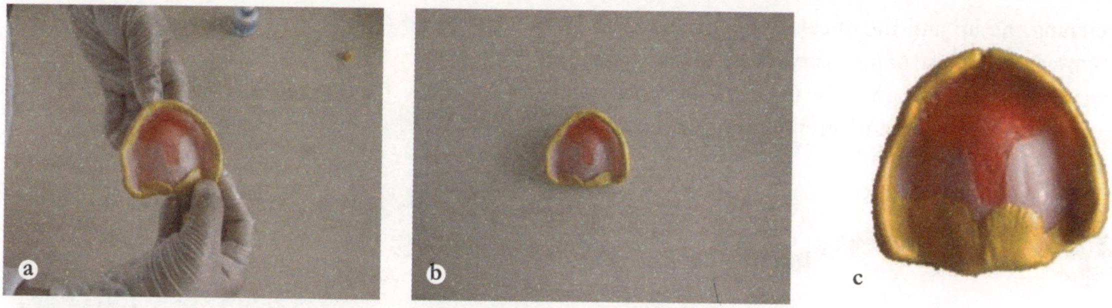

Fig. 10.8 a and b. Mixed impression material is shaped into a rope and placed along the borders of the custom tray. c. Border moulded tray-maxillary

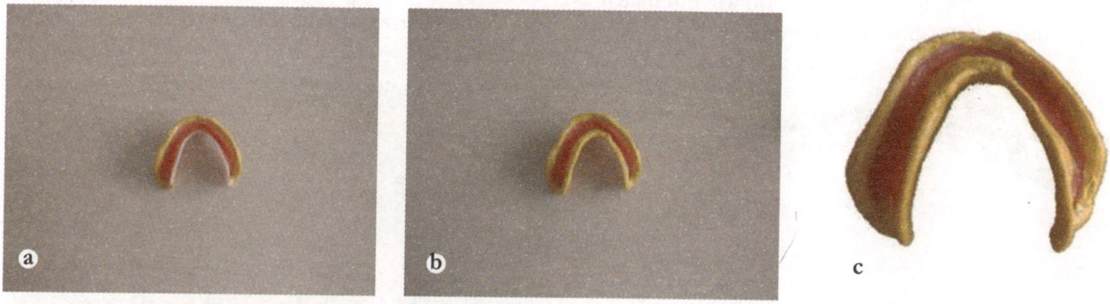

Fig. 10.9 a. and b. Mixed impression material is shaped into a rope and placed along the borders of the custom tray c. Border moulded tray-mandibular.

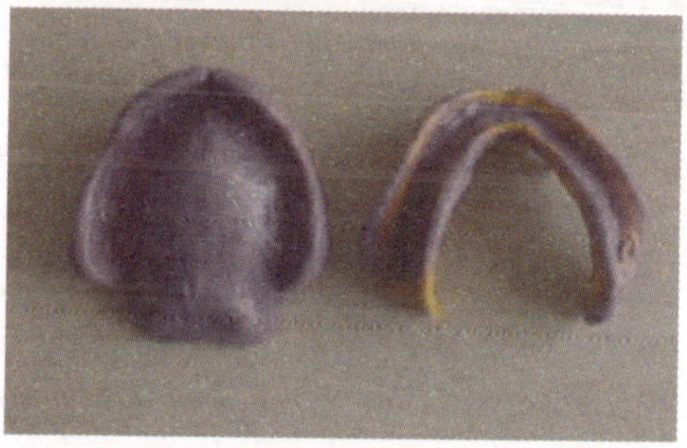

Fig. 10.9 Secondary impression recorded using light body polyvinyl siloxane

it should not unseat the denture. Creation of a vacuum is also indicated. To achieve all the above, borders should be moulded with the help of tissues by simulatory movements such as stretching the lips and cheeks and by moving the tongue. Operator can assist in simulating the movement of cheek and lips where as the tongue movements can only be done by the patient.

Border moulding and secondary impression

For the purpose of border moulding two materials can be used (1) putty silicone, (2) green stick compound. To get effective border moulding there must be space of minimum 2mm between the sulcus and the border of the tray when the functional movements are simulated. When green stick is used borders are moulded in sections. The maxillary borders are moulded starting from the posterior region. When the posterior sections are completed on both sides, the tray should be able to stabilize itself. In the mandibular tray buccal shelves are completed first and this will ensure stability for the tray. Border moulding of the external sulcii is achieved by stretching the lip and the cheek outward and then downward in the case of maxillary tray and upward in the case of mandibular tray. The third stage in border moulding will be an inward stretching of the lip and

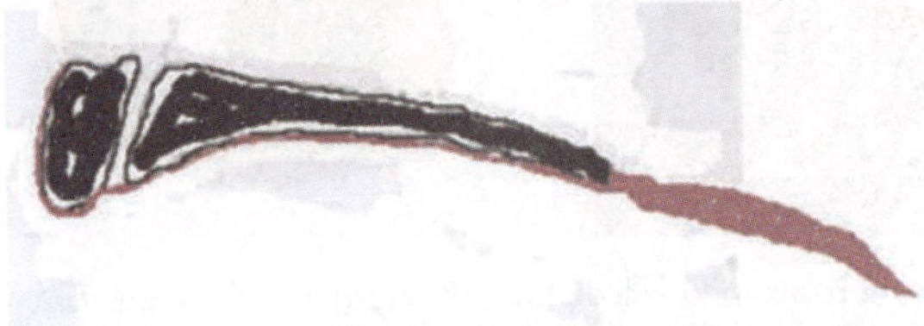

Fig. 10.10 Hard and soft palate relation. Is generally interpreted as in the figure. This relation will not match with the definition of posterior palatal seal.

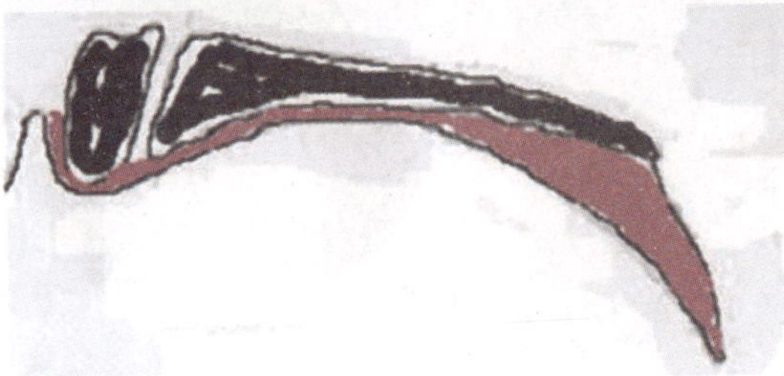

Fig. 10.11 Figure shows the correct relationship of hard and soft palate which can accommodate the definition of posterior palatal seal.

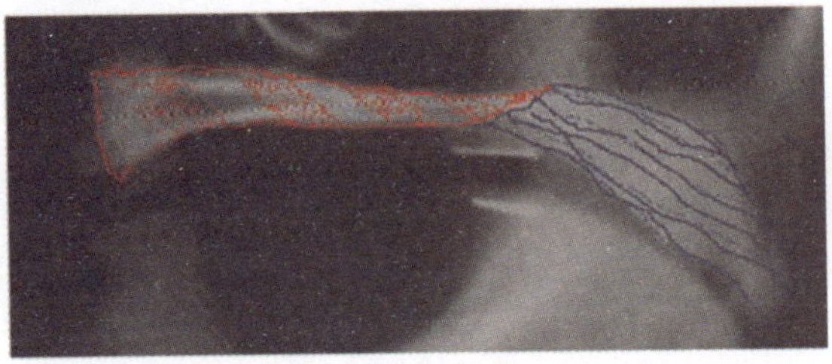

Fig. 10.12 Hard and soft palate relation identified on a radiograph. Wire markers indicate the most posterior extension of the denture

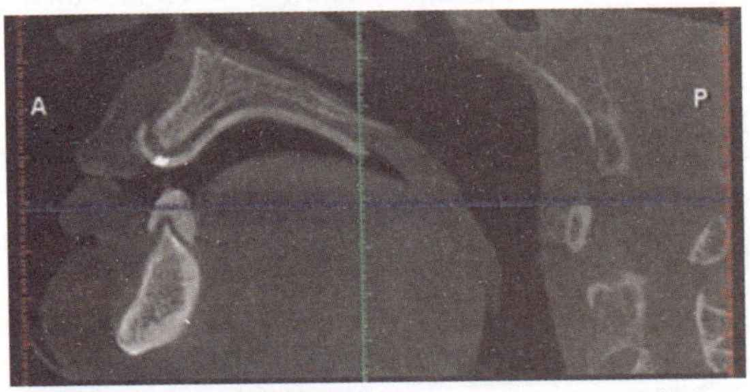

Fig. 10.12a Hard and soft palate relation as seen in conebeam CT image

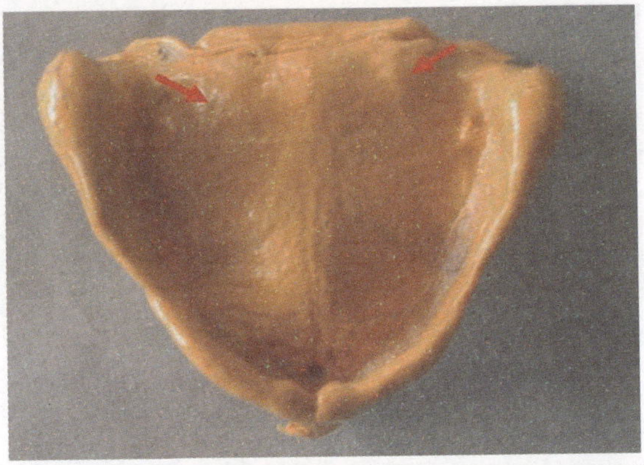

Fig. 10.13 Arrows indicate bulged posterior palatal seal area

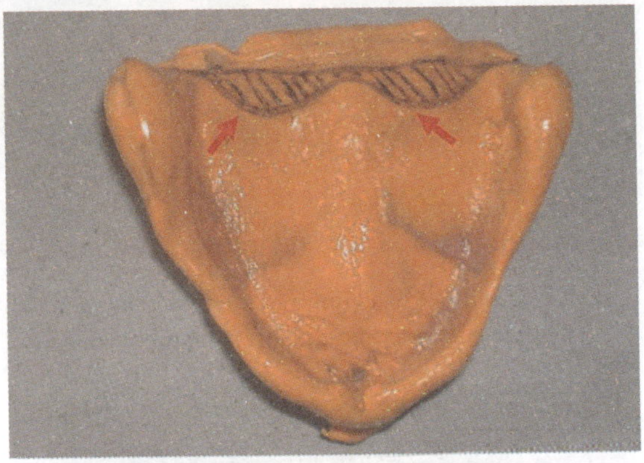

Fig. 10.14 Posterior palatal seal area marked

cheek. The first action will ensure the correct height where as the second and third action will ensure the width of the border. While stretching the lip and the cheek inward it is desirable to apply continuous finger pressure at the borders. When putty silicon is used border can be moulded either in sections or in one step. Maxillary border moulding is done in single stage. If it has to be done in two stages, it is better to do the palatal seal area seperately. Mandibular border moulding is done in two stages – labial and buccal in one stage and lingual subsequently. In highly compromised ridges, the spacer wax is removed and the entire tray is filled with silicone putty and the border moulding is done. Then the central region is cut off leaving the borders intact. When silicone is used, tray should be treated with adhesive. 10.5d (fig 10.6 - 10.9)

While doing the border moulding five areas are to be given special attention

1. Posterior palatal seal
2. Coronoid impression
3. Lingual crescent area
4. Retro mylohyoid area
5. Masseteric notch

Posterior palatal seal area: This is an area where the posterior border of the maxillary denture terminates. By copying this area we determine the posterior extension and provide a seal for the denture. The posterior border is determined by observing the movement of the soft palate. The patient is instructed to say "ah" gently while the soft palate moves upwards. When it comes back again the patient can be instructed to do the same. By repeatedly doing this, a line can be visualized at the junction of the hard and soft palate which is otherwise known as the posterior vibrating line. Then the patient is instructed to blow air through the nose with the nostrils closed. This will make the soft palate as well as the soft tissues attached to the posterior region of the hard palate to curl forward and form a definitive line. This process is known as valsalva maneuver which will help in identifying the anterior vibrating line. The anterior vibrating line can be further verified if "ah" is pronounced in short forceful bursts. The tissue present between the vibrating lines is compressed to obtain the posterior palatal seal. The compression is desired to be obtained through the border moulding material i.e., the green stick or the putty silicone and it should be within the physiologic limit. If an area can be compressed by an instrument by two millimeter for the purpose of posterior palatal seal, only one millimeter need be compressed to ensure adequate seal and this will not restrict the blood supply. If blood supply is not ensured during denture wearing, ulceration may result. When posterior palatal seal is incorporated the tray will have positive retention when it is pulled away from the fitting surface. To place the border moulding material i.e., green stick or putty silicone exactly in the seal region, it is desirable to copy the lines - anterior and posterior vibrating lines on the tray before placing the material in between. (fig 10.10 - 10.14)

Coronoid impression – While copying the sulcus at the tuberosity region the border moulding material should be placed on the external surface of the tray also. The patient is instructed to move the mandible laterally so that the coronoid process of the mandible will make a positive impression on the border moulding material. This is to get an idea of the possible thickness of the denture base which can be used safely with out causing injury to the soft tissue that could be trapped between the denture base and the coronoid process.

Lingual crescent area – The depth and width of the lingual crescent is to be moulded by specific tongue movements. The depth of the area is determined by instructing the patient to raise the tongue and reach for the upper lip from one angle of the mouth to the other while the mouth is kept open. The width of the crescent area is moulded by protruding the tongue horizontally forward. Lingual crescent area should never be moulded by asking the patient to roll back the tongue.

Retromylohyoid area – The lingual border of the mandibular denture is appropriately moulded where it is against the mylohyoid muscle but beyond the mylohyoid muscle in the retromylohyoid region, the muscular element that has got moulding capacity is the palatoglossus contained in the retromylohoid curtain which can be activated by protruding the tongue. Very often operators tend to over extend this region with out causing displacement to the tray and may reach up to the superior constrictor muscle. This can cause swallowing difficulties to the denture wearer at a later stage. It requires much experience on the part of the operator to decide on the correctness of extension of the border moulding in the retro mylohyoid region.

Masseteric notch – This is a depression caused at the external border of the mandibular denture in the posterior region by the anterior border of the masseter through buccinator muscle. This area is moulded by keeping the mouth open, with trays in position and asking the patient to close against force. The operator has to apply finger pressure downwards while the patient attempts to close the mouth.

Border moulding is to be accomplished with the cooperation of the patient while stretching the lips and cheeks. A minimum of 30 sec should be allowed for the moulding of impression material. Vigorous movements do not produce the desired moulding because it is multi directional.

Once the border moulding is completed the wax spacers are removed completely and the over flown border moudling material into the inner aspect of the tray is removed. Either Zinc oxide eugenol impression paste or rubber base (light body, regular body / mono phase) can be used for secondary impressions. The authors do not recommend the use of green stick border moulding and zinc oxide eugenol lining impressions. One perforation in maxillary tray in the palatal slope will avoid possible air trap. Rubber base impression requires adhesive to be painted on the tray surface. Adhesive must be dried for a minimum of 3 minutes. Impression material is mixed and spread uniformly over the tray surface including the borders. Then the tray is placed inside the mouth and pressure is applied over the ridges where platforms are made for the fingers of the operator to rest. When all the borders show the excess impression material flowing out and when the operator is convinced that the tray is seated fully further loading can be stopped and a repeat act of border moulding should be carried out. When the maxillary impression is taken, the patient can be instructed to bend the head forward and to protrude the tongue out for 30 seconds. Once the impression material is set, the tray can be removed gently. The maxillary tray very often does not get separated. In that case first the lips must be pulled up and the seal is broken. In a closed position the patient can also drive air between the tray and tissue to facilitate the removal. The mandibular trays do not pose problem except in cases of bilateral lingual undercuts. Instead of pulling the tray out if the tray is gently pushed inside the removal becomes easier. In the case of maxillary undercuts it is desirable to have elastic materials for both border moulding and for lining impression. Well formed casts are obtained from this impression by appropriate techniques of beading and boxing.

Suggested Reading

1. Fisher RD.*Six fundamental rules for making full denture impressions.*J Prosthet Dent. 1951;Jan-Mar1(1-2):135-44
2. Russell, A. F. *The reciprocal lower complete denture.* J Prosthet Dent 1959;9:180-190
3. Raybin, N. H. *The polished surface of complete dentures.* J Prosthet Dent 1963;3:236-239
4. Schiesser, F. J. Jr. *The neutral zone and polished surfaces in complete dentures.* J Prosthet Dent 1964;14:854-865.
5. Stromberg, W. R. and Hickey, J. C. *Comparison of physiologically and manually formed denture bases.* J Prosthet Dent 1965;15:213-226.
6. Lott, F. and Levin, B. *Flange technique: An anatomic and physiologic approach to increased retention, function, comfort and appearance of dentures.* J Prosthet Dent 1966;16:394-413.
7. Wright, C. R. *Evaluation of the factors necessary to develop stability in mandibular dentures.* J Prosthet Dent 1966;16:414-430.
8. Marmor D, Herbertson JE.*The use of swallowing in making complete lower impressions.*J Prosthet Dent. 1968; Mar19(3):208-18
9. Arbree, N. S., Yurkstas, A. A. and Kronman, J. H. *The coronomaxillary space: literature review and anatomic description.* J Prosthet Dent 1987;57:186-190.
10. Razek, M., Abdella, F., *Two dimensional study of the neutral zone at different. occlusal vertical heights.* J Prosthet Dent 1981;46:484-89.
11. Fahmy, F.M., Kharat, D. *A study of the importance of the neutral zone in complete dentures.* J Prosthet Dent 64:459-65.
12. Nikoukari H.*A study of posterior palatal seals with varying palatal forms.* J Prosthet Dent. 1975;Dec34(6):605-13
13. LaVere AM, Freda AL.*An individualized impression tray utilizing the patient's existing denture.*J Prosthet Dent. 1976 Sep; 36(3):334-6.

14. Beresin, V.E., Schiesser, F.J, *The Neutral Zone in Complete Dentures.* J Prosthet Dent 1976;36:356-65.
15. Schwarz WD.*One-step border molding of complete denture impressions using a polyether impression material.*J Prosthet Dent. 1980 Jan;43(1):117
16. Klein IE, Goldstein BM.*Physiologic determinants of primary impressions for complete dentures.*J Prosthet Dent 1984 May;51(5):611-6.
17. Kinderknecht KE, Dominici JT, Clark EP.*Preliminary silicone putty casts: diagnosis to final impression for complete dentures.*J Prosthet Dent. 1996 Apr;75(4):453-6.
18. Chaffee NR, Cooper LF, Felton DA.*A technique for border molding edentulous impressions using vinyl polysiloxane material.*J Prosthodont. 1999 Jun;8(2):129-34
19. Massad JJ, Cagna DR.*Vinyl polysiloxane impression material in removable prosthodontics. Part 1: edentulous impressions.* Compend Contin Educ Dent. 2007; Aug;28(8):452-9
20. Devan MM. *Basic principles in impression making.* J Prosthet Dent 1952;2:26-35.
21. McCord J F,Tyson K W, *A conservative prosthodontic option for the treatment of edentulous patients with atrophic (flat) madibular ridges,* Br Dent J 1997; 182(12): 469-72
22. Tyson K W, McCord J F, *Chairside options for the treatment of complete denture problems associated with the atrophic (flat) mandibular ridge,* Br Dent J 2000; 188: 10-14
23. Lynch C D and Allen P F, *Management of the flabby ridge : using contemporary materials to solve an old problem.* Br Dent J 2006; 200: 258-61
24. Crawford W I and Walmsley, *A review of prosthodontic management of fibrous ridges.* Br Dent J 2005; 199: 715-19
25. Hasanreisoglu Ufuk et al, *Evaluation of reproducibility of the peripheral tissues in edentulous patients,* Tr.J. of Medical sciences, 1998; 28: 291-94
26. Komiyama Osamu et al, *Effects of relief space and escape holes on pressure characteristics of maxillary edentulous impressions,* J Prosthet Dent 2004; 91:570-6
27. Al-Ahmad Adel et al, *Pressure generated on a simulated mandibular oral analog by impression materials in custom trays of different design.* J Prosthdont 2006;15:95-101
28. Duncan P Jacqueline et al, *A selective impression technique for the edentulous maxilla,* J Prosthet Dent 2004; 92:299-301
29. Smith Dale et al, *One step border molding of complete denture impressions using a polyether impression material,* J Prosthet Dent 1979; 41 :347-51

11

Jaw relations

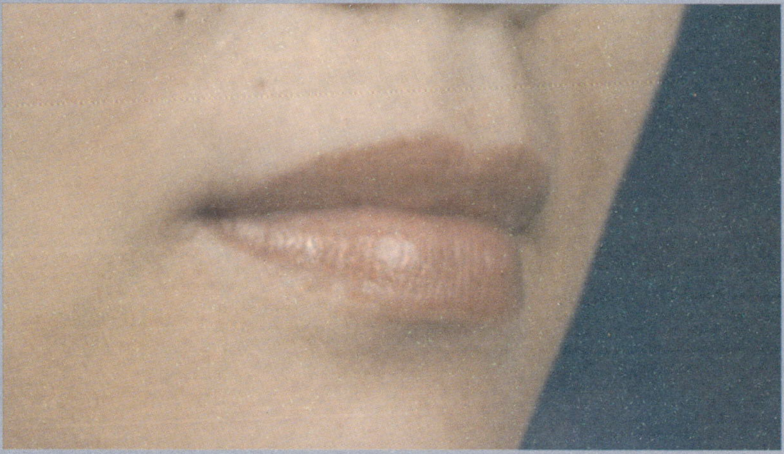

Jaw relations are relevant because dentures are fabricated outside the mouth

Dentures are made outside the mouth. The first requirement is the replica of the foundation on which the dentures are to be fabricated. This is obtained by making casts. If the dentures fit onto the casts, they should definitely fit on to the residual ridges. Now the teeth have to be arranged – fourteen teeth on to the maxillary denture and fourteen teeth on to the mandibular denture. The maxillary and mandibular teeth have to be aligned in an occlusal relationship. This arrangement can be made outside the mouth only if the casts are related mutually as they appear in the patient's mouth. Hence it becomes necessary to relate the upper and lower residual ridges and transfer that relationship to an instrument which can maintain the relationship while arranging the teeth. The upper and lower teeth are arranged into an occlusal relationship using that instrument and when the denture is transferred to the patient's mouth, the same occlusal relationship should be maintained. The stage of relating the upper and lower residual ridges is known as "registration of jaw relations". This relationship is transferred to a simulating device and it is known as articulator. With the aid of the registered relations, the upper and lower casts can be mounted on to the articulator and afterwards the articulator will function almost similar to the human jaws.

The upper jaw is fixed to the skull and a positional relationship between the skull and maxillary residual ridge can be transferred to the articulator through a face bow. Now the relationship between the upper and lower residual ridges has to be copied. The mandible moves in relation to the maxilla both in vertical and horizontal directions. Hence a standard position of the mandible has to be identified, recorded or registered and transferred to the articulator. Which is the standard or correct position of the mandible? The position of the mandible, the individual maintained when he had his dentition and which is kept at occlusion is the correct position. But now the individual is completely edentulous. So a guess work has to be employed which has ration and logic behind it.

First we have to think of the vertical relation between the maxillary ridge and the mandibular ridge. If the patient had posterior teeth, a reasonable measurement could have been made through radiographs and the same distance between the jaws could be copied in the dentures. But in an edentulous individual, the vertical distance between the jaws is established through an assumption that the rest position of the mandible remains the same irrespective of the dentulous or edentulous state. In the dentulous state, the space between the residual ridges was occupied by the teeth and the free way space. If the free way space is assigned a distance of 3 or 4 mm, the calculation becomes easier in the edentulous state. Our aim is to find out the vertical distance between the upper and lower ridges at occlusion when the patient had all the teeth. In the edentulous state, if the distance between the ridges at rest position of mandible is found out; the vertical distance at occlusion can be calculated by deducting the free way space from it. Occlusal rims are placed over the ridges, adjusted for height and then united by sealing. The sealed occlusal rims will act as an aid to relate the casts.

Measuring the inter arch distance inside the mouth is not a realistic proposal. Because the moment lips are parted, the lower jaw will drop down. Hence two points are selected extra orally – one representing the maxillary ridge is placed either on the tip of the nose or near the anterior nasal spine, close to the columella and one representing the mandibular ridge is placed over the chin, an area which is not easily stretched by the movements of the lower lip. On the selected areas, markers are fixed and measurements are made between them. First measurement is to find out the rest position distance between the markers. The patient is allowed to sit upright, relaxed and without head rest. This will bring the head to a natural position. The lower occlusal rim is placed over the mandibular ridge and the patient is asked to keep the lips in gentle contact. After a few minutes, the mandible will attain rest position. This is measured. The patient can be asked to pronounce 'M' repeatedly and to maintain a relaxed position. Measurement can be repeated. The exercise can be repeated a few times till congruent results are obtained. After this the maxillary occlusal rim is placed and the patient is asked to occlude the rims. The occlusal rim designing is explained in the subsequent section. At the occluded state, the measurement is taken again and the rim height is adjusted till the second measurement becomes lesser than the first measurement by 4mm (free way space measurement). Once this is achieved, patient is asked to pronounce 'S' repeatedly and during this act, one millimeter space (closest speaking space) should appear between the rims. If it is not present, height has to be reduced till that is obtained. At this stage, the vertical height between the ridges is correctly established with both free way space and closest speaking space maintained. The upper and lower occlusion rims should meet each other on a perfect plane.

Once the vertical relationship is established, the horizontal relationship has to be registered. In the horizontal plane, the mandible moves forward and to both sides. After that the mandible goes back to its original position. When the mandible moves back, the condyles are placed in an anterior and superior position in the glenoid fossa. This particular position is known as centric relation and which is registered as the correct position in the horizontal plane. During the posterior movement we do not know whether the condyles are in the centric relation position. Hence the manifestations of the position are taken into consideration. The classic manifestation is repeatability of the position. If the patient can bring back the mandible repeatedly to the same position, it can be presumed that centric relation is achieved. At the same time the condyles can be palpated just in front of the tragus to find out the movement. Patients can easily achieve the centric position by rolling back the tongue back to reach for the posterior border of the base and by reclining back by 45 degrees. This position if registered will relate the casts in the horizontal direction.

The maxillary and mandibular casts related vertically and horizontally can now be mounted in the articulator and from this point onwards the articulator movements are expected to simulate the mandibular movements. In order to achieve this a few more conditions are to be satisfied. One is that the articulator should have dimensions almost comparable to the human system. One example is the inter condylar distance which should approximately be 110 mm. For the opening and closing movements the mandible makes use of an axis. The articulator should also have a similar axis. The casts when mounted on the articulator must maintain a distance from the said axis of the articulator which should be comparable to that present in the patient. If this is not achieved, the occlusion generated in the articulator will not faithfully follow a relationship in the arc of closure. This is the reason why the maxillary cast is first fixed in the articulator using a face bow.

The Procedure

The casts obtained from the final impression are trimmed so that the sulcus is clearly visible and at the same time well supported by the land. A line is drawn with an indelible pencil along the fornix of the sulcus. This line would limit the extension of the transfer base. A base prepared on the cast and that can be transferred to the mouth and back to the cast is termed as transfer base or record base. Maxillary base can be prepared either in shellac base plate or in autopolymerising resin in routine clinical situations but the mandibular one should preferably be prepared in auto polymerising acrylic resin. The maxillary base is wide and has sufficient area to provide strength whereas the mandibular base is narrow and shellac base plate would get distorted easily during the operation and transfer. Transfer bases prepared in autopolymerizing resin are far superior to those prepared in shellac base plates in preventing warpage that would occur during the operations both in the clinic and in the lab. Areas of undercuts of more than 1 mm should be blocked out with wax to make the placement of the bases easier. Undercuts are usually present in the maxillary tuberosity region, labial region, mandibular mylohyoid region and in the lingual crescent region. If the undercuts can be managed by altering the path of insertion, it would always improve the retention. Unmanageable undercuts are always corrected surgically during the preparation stage.

Once the bases are prepared, occlusal rims

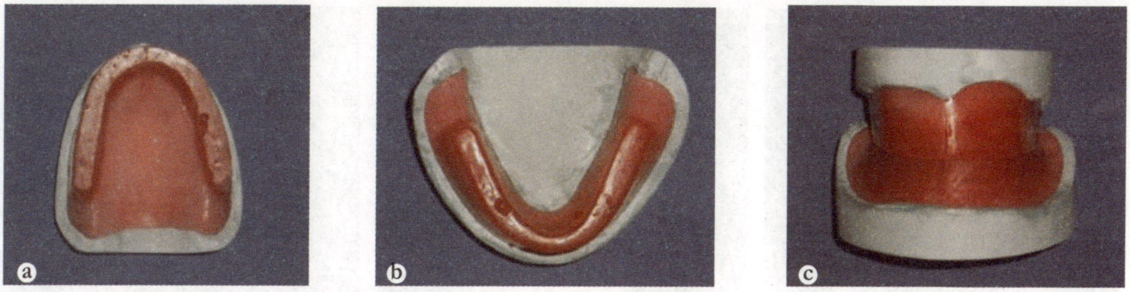

Fig. 11.1 a,b,c Upper/lower occlusal rims

are made in modelling wax. Wax should be rolled after softening it and care should be taken to avoid entrapment of air and pieces of separating paper. The rims should have a width of 4mm in the anterior region 5mm in the premolar region and 6 mm in the molar region. Mandibular occlusal rim is prepared first. The occlusal rim formed should follow the arch form of the mandibular ridge. Initially the crest of the posterior ridge is identified and a line is drawn with a pencil from the anterior border of the retro molar pad to the premolar region. This line is projected anteriorly and posteriorly to the land of the cast. The record base is then placed over the cast and posterior occlusal rim is made so that the midline of the occlusal rim coincides with the line previously extended to the land of the cast. In other words the occlusal rim will have a width of 3 mm on either side of the line. The posterior extension should be limited to 2mm short of the anterior border of retro molar pad. The height of the occlusal rim is adjusted to the midpoint of the retro molar pad. Posterior occlusal rims are prepared on both sides first. Then it is connected by the anterior occlusal rim, which should follow the anterior arch form of the ridge. The labial surface of the occlusal rim should not be made beyond the middle point of the labial sulcus. The height is limited to 18mm from the sulcus. Once this is completed, the occlusal rim is finished and polished. (fig. 11.1)

The maxillary occlusal rim should follow the arch form developed for the mandible. Maxillary occlusal rim is made in one stretch following the dimensions mentioned earlier. The labial surface of the occlusal rim should be placed 8 mm anterior to the midpoint of the incisive papilla. In order to ascertain this point, a line is drawn on the cast through the midpoint and extended across to the land area. The labial surface of the maxillary rim is positioned 8 mm anterior to this line. The height of the occlusal rim in the anterior region measured from the labial sulcus should be limited to 22mm. The full arch occlusal rim is made and on completion it will have a slope of nearly 3 mm antero posteriorly.

The completed maxillary occlusal rim should have a labial proclination where as posteriorly the buccal surfaces should incline in a palatal direction. Labial surface of the mandibular rim is made vertical and the buccal surfaces are inclined lingually. The height and labial positioning of the occlusal rims are subjected to variation during the clinical process.

Instruments and materials required:

1. Prepared occlusion rims
2. Modelling wax
3. Wax knife
4. Flat surfaced metallic wax trimming instrument
5. Calipers / Willi's gauge
6. Bowl of cold water
7. Denture adhesive
8. Staple pins / bite registration paste /alu wax

The patient is seated erect with the head unsupported. Two triangular pieces of adhesive plaster are placed - one at the tip of the nose and the other at the chin with the apices facing each other. The mandibular occlusal rim is then placed inside the mouth and the patient is asked to sit relaxed. The distance between the apices of the triangles is measured with a caliper. Then the patient is instructed to breath

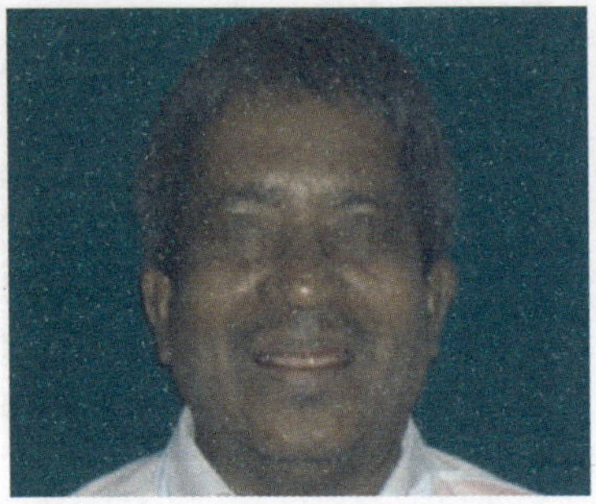

Fig. 11.2 Visibility of occlusion rims on smiling

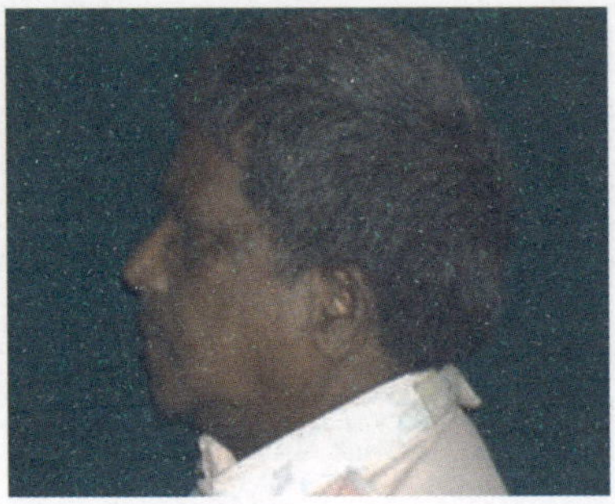

Fig. 11.3 Soft tissue support obtained with occlusion rims

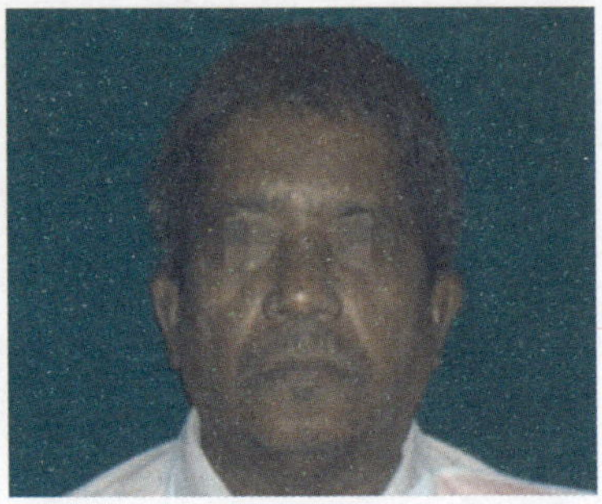

Fig. 11.4 Soft tissue support and adequate visibility of the vermilion borders

deeply and relax. In the relaxed state the upper and the lower lips should just meet. The measurement is again repeated. This measurement indicates the mandibular position at rest. By keeping the mandibular occlusal rim, it is presumed that the gravitational forces will keep the mandible in a near dentulous state. After this, the mandibular occlusal rim is adjusted. The height in the anterior region is placed just below the level of the dry wet junction of the lower lip. Then the patient is instructed to sit relaxed and an instrument is passed through the angle of the mouth to ascertain whether it touches the occlusal surface of the rim. The height of the occlusal rim at the angle of the mouth is thus

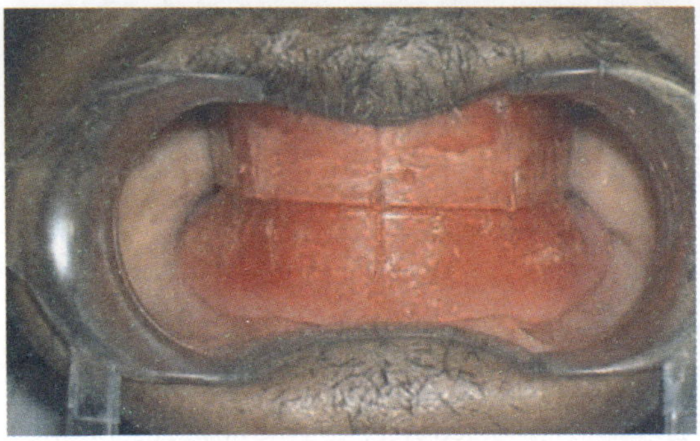

Fig. 11.5 Adjusted rims at occlusion

determined. There is a possibility of committing mistakes in this stage if the mandibular denture base is not retentive and if it is not seated close to the ridge. Now the posterior occlusal rim height is adjusted from the angle of the mouth to the mid point of the retro molar pad. Once this is done the mandibular rim is placed back on to the cast. At this stage, the anterior portion of the occlusion rim can be cut and removed so that in the subsequent stages intra oral visual examination becomes easier. This portion can be added later while registering the relation.

The maxillary rim is then placed inside the mouth and the first thing to be ascertained is the soft tissue support, ie. the contour of the upper lip. If the upper lip is not adequately supported, visibility of the vermillion will not be adequate. Nasiolabial angle will be more than 95 degrees in edentulous individuals. This can be appreciated by observing the profile view of the face. The nasiolabial folds will become deepened in the edentulous state. However attempts should not be made to obliterate the fold completely. Experience in the assessment can be obtained by observing the facial features of dentate

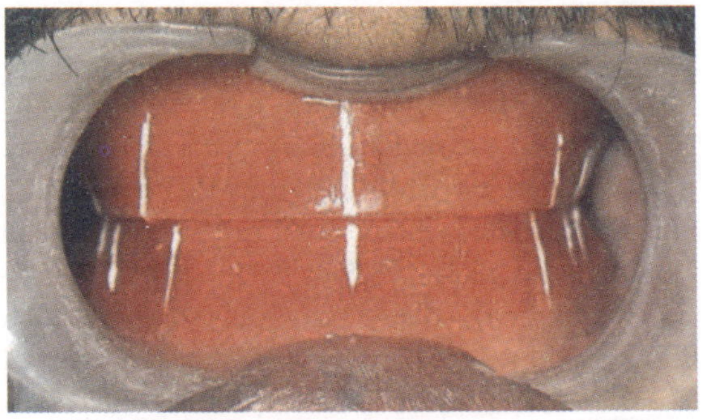

Fig. 11.6 Mid lines and canine lines marked with white crayons

individuals over a period of time. Once the soft tissue support is obtained, the patient will get a dentulous appearance. Visibility of the occlusal rim is checked at rest and during action of the upper lip viz smile. (fig. 11.2-11.4) It is then trimmed perpendicular to the midsagittal plane or parallel to the inter papillary axis. At rest 1 mm visibility is desired and as age advances, the visibility gets reduced. When the patient is asked to smile, the lips should go up as a

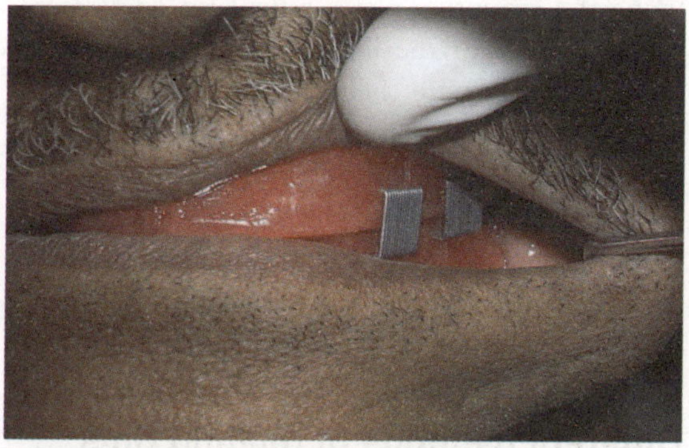

Fig. 11.7 Occlusion rims united with staple pins

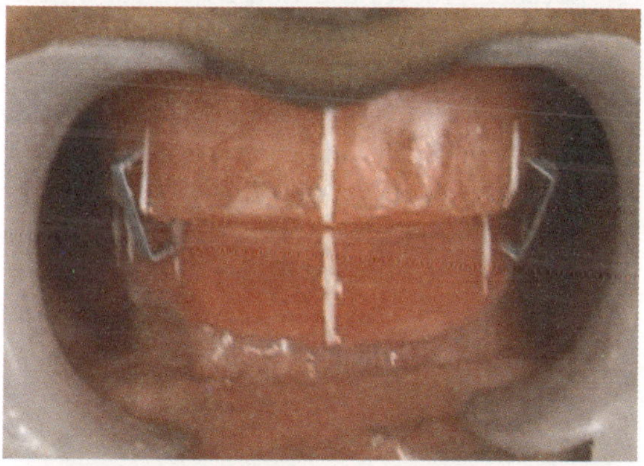

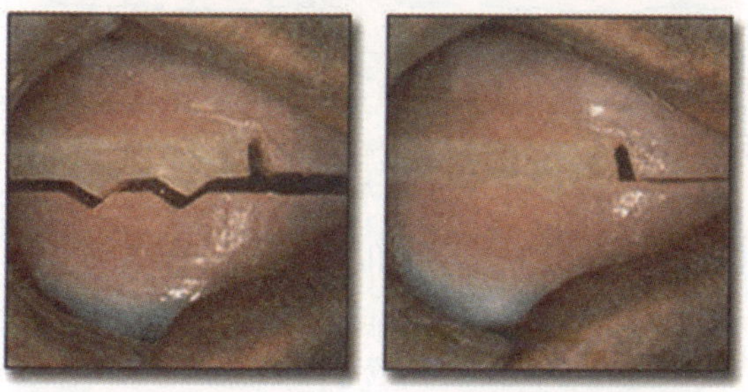

Fig. 11.8 Alu wax can also be used to record centric

curtain showing the possible dimensions of anterior teeth. In most of the cases the gingival portion of teeth will not be visible. This will act as a guide in arranging the teeth. Considering this factor the anterior occlusal rim is shaped and adjusted. The posterior occlusal rim height is adjusted to ala-tragal line. This line is marked between the root of the ala of the nose and the upper border of the tragus. In younger individuals the middle point of the tragus is usually selected. Orientation of the plane can be ascertained by an instrument called Fox's occlusal plane indicator. It is a metallic or plastic plate which when held against the occlusal rim would help in comparing the parallelism of occlusal plane with ala-tragal line. Orienting the occlusal plane parallel to the ala-tragal line, helps the operator to start with the jaw relation procedures. However this should not be confused with the occlusal plane he/she is going to generate at a later stage. The teeth need not necessarily be arranged in this plane but it is a valid starting point especially to the novice. (fig. 11.5)

Once the occlusion rims are adjusted for its shape, height, and the soft tissue support and for close approximation of the upper and lower rims, a verification method on the height is to be administered. This is by way of phonation. The patient is asked to pronounce 'S' repeatedly and the operator has to observe for an one millimeter gap between the occlusion rims. While phonation, if the occlusion rims are coming into contact the height of the mandibular rim should be reduced so that the closest speaking space appears during speech. Another phonation test administered is the pronunciation of 'F' and 'V' and during phonation the lower rim should gently contact the upper lip. But this becomes more relevant in the trial stage because it is concerned with the position of the maxillary anteriors and their relationship with lower lip. A sharp line is now marked in the midline coinciding with the mid sagittal plane of the face. The tubercle of the philtrum can provide a guide line in identifying the mid sagittal plane of the face but the visual perception of the operator should determine the coincidence of the mid sagittal plane and the mark made on the maxillary occlusion rim. Patient is then instructed to close the mouth in centric relation. An instruction to roll back the tongue and to reach for the posterior border of the maxillary record base will automatically position the mandible in the centric relation position. At this point the mid line is extended over to the mandibular occlusion rim. Another line is marked vertically in the canine region on both sides. Similarly sloped double lines are marked in the molar region. These markings will help the operator to verify the mandibular position repeatedly. (fig. 11.6). Once the mandibular position i.e. the centric relation is ascertained, the maxillary and mandibular rims are to be united in order to register the relation. Most of the operators prefer to unite the occlusal rims using a heated instrument. For a beginner this is not a safe method because of the chances of burning the soft tissue. If proper care is taken to retract the lips and cheeks with one hand and to take a finger rest while moving the heated instrument, problems can be avoided. A beginner can try to seal the occlusal rims with heated staple pins. (fig. 11.7)

After sealing the rims, time must be allowed for the molten wax to harden. Making 'V' cuts on the occlusal surfaces and troughs to accommodate bite registration paste is an alternate method of bite registration. Then the sealed occlusion rims are removed in one piece or two pieces. In case of restricted opening alternate techniques of sealing should be thought of. Outside the mouth the sealing is once again reinforced and the rims are chilled in cold water. The casts are then repositioned on the record bases. Care should be taken to seat the record bases properly so that the casts and transfer bases maintain a clearance of 3 mm at the heels. Heels of the mandibular cast are to be trimmed on most of the occasions. Record bases and the casts are then united using sticks and super glue. When semi adjustable articulators are used, the maxillary casts are mounted initially in the articulator by face bow transfer and hence mounting the mandibular cast is easier. In fixed path articulators the occlusal plane is made to coincide with the horizontal mid plane of the articulator while mounting the casts. Before fixing the mounting plates articulator adjustments especially that of the incisal guide pin should be made. The casts are then connected to the upper and lower members successively. By this process, the casts are related vertically and horizontally as in the patient and the articulator now starts performing as the human system. The teeth are now arranged in the articulator and the occlusion generated will be faithful in the patient's mouth.

Different methods of relating rims

1. Locating grooves and troughs are cut on the occlusal surfaces and smear the wax surface with vaseline. Fill it with zinc oxide eugenol paste/ elastomer/bite registration paste/alu wax. (11.8)
2. Make sure that the rims approximate evenly and then unite them with pins
3. After cutting locating grooves and smearing with vaseline, softened wax wafer is placed in between and the patient is asked to bite on it. More than one record can be made with this technique

Suggested Reading

1. Kingery, R. H. *A review of some problems associated with centric relation.* J Prosthet Dent 1952; 2:307-319.
2. Kapur, K.K. and Yurkstas, A. *An evaluation of centric relation records obtained by various techniques.* J Prosthet Dent 1957;7:770-86
3. Lucia, V. 0. *Centric relation - theory and practice.* J Prosthet Dent 1960;10:849-856.
4. Lucia, V. 0. *A technique for recording centric relation.* J Prosthet Dent 1964;14:492-505.
5. Hickey, J. A. *Centric relation - A must for complete dentures.* Dent Cli N Am 1964 Nov:587-600.
6. Atwood, D.A. *A critique of research of the posterior limit of the mandibular position.* J Prosthet Dent 1968;20:21-36.
7. Roraff, A. R. and Stansberry, B. E. *Errors caused by dimensional change in mounting material.* J Prosthet Dent 1972;28:247-252.

8. Kantor, M. E., Silverman, S.I. and Garfinkel, L. *Centric relation recording techniques. A comparative investigation.* J Prosthet Dent 1972;28:593-60. J Prosthet Dent 1973;30:604-606.
9. Lundeen, H. *Centric relation records: The effect of muscle action.* J Prosthet Dent 1974; 31:244-25.
10. Moss, M. L. *A functional cranial analysis of centric relation.* Dent Cli N Am 1975;19:431-442.
11. Levy, *P. H. Clinical implications of mandibular repositioning and the concept of an alterable centric relation.* Dent Cli N Am 1975;19:543-570.
12. Shafagh, I., et al. *Diurnal variance of centric relation position.* J Prosthet Dent 1975;34:574-582.
13. Guichet, N. F. *Biological laws governing functions of muscles that move the mandible. a. Part I: Occlusal programming.* J Prosthet Dent 1977;37:648-656. *b. Part II: Condylar position.* J Prosthet Dent 1977; 38:35-41. *c. Part III: Speed of closure - manipulation of the mandible.* J Prosthet Dent 1977;38:174-179. *d. Part IV: Degree of jaw separation and potential for maximum jaw separation.* J Prosthet Dent 1977;38:301-310.
14. Meyers, M. *Centric relation records - historical review.* J Prosthet Dent 1982;47:141-145.
15. Gilboe, D. R. *Centric relation as the treatment position.* J Prosthet Dent 1983; 50:685-689.
16. Dawson, P. E. *Optimum TMJ condylar position in clinical practice.* Int J Perio Rest Dent 1985;3:11.
17. Woelfel, J. B. *New device for accurately recording centric relation.* J Prosthet Dent 1986; 56:716-727.
18. Wood, G.W. *Centric relation and the treatment position in rehabilitating occlusions: A physiologic approach. Part I: Developing optimum mandibular posture.* J Prosthet Dent 1988;59:647-65.
19. McCord JF, Grant AA.Registration: *stage II—intermaxillary relations.*Br Dent J. 2000 Jun 10;188(11):601-6.
20. Agarwal A, Howlett JA, Howell PG.*A biometric guide to prosthetic tooth positioning investigated in subjects with Class II division 2 incisor relationships.* Eur J Prosthodont Restor Dent. 2000 Dec;8(4):127-9.
21. Shanahan *TE. Physiologic jaw relations and occlusion of complete dentures.* 1955.J Prosthet Dent. 2004 Mar;91(3):203-5.
22. Williamson RA, Williamson AE, Bowley J, Toothaker R. *Maximizing mandibular prosthesis stability utilizing linear occlusion, occlusal plane selection, and centric recording.*J Prosthodont. 2004 Mar;13(1):55-61.
23. Boulos PJ.*Simplified method for recording maxillomandibular relations in complete dentures.* N Y State Dent J. 2007 Apr;73(3):24-7.
24. Daher T, Dermeṇdjian S, Morgano SM. *Obtaining maxillomandibular records and definitive impressions in a single visit for a completely edentulous patient with ahistory of combination syndrome.*J Prosthet Dent. 2008 Jun;99(6):489-91.
25. Al-Ansari A. *Predicting successful outcomes of complete denture therapy.*Evid Based Dent. 2010;11(2):47.

12

Articulators

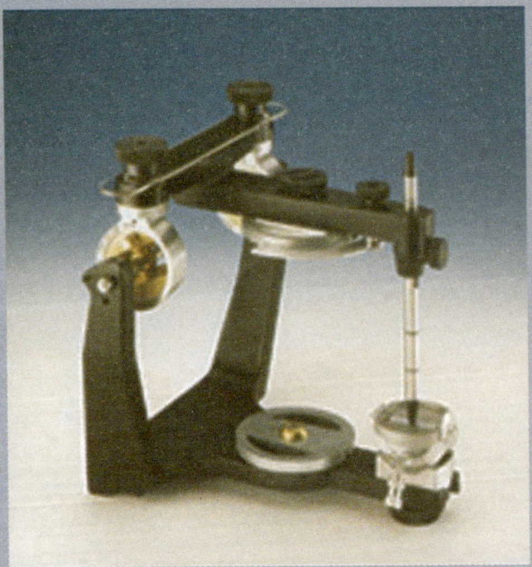

Dentures are fabricated outside the mouth. Hence an articulator that simulates the human system is necessary.

The maxillary and mandibular residual ridges are related in the desired position during the jaw relation stage. Further stages of the fabrication of complete dentures has to be done outside the mouth. For this purpose the maxillary and mandibular casts are first related using the jaw relation record and then the entire assembly is mounted in an instrument that represents the jaw members as well as the temporomandibular joint. Articulator is the instrument of choice and it will act as the patient in his absence. Articulator has to simulate all the functional movements of the jaws but very seldom it is fully achieved. Three different types of articulators are mainly used in Prosthodontics viz. non adjustable articulators, semi adjustable articulators, fully adjustable articulators.

International Prosthodontic Workshop on complete denture occlusion has accepted a classification system for articulators comprising of four classes.

Class I. A simple holding instrument capable of accepting a single static registration. Vertical motion is possible.

Subdivision A: Vertical motion is possible, but only for convenience. Examples: The Corelator and The Verticulator (Fig 12.1a)

Subdivision B: Vertical motion is joint related. Example: The Centric Relator (Fig 12.1b)

Class II. An instrument that permits horizontal as well as vertical motion but does not orient the motion to the temporomandibular joints.

Subdivision A: Eccentric motion permitted is based on average or arbitrary values.Examples: Gysi Simplex, Shofu Handy II (Fig 12.2a)

Subdivision B: Eccentric motion permitted is based on theories of arbitrary motion. Example: The Monson Maxillomadibular articulator (Fig. 12.2c)

Subdivision C: Eccentric motion permitted and is determined by the patient using engraving methods. Examples: The Gnathic Relator, The House articulator

Class III. An instrument that simulates condylar pathways by using averages or mechanical equivalents for all or part of the motion. These instruments allow for orientation of the cast relative to the joints and may be arcon or nonarcon instruments. (Arcon articulator - An articulator that maintains anatomic guidelines by the use of condylar analogs in the mandibular element and fossa assemblies in the maxillary element.)

Subdivision A: Instruments that accept static protrusive registrations and use equivalents for the rest of the motion. Examples: Hanau Model H, Dentatus, Bergstrom articulator. (Fig. 12.3a)

Hanau Model H was designed by Rudolph Hanau in 1923. This articulator accepts face-bow transfer and the horizontal condylar inclinations are set by means of a protrusive interocclusal record. This articulator is non arcon type with the condylar elements fixed to the upper member. The Bennett angle (L) is calculated from the horizontal condylar inclination (H) by means of Hanau's equation $L=(H/8)+12$.

Dentatus was designed by Beyron in 1944 in Sweden. This articulator is unique in that the relationship between the upper and lower members can be standardized with a "gauge block", so that casts can be transferred from one articulator to another and still maintain the relationship.

Subdivision B: Instruments that accept static lateral protrusive registrations and use equivalents for the rest of the motion. Examples: Denar Mark II, Whip Mix,Case Articulator, Gysi Trubyte articulator, Hanau Kinoscope, Stansbury tripod, Ney articulator, Panadent. (Fig. 12.3b)

The Ney articulator was designed by De Pietro in 1960 and was the first instrument to have condylar housing that contained adjustable rear, medial, and top walls in one assembly.

The Panadent articulator was designed by Robert Lee and utilizes interchangeable preformed curved analog fossae for condylar pathways. These preformed analogs which were developed from research that demonstrated the lateral condylar pathways, were quite similar in curvature except for steepness of the horizontal condylar inclination and the measure of immediate side shift.

Class IV. These instruments can accept three dimensional dynamic registrations. Class IV articulators allow for orientation of the cast to the temporomandibular joints and replication of all mandibular movements.

Subdivision A: The cam representing the condylar paths are formed by registration engraved by the patient. Example: TMJ articulator (fig. 12.4a)

Subdivision B: Instruments that have condylar paths that can be angled and customized either by selection from a variety of curvatures, by modification, or both. Examples: Stuart Gnathological Computer, Denar Model 5A (Fig. 12.4b).

These articulators are the instruments of choice for complete reconstructions and as teaching aids for advanced occlusal studies.

Awni Rihani in 1980 proposed a classification of articulators that appears to be the accepted terminology to date. The classifications were based on the acceptability of the following records:

1. Face-bow record
2. Centric jaw relation record
3. Protrusive record
4. Lateral records
5. Intercondylar distance

A nonadjustable articulator can accept one or two of the following records: Face bow, centric jaw relation or protrusive record (Fig. 12.5).

A semi adjustable articulator can accept all three of those records. (Fig. 12.6)

A fully adjustable articulator can accept the following five records: Face bow, centric jaw relation, protrusive, lateral records, and intercondylar distance record. (Fig. 12.7)

- A class I articulator is a nonadjustable articulator.
- A class II or III articulator is a semiadjustable articulator.
- A class IV articulator is a fully adjustable articulator.

For prosthodontic purposes, generally semi adjustable articulators are made use of. These can be of two types namely arcon and non arcon. In arcon type articulators, the condylar element is fixed to the lower member where as in the non arcon articulators, the condylar element is attached to the upper member. On opening the articulator, the angle between the condylar inclination and the occlusal plane remain stationary in the arcon type whereas the angle varies in the non-arcon articulator. The term arcon was coined by Bergstrom from the words articulator and condyle. (Fig. 12.8, 12.9)

Requirements of an articulator

1. Once adjusted the upper and the lower members of the articulator should maintain the horizontal and the vertical relationship between the upper and lower casts precisely. This would ensure the maintenance of the centric position.
2. The articulator should have provisions to allow easy mounting and detachment of the casts.
3. An incisal guide pin is fixed preferably to the upper member and it should stop on an incisal guide table to maintain the vertical relationship. Both the pin and table should have adjustability.
4. The articulator should open and close in a hinge fashion whenever required.
5. The articulator should receive a face bow so that the casts can be mounted in relation to the intercondylar axis as seen in the patients head. A face bow transfer should ensure the position of the cast in all the three dimensions namely vertical, lateral and anteroposterior in relation to the opening axis.
6. The articulator should provide an unhindered vision from all directions so that the operator can observe the occlusal relationship from both the buccal and the lingual positions.
7. The condylar elements should have adjustability for horizontal condylar inclination and for Bennett movement.
8. The articulator should be sturdy and should resist wear on continued use. For making complete dentures it is always preferred to use an articulator that has got similarity in dimensions to the human system. In olden times a small hinge articulator was always used. Its dimensions had no similarity to the human head dimensions. An average value articulator is much better than a hinge articulator because of its similarity to human system.

When the dentures are made in a hinge articulator the distance between the opening axis and the mounted casts is too short when compared to that present in the human head. The opening arc of the articulator and that of the human system are not similar and

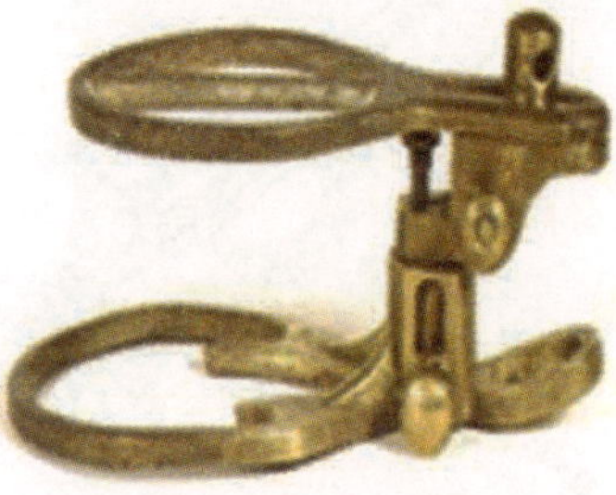

Fig. 12.1 a. Hinge articulator –Class I Subdivision A: Vertical motion is possible, but only for convenience.

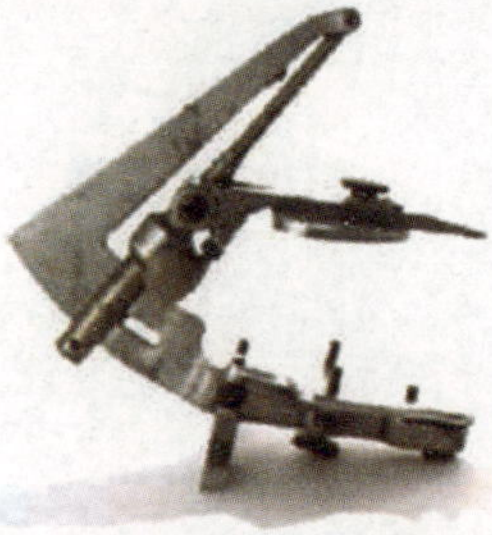

Fig. 12.2 b. The Monson Maxillomandibular articulator-ClassII -Subdivision B: Eccentric motion permitted is based on theories of arbitrary motion

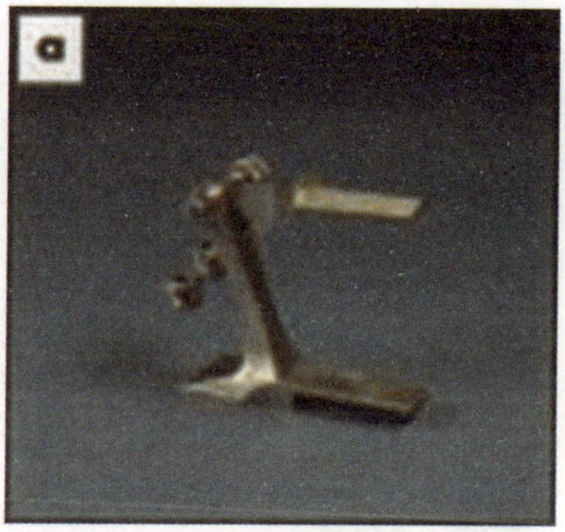

Fig. 12.1 b. Hinge articulator- Class I Subdivision B: Vertical motion is joint related

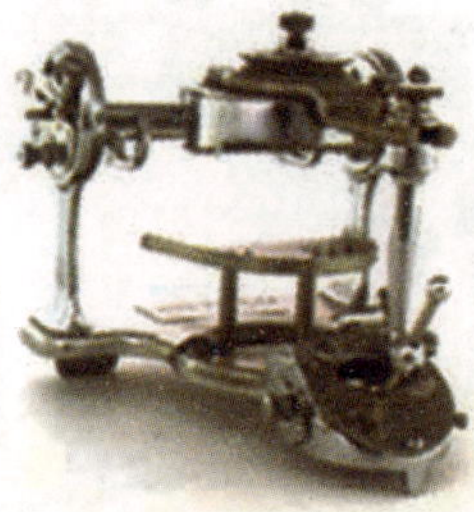

Fig. 12.2 c. The Gnathic Relator :ClassII Subdivision C: Eccentric motion permitted is determined by the patient using engraving methods

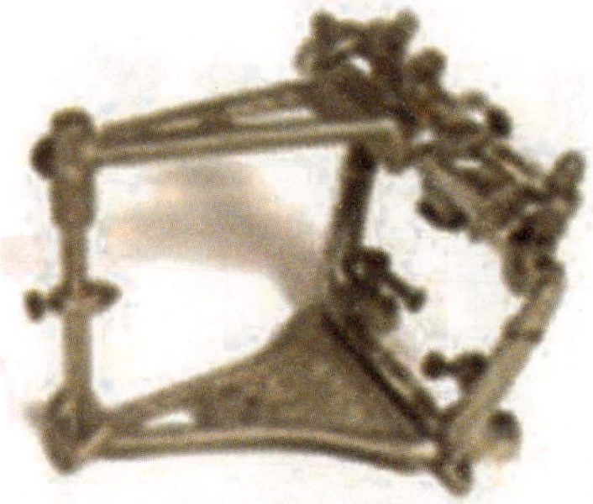

Fig. 12.2 a. Gysi simplex: Class II-Sub division –A: Eccentric motion permitted is based on average or arbitrary values.

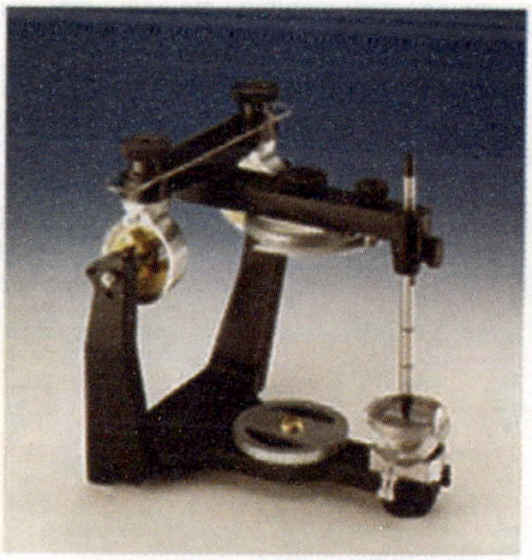

Fig. 12.3 a. Hanau Wide Vue articulator: Class III Subdivision A: Instruments that accept static protrusive registrations and use equivalents for the rest of the motion.

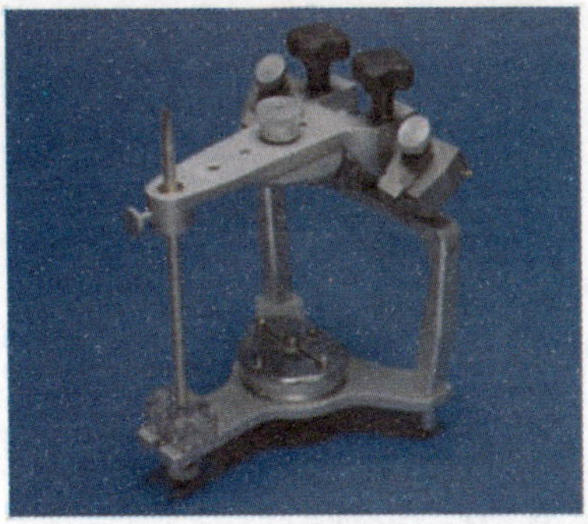

Fig. 12.3 b. WhipMix articulator: Class III Subdivision B: Instruments that accept static lateral protrusive registrations and use equivalents for the rest of the motion.

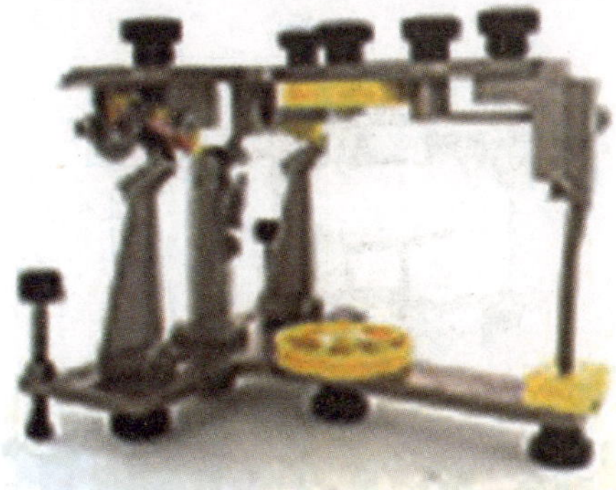

Fig. 12.4 a. TMJ articulator: Class IV Subdivision A: The cam representing the condylar paths are formed by registration engraved by the patient.

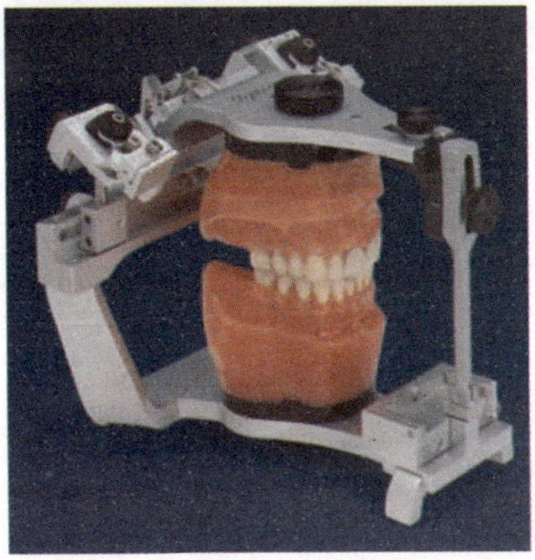

Fig. 12.4 b. Denar Model 5A ClassIV Subdivision B: Instruments that have condylar paths that can be angled and customized either by selection from a variety of curvatures, by modification, or both.

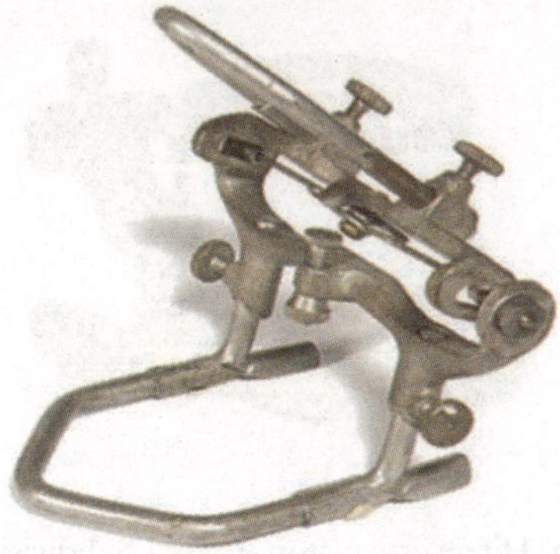

Fig. 12.5 Non adjustable articulator - Gritman articulator

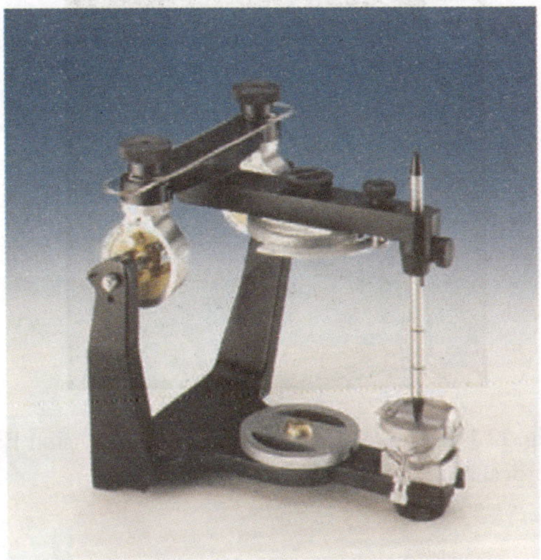

Fig. 12.6 Semi adjustable articulator - Hanau Wide Vue

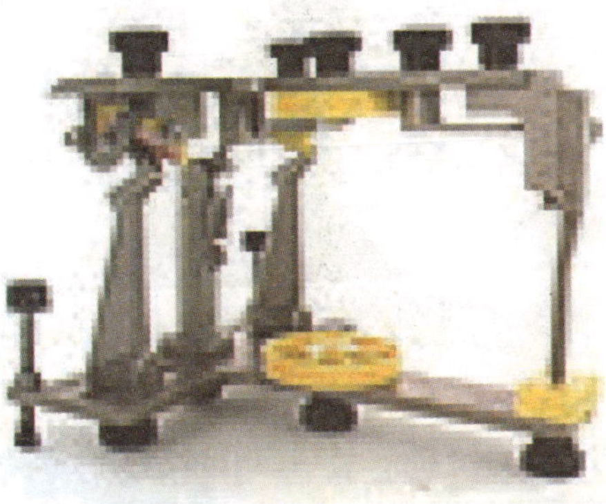

Fig. 12.7 Fully adjustable articulator - TMJ articulator

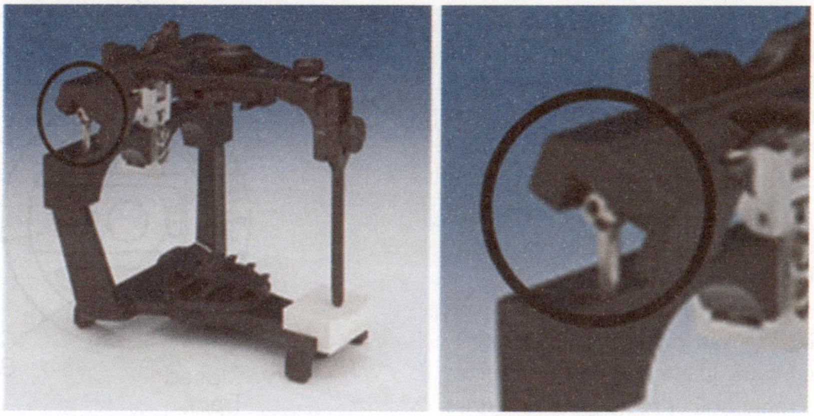

Fig. 12.8 Arcon articulator-condylar housing in the upper member and condylar element attached to the lower member

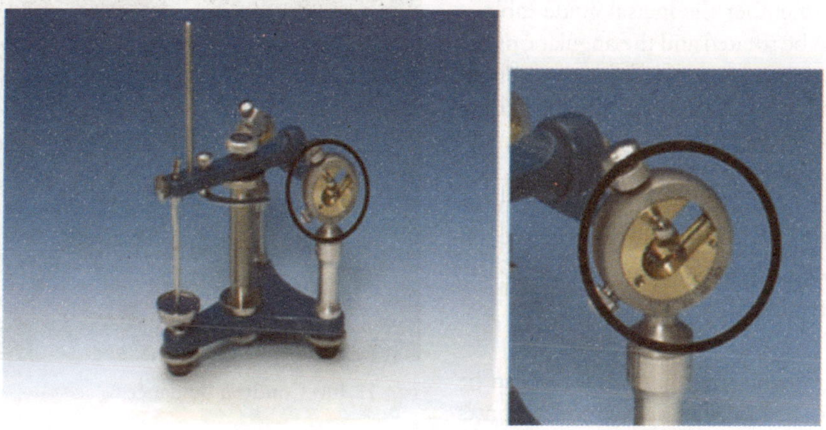

Fig. 12.9 Non-Arcon articulator-condylar housing in lower member, and condylar element attached to the upper member

on most of the occasions a premature contact is observed at the posterior region. Similarly the lateral excursive movements will also be affected if such an articulator is used. Use of a semi adjustable articulator which can receive a face bow transfer will produce jaw movements which is almost similar to the human system and the occlusion generated in the articulator will be faithful in patients.

Dentatus Articulator ARH

This is a semi adjustable articulator that consists of an upper jaw member and a lower jaw member. The lower jaw member is triangular in shape and at the posterior angles two condylar posts are positioned. On top of the condylar posts is a condylar assembly holder. The condylar housing has a circular frame in which the condylar track assembly is positioned. The assembly has a slot known as condylar track in which the condylar sphere moves. The condylar track assembly can be rotated within the circular frame of the condylar assembly holder. The rotation is done around the opening axis of the articulator. The condylar track assembly can be adjusted to desired positions by a set screw and thereby the horizontal condylar inclination can be fixed. The circular frame of the condylar holder is slotted in the anterior portion to accommodate stop screws for the condylar spheres. The condylar track assembly is also provided with an auditory pin to hold the ear piece face bow. The circular frame of the condylar track assembly holder has got markings in degrees to indicate the horizontal condylar inclination. The condylar track assembly is provided with a line marked along the radius which when coincides with an angulation – marking, provides an information on horizontal condylar inclination. The assembly is also provided with a lock screw which when tightened will lock the condylar sphere but it will allow the condylar axis pin to rotate. On locking, the articulator will work like a hinged instrument. The condylar assembly holder can rotate around a vertical axis on the condylar post. This is to allow for the Bennet angle settings. Angles are marked on top of the condylar posts. At the anterior part of the lower jaw member the incisal guide table is attached. This can be rotated and the angulations are calibrated. Lock nuts are provided for the Bennet angle settings and the incisal table settings. These lock nuts will also serve as legs for the instrument. The upper jaw member is a flat rod which is attached to the condylar axis rod. At the anterior portion the upper member is provided with three attachments-

1. Orbital axis plane indicator
2. Support rod for upper jaw member
3. Incisal pin

Both the incisal pin and the orbital axis pin can be tightened with lock nuts. The incisal guide pin is provided with a calibration on top and a curvature in the upper half. The calibrations help the operator to reposition the incisal pin accurately. The curvature allows the upper member to move up and down so that on tightening the tip of the incisal guide pin will always be at the center of the incisal guide table, ensuring the centric position.

The upper and lower members are provided with mounting plates which are attached to the members through screws. This system allows an operator to use the same instrument for more than one patient provided separate mounting plates are procured.

Hanau Wide Vue

The Hanau Wide-Vue Articulators are classified as semi-adjustable, based on arcon principle. The condyle of the articulator is a part of the lower member and functions as the condyle of the patient's mandible.

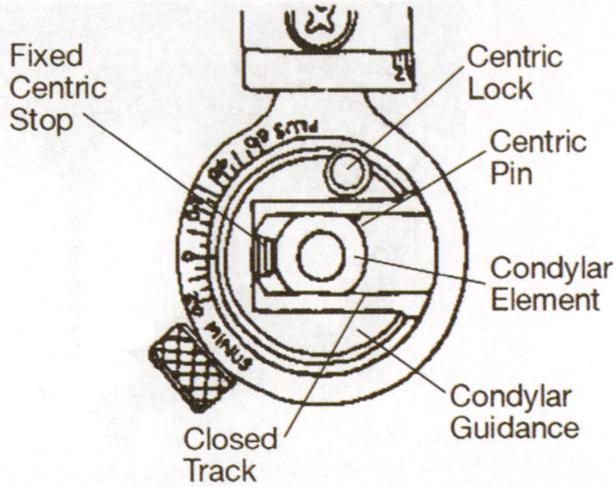

Fig 12.10a Condylar guidance

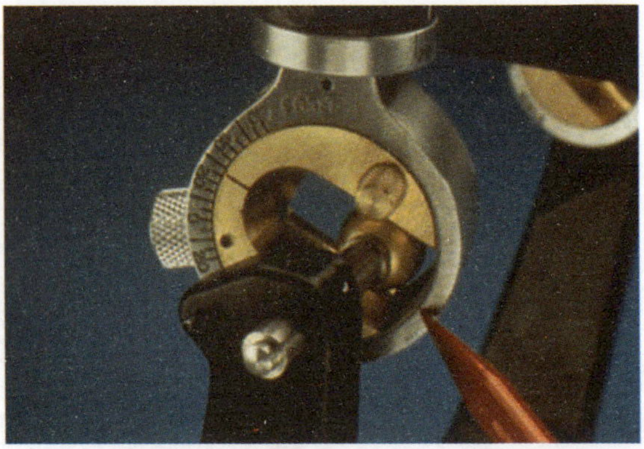

Fig 12.10b Condylar guidance

Condylar guidance: The condylar guidances are the control centers of the articulator and they adjustably assimilate the multiple function of the glenoid fossa (Fig 12.10a,b).The condylar track may be adjustably inclined on the horizontal transverse axis from a "zero" to a plus 60 degree or to a minus 20 degree. These inclinations are termed the protrusive inclination and simulate the patient's superior wall of the fossa.The Condylar track may also be adjusted on the vertical axis from a "zero" sagittal to 30°. This angle is termed the progressive Bennett angle and corresponds to the medial wall of the patient's fossa.

Closed condylar track: The condylar guidance track rotates in an enclosed housing which stops the condylar element, preventing the accidental

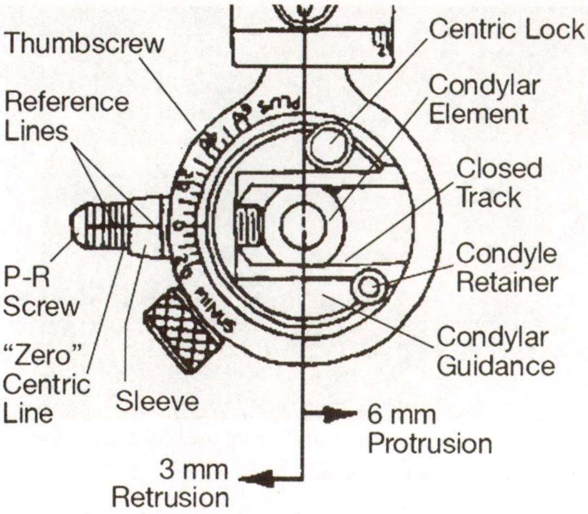

Fig 12.11 Closed condylar track with centric stop and PR screw

disengagement of the upper member (Fig 12.11).

Fixed centric stop: A centric stop at the posterior end of the track limits the anterior movement of the condylar element. When the element rests against the stop it is at centric, the point from which the protrusive or Bennett angles both emanate.

Adjustable protrusive-retrusive: The micrometer adjustment permits the condylar element to be protruded 6 mm from centric or to be retruded 3 mm from centric. An axial reference line transcribes the one mm spaced lines on the P-R Screw and a similar line appears on the sleeve of the guidance. Protrusion or retrusion of the condylar element can be fractionally adjusted by selective rotation of this P-R Screw. One full turn of the one millimeter pitch screw equals 1 mm. protrusion or retrusion. This adjustment is secured by tightening the thumbscrew lock at the medial of the guidance. The micrometer adjustment may be returned to this exacting centric position at any time.

Centric lock: Engagement of a centric lock depresses a centric pin, causing it to arrest the condylar element at the centric position. When locked, the upper member is restricted to an opening and closing movement only. Releasing the centric lock two full turns will disengage the centric pin and return the element's freedom of movement in the condylar track.

Condylar shafts: The condylar shafts adjustably slide in the "wings" of the lower member (Fig 12.12a,b). They have been factory fixed by setscrews when their brass shoulders rest against the flatted sides of the condylar elements at the "zero" centric position. A resilient bumper will protectively stop the upper member and rest against the "wing" of the lower member when fully opening the articulator.

Dual-end incisal pin: Coinciding with these condylar shaft adjustments is an alignment of the

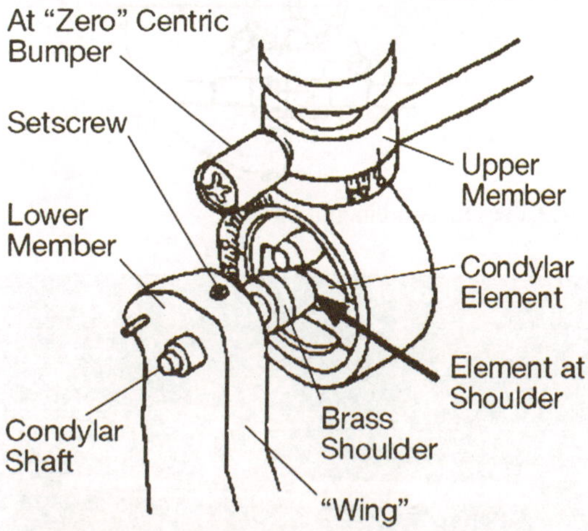

Fig 12.12a Condylar shaft attached to the lower member

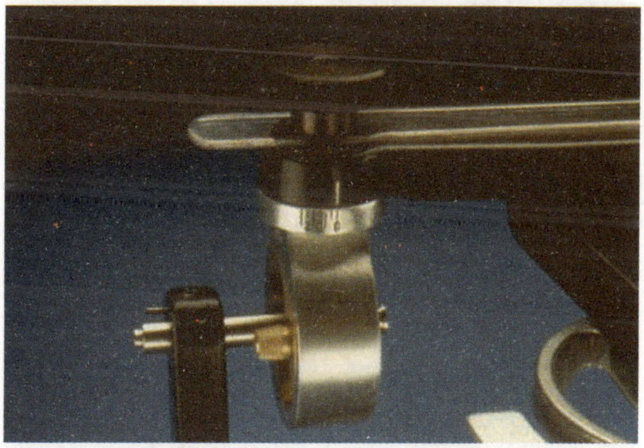

Fig 12.12b Condylar shaft attached to the lower member

chisel edge of the incisal pin with the central table of the Incisal Guide. The Incisal Pin serves as the forward control of the articulator. It maintains a vertical stop and provides a stylus contact for the excursive movements of the Articulator against the various inclined guiding surfaces of the Incisal Guide.(Fig 12.13a). A mid-line groove is cut in the

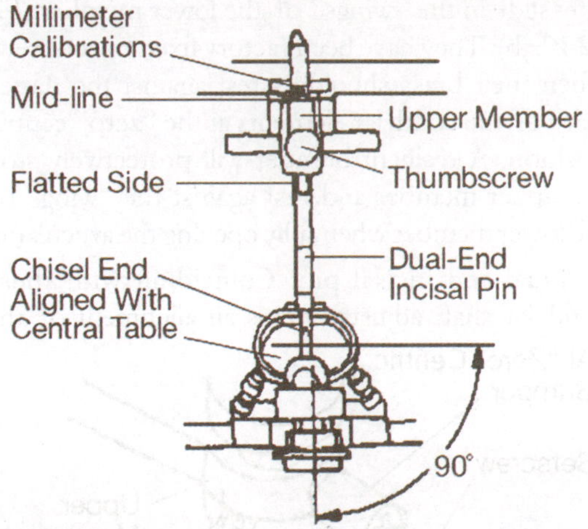

Fig 12.13a Dual end incisal pin

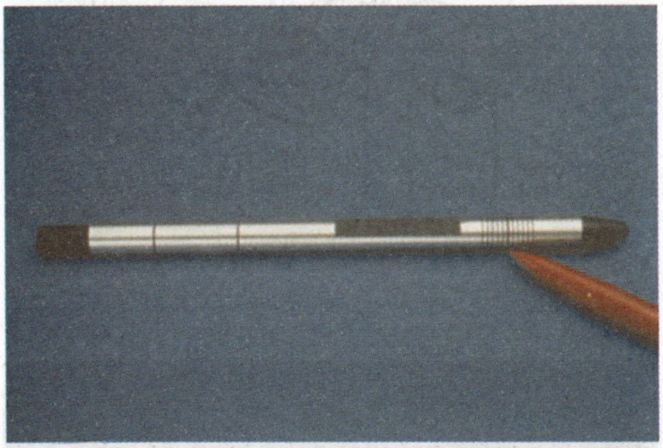

Fig 12.13b Dual end incisal pin

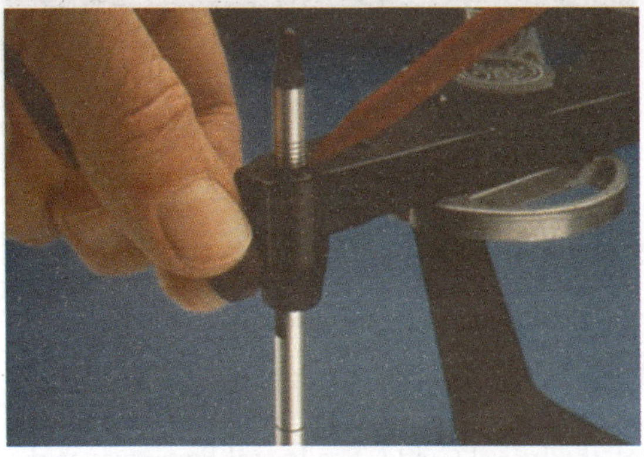

Fig 12.13c Wider groove in flush with upper member

incisal pin about one inch from the spherical tip.(Fig 12.7b). Five additional lines calibrated in millimeters extend on either side thereof. These lines are used

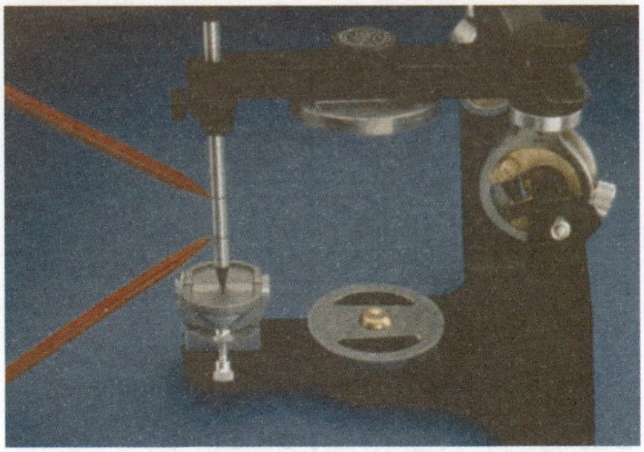

Fig 12.13d Two grooves at 37 mm and 54 mm below Frankfurt horizontal plane

for recording or altering the vertical dimension. The Incisal Pin is inserted into, and the wider mid-line of these metric grooves is aligned with, the top edge of the Upper Member (Fig 12.13c). It is secured by the Thumbscrew bearing against the flatted side on the pin. This adjustment places the chisel end at 90 degrees to and in contact with the central table of the Incisal Guide and provides a parallelism of the Upper Member to the Lower Member.

Two annular grooves, (Fig 12.13d) appear on the Incisal Pin at 37 and 54 mm below the Frankfort Horizontal Plane. These grooves form arbitrary vertical landmarks for alignment of the incisal edge of the maxillary centrals when making a Facebow transfer. The 37 mm. line is based in part on the Bonwil Triangle and results in a generally horizontal appearing plane of occlusion.

The 54 mm line forms an average landmark for alignment of the incisal edge of the upper centrals when making a facebow transfer. The incisal pin extends beyond the top of the upper member and provides a third point of stability when inverting the articulator for mandibular cast mounting. The spherical tip of this incisal pin serves as the dual-end and is useful for fabricating customized acrylic anterior guide tables.

Adjustable incisal guide: The adjustable incisal guide provides an independent adjustment of anterior guidance. It cooperates with the incisal pin and condylar guidances to present a stable, three-dimensional programmed guide pattern for the mounted casts. (Fig 12.14a) The incisal guide rotates

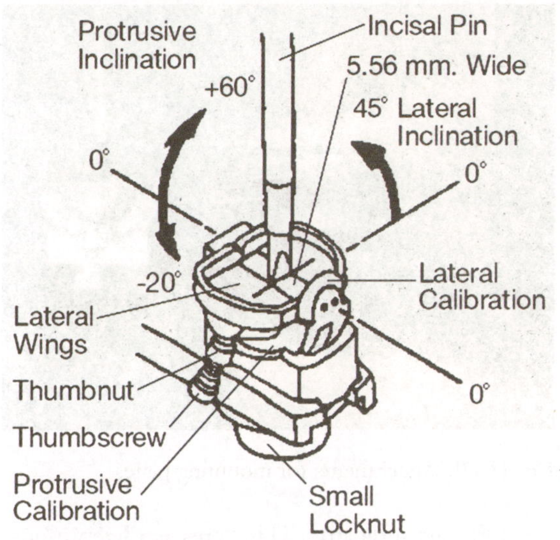

Fig 12.14a Adjustable incisal guide

antero-posteriorly from a horizontal "zero" degree to a 60 degree positive inclination of protrusion which is then secured by the small locknut (Fig 12.4b).

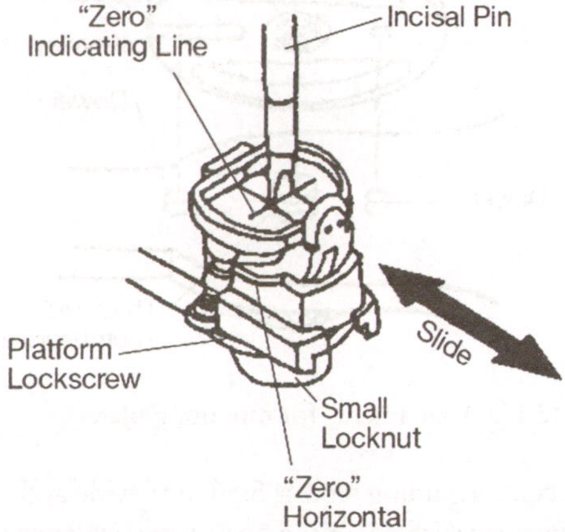

Fig 12.15a Slot for repositioning incisal guide table

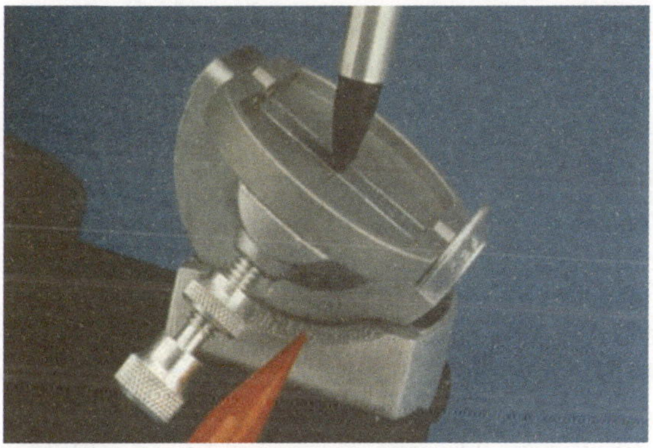

Fig 12.14b Incisal guide table rotated anteroposteriorly

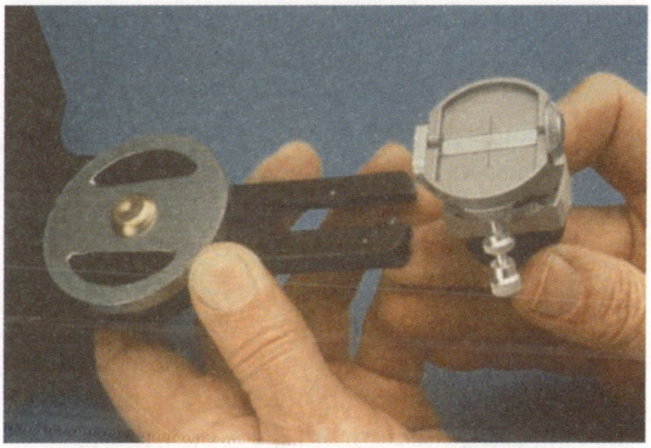

Fig 12.15b Slot for repositioning incisal guide table

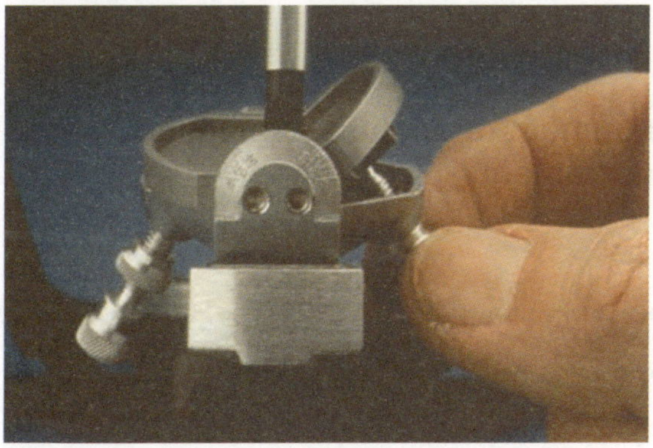

Fig 12.14c Adjustable lateral wings

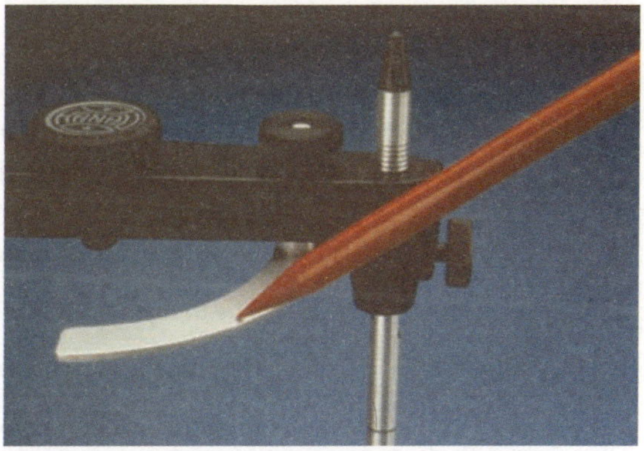

Fig 12.16 Cresent for anterior reference mark

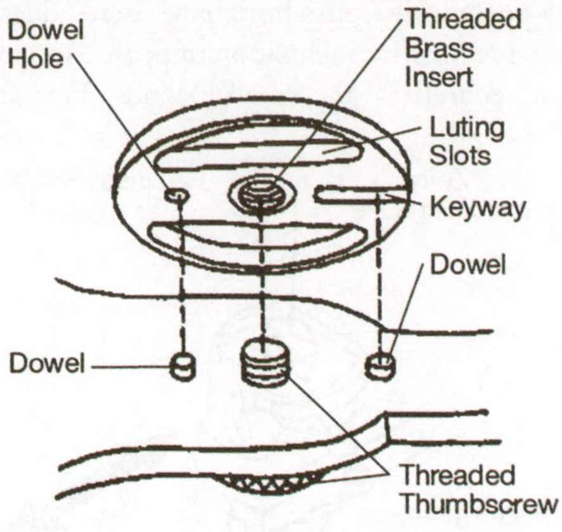

Fig 12.17a Attachments for mounting plates

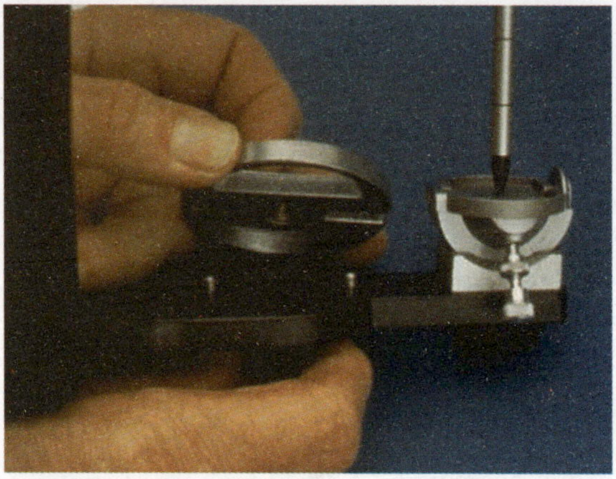

Fig 12.17b Attachments for mounting plates

The central guiding table is 5.56 mm. wide and forms the inclined surface for the protrusive guidance of the incisal pin. Separately adjustable lateral wings elevate by a thumbscrew from a "zero" horizontal to a 45 degree incline and are fixed by a thumbnut (Fig 12.14c). The calibrations are very small and serve only as a reference. An anterior slot, Fig 12.15a,17.15b in the lower member, allows repositioning of the incisal guide. Adjust and lock the guide at a "zero" horizontal and slightly loosen the platform lockscrew. Slide the platform antero-posteriorly to align the chisel end of the incisal pin with the "zero" indicating line on the lateral wings. This adjustment will place the incisal pin contact on the rotational center of the guide, thereby maintaining the vertical dimension when adjusting the inclination for protrusion.

Orbitale indicator: This "crescent" represents the patient's infra-orbitale notch and is the anterior reference landmark of the frankfort horizontal plane (Fig 12.16). When used with an orbitale pointer on a facebow it provides an anatomical vertical orientation for the upper arch, obviating the use of any average reference lines on the incisal pin.

Mounting plates: Mounting plates are used to lute the upper and lower casts to the upper and lower articulator members by the means of a gypsum material. At their center is a domed brass insert which is internally threaded for attachment to the upper or lower member. Longitudinally disposed to the luting slots and on the center plane of the insert is a keyway and a dowel hole which register over two dowels in the upper and lower member (Fig 12.17a, 12.17b).

A chronological table of the development of occlusal concepts and occlusal instruments

1805	Gariot	Develop a plaster articulator
1840	Cameron Evens	The first patented mechanical articulator.
1854	Bonwill	Proposed a Bonwill's triangle.
1859	Bonwill	Proposed a Three points contact occlusion.

1859	Bonwill	Develop the anatomical articulator which becomes the archetype of the condylar articulator.
1866	Balkwill	Proposed a Balkwill angle and described the forwards and downwards movement of the condyle
1890	Spee	Propose the theory of the Spee's curve.
1896	Walker	Measure a human mandibular movement for the first time, and recognize the need which gives an Articulator a Sagittal condylar path.
1896	Walker	Develop the first adjustment Articulator of the arcon type.
1899	Snow	Develop a face bow.
1901	Gysi	Introduced a gothic arch tracing method.
1901	Christensen	Introduced a Christensen phenomenon. Developed a check bite technique.
1907	Angle	Introduced the Angle classification (Angle's Key to occlusion).
1908	Bennett	Described the bodily shift movement of the mandible (Bennett movement)
1908	Gysi	Developed The Gysi Adaptable Articulator.
1912	Zsigmondy	Measured a path of masticatory movement and described the 3 phase theory of mastication.
1919	Monson	Developed a Monson Articulator.
1920	WadsWorth	Developed The WadsWorth Articulator. The general idea of the lateral incisal guide table that split in two was adapted in this Articulator.
1920	Monson	Proposed Monson's spherical theory.
1920	Hall	Proposed Hall's conical theory. developed the Automatic Anatomic Articulator in 1921, the Arbitrary Articulator in 1924, and a three-dimensional Articulator in 1926 .
1921	McCollum,Stallard	introduced Gnathology
1921	Hanau	Developed Hanau-model H articulator.
1926	McCollum	Described a hinge axis locating method.
1926	Hanau	"Hanau Quint".
1929	McCollum,Stallard	Established The California Gnathological Society.
1929	Gysi	proposed that an average inclination of sagittal condylar path is 33 degrees based on the Camper's line.
1930	McCollum	Developed The Gnathograph (the archetype of the Pantograph).
1934	McCollum	Developed The Gnathoscope Articulator.
1941	Payne	Proposed a modified teeth set-up method.

1944	Beyron	Developed The Dentatus Articulator.
1949	Stallard,Stuart	Introduced mutually protected occlusion.
1950	Thomas	Described the Cusp to fossa waxing technique (wax corn technique) and Tripodism which aimed to fulfill the Organic occlusion.
1955	McCollum	Proposed a balanced occlusion as an ideal occlusion for rehabilitation in natural dentition.
1955	Stuart	Developed Stuart computer.
1958	Gysi	Proposed that there is a difference in sagittal condylar element of the protrusive movement and the lateral movement.
1958	Hanau	Developed Hanau H2-O Articulator.
1958	D'Amico	Emphasized the role of the canine tooth in lateral excursion of the mandible. "canine protected occlusion"
1959	Meyer	Introduced the Functionally Generated Path technique
1961	Schuyler	Propose group functioned occlusion.
1962	Payne	Described the Cusp to marginal ridge waxing method.
1962	Posselt	described an envelope of mandibular movement which is a three-dimensional figure which is named "Posselt Diagram"
1965	Stuart	Developed Whip-Mix Articulator.
1966	Pound	Introduced the phonetic method for measuring occlusal vertical dimension of occlusion and proposed the anterior tooth arrangement method in complete denture.
1968	Swanson,Wipf	Developed the TMJ Articulator.
1968	Granger	Developed the Simulator Articulator.
1970	Mitsuya,Yamasita	Developed the Cosmax Articulator.
1973	Lundeen	Proposed that the inclination of sagittal condylar path is about 45-50 degrees based on the Frankfort plane.
1973	Pound	Proposed a lingualized occlusion for complete denture
1974	Dawson	Proposed anterior group functioned occlusion.
1974	Guichet	Developed Denar D5A Articulator.
1975	Guichet	Develop Denar Mark II Articulator.
1975	Lee	Developed Panadent Articulator.
1976	Broadrick	Developed the Broadrick occlusal plane analyzer

Suggested reading

1. Starcky EN, *The history of articulators: The appearance and early history of facebows.* J Prosthodont 2000;9:161-165
2. Starcky EN, *The history of Articulators: A Critical history of articulator based on geometric theories of mandibular movement, part I.* J Prosthodont 2002;11:134-1, part II: Rupert Hall's Conical theory. J Prosthodont 2002;11:211-222,
3. Starcky EN, *The history of articulators: Early attempts to reproduce mandibular movement.* J Prosthodont 2000;9:51-56, *part II.* J Prosthodont 2000;9:110-112, *part III: Searching for the solution to a puzzle.* J Prosthodont 2000;9:217-221.
4. Starcky EN, *The history of articulators: From facebows to the gnathograph, a brief history of early devices developed for recording condylar movement: part I.* J prosthodont 2002;10:241-248, *part II.* J prosthodont 2002;11:53-62
5. Starcky EN, *The history of articulators: A perspective on the early years, part I.* J Prosthodont 1999;8:209-211, *part III.* J Prosthodont 1999;8:277-280
6. Starcky EN, *The history of articulators: Unusual concepts or it seemed to be a great idea at the time* J Prosthodont 2001;10:170-180
7. Starcky EN, *The history of articulators: pursuing the evolution of the incisal-pin and guide.* J Prosthodont 2001;10:52-60, part II. J Prosthodont 2001;10:113-121
8. Celenza FV, *An analysis of articulators* Dent Clin North Am 1979;23:305-326
9. Mitchell DL, *Articulators through the years, part II - From 1940.* J Prosthet Dent 1978;39:451-458
10. Weinberg LA, *An evaluation of basic articulators and their concepts, part I: Basic semiadjustable articulators,* J Prosthet Dent 1963;13:645-663
11. The Academy of Prosthodontics -1999, *The Glossary of Prosthodontic Terms.* J Prosthet Dent 1999;81:41-110
12. Becker CM, Kaiser DA, *Evolution of occlusion and occlusal instruments.* J Prosthodont 1993;2:33-43
13. Schwartz H, *Occlusal variation for reconstructing the natural dentition,* J Prosthet Dent 1986;55:101-105
14. Wipf HH, *Pathways to occlusion: TMJ stereogrphic analog and mandibular movement indicator,* Dent Clin North Am 1979;23(2):271-287
15. Iven Klineberg, *Occlusion:Principles and Assessment,* Wright, Oxford, pp.163-186
16. Mohl ND, Zarb GA, Carlsson GE, *A textbook of occlusion,* Quintessence Publ Co., 1991, pp.161-171
17. Gerber A, Steinhardt G, *Dental occlusion and the temporomandibular joint,* Quintessence Publ Co., 1990, pp.9-20
18. Santos JD, *Occlusion:Principles and concepts,* Ishiyaku Euro America Tokyu Inc. 1985, pp.170-196
19. Thomas CJ, *A classification of articulators,* J Prosthet Dent 1973;30:11-14
20. Levin B, *A reevalution of Hanau's Laws of Articulation and the Hanau Quint,* J Prosthet Dent 1978;39:254-258
21. Isaacson D, *A clinical study of the bennett movement,* J Prosthet Dent 1958;8:641-649
22. Schwartz H, *Occlusal variations for reconstructing the natural dentition,* J Prosthet Dent 1986;55:101-105
23. D'Amico A, *The canine teeth- normal functional relation of the natural teeth of man,* J South Calif Dent Assoc 1958;26:6-23,49-60,127-142, 175-182,194-208,239-241
24. Fereday RC, *Francis Balkwill and the physiology of mastication,* Br Dent J 1994;176(10):386-393
25. Von Spee FG, *The gliding path of the mandible along the skull.* Archiv Anat Phys 1890; 16:285-294. (Translated by Biedenbach MA, Hotz M, Hitchcock HP, J Am Dent Assoc 1980; 100:670-675).
26. Rihani A, *Classification of articulators, J Prosthet* Dent 1980;43:344-347
27. Winkler S, *Essentials of complete denture prosthodontics,* 2nd ed 1972, pp.142-182
28. Hobo S, Ichida E, Garcia LT, *Osseointegration and occlusal rehabilitation,* Quintessence Publ Co., 1990, pp.291-296, 361-381
29. Rosenstiel SF, Land MF, Fujimoto J, *Contemporary fixed prosthodontics,* Mosby Inc.,St. Louis, 2001, pp.25-58

13

Face bow transfer

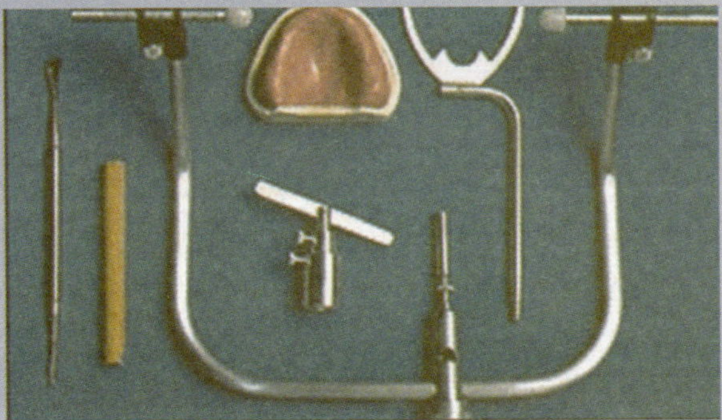

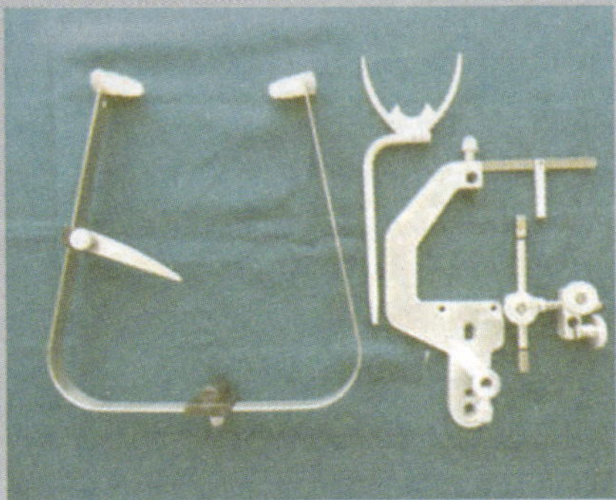

Face bow transfer make the articulator a realistic simulator of the human system

Mandible moves around three different axes. The opening and the closing movements, that occur within 12 mm of inter incisal opening, is around an axis passing through the condyles. Existence of a singular axis is disputed but for all practical purposes it is desirable to consider, that mandible moves around a singular axis. While relating the maxilla to the mandible, it is desirable to relate the opening axis also. In simpler terms the axis passing through the condyles conventionally known as hinge axis is to be related to the maxilla. The term relation is explained as a spatial relation. Maxilla when related to the axis in space, the distance between them is to be ascertained in three dimensions. The first one is the distance between the hinge axis and the maxilla in the anteroposterior direction. The second one is in a lateral direction. The mid sagital plane is considered as the reference plane and this is made to coincide with the mid plane of the articulator. If there is provision to adjust the distance between the condylar posts of the articulator to match the inter condylar distance of the mandible, mid sagital plane reference can be avoided. By recording these two relationships, the position of the maxilla in relation to the hinge axis in the horizontal plane is determined. Now maxilla has to be positioned according to the third dimension ie. in the vertical direction. For this purpose, the plane connecting hinge axis to orbitale is taken as the reference. This plane is presumed to be related to Frankfort horizontal plane but that is disputed. However this plane serves as a valid reference, that the maxillary cast can be related to the articulator in the vertical direction similar to that in the skull. Relating maxilla to the mandibular hinge axis helps the operator in relating the maxillary cast to the articulator hinge axis. By simulating the relationship, the opening and closing arc of movement of the mandibular teeth can be made equivalent both in the mouth and in the articulator. If the articulator is smaller in dimensions, the arc becomes comparatively smaller having greater curvature and that will not match in the mouth where the arc is comparatively flatter because of a bigger radius. Hence it is always desirable to relate the maxilla with the hinge axis when it occupies the terminal position, so that the occlusion generated in the articulator will function identically with in the human system. Relating the maxilla with the hinge axis is done by a caliper like device which is known as the face bow. A typical face bow has three functions.

a. to relate the maxilla to the terminal hinge axis of the condyles.
b. to relate the occlusal plane to the skull in the horizontal direction – preferably to frankfort horizontal plane.
c. to facilitate mounting the casts onto an articulator.

There are two main types of face bows.

1. Arbitrary face bow.
2. Kinematic face bow.

In general clinical practice the former is always used.

Arbitrary face bow

This type is considered adequate for prosthetic work. It basically consists of a U-shaped frame with condylar rods located at the ends of the frame. To the frame a fork is attached which is related to the upper plane. There are two types of arbitrary face bows.

a. **Fascia type face bow:** The condylar rods are located arbitrarily by making a point 13mm anterior to the most posterior part of the tragus on a line connecting the outer canthus of the eye and the external auditory meatus. (cantho meatal line). In the articulator the condylar rods of face bow are connected to the condylar shaft of the articulator (axis). (fig 13.1)
b. **The earpiece bow:** This has the condylar rods located in the external auditory meatus. On being transferred to the articulator the condylar rods are connected to a post present behind the articulator hinge axis.

If great accuracy on the location of the mandibular hinge axis is necessary, a kinematic record is preferred. This has a fork which is fixed to the lower occlusal rim. This fork is attached to a frame with adjustable condylar pins which can be positioned arbitrarily over the condyles. The patient is asked to make small opening and closing movements and the pointers are adjusted until no translation occurs i.e., there is purely rotational movement for the pins. This hinge axis is marked with a skin marking pencil and the face bow is used in a regular manner as in the former case.

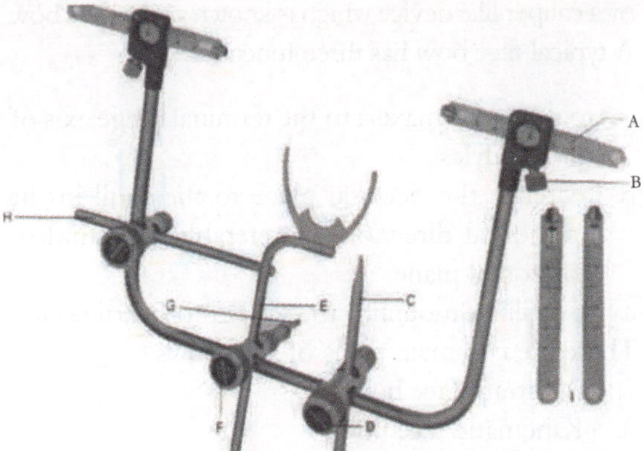

A. Calibrated condylar rod
B. Set screw for calibrated condylor rod
C. Orbital pointer pin
D. Locking clamp for orbital pointer pin
E. Bite fork
F. Locking clamp for orbital pointer pin
G. Anterior jack screw
H. Calibrated condylar rods

Fig. 13.1 Ear piece face bow(arbitrary)

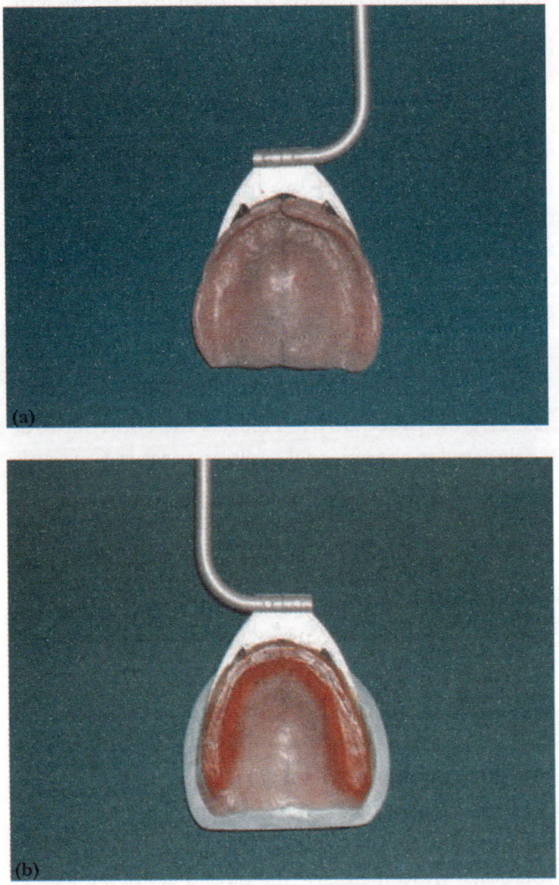

Fig. 13.2 a,b-Fork attached to the occlusal rim.Yoke should be parallel to the midline

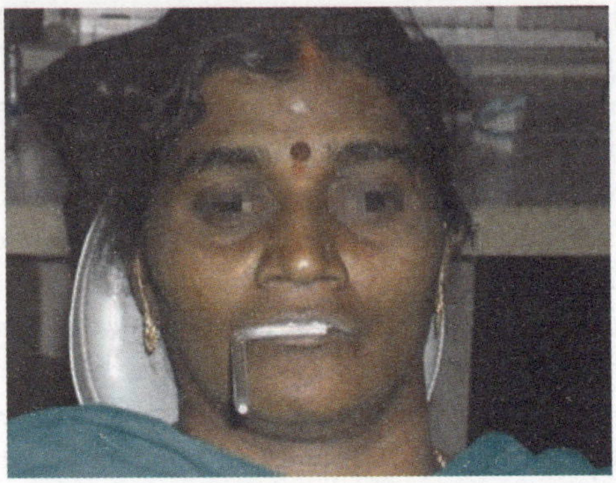

Fig. 13.3 While attaching the fork short portion of the yoke should be perpendicular to the mid saggital plane and parallel to the interpupillary line

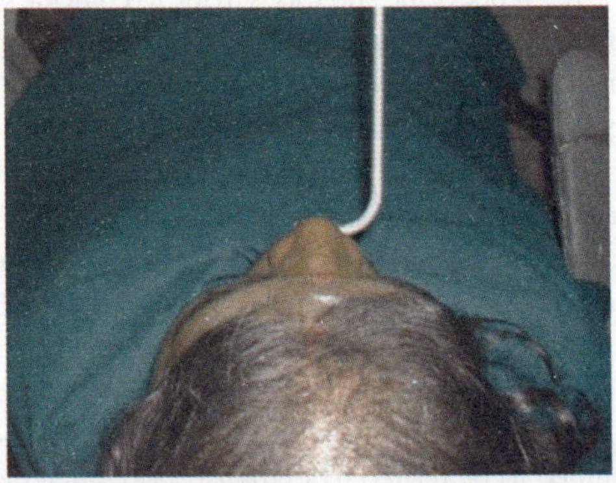

Fig. 13.4 Long portion of the yoke should be parallel to the mid saggital plane

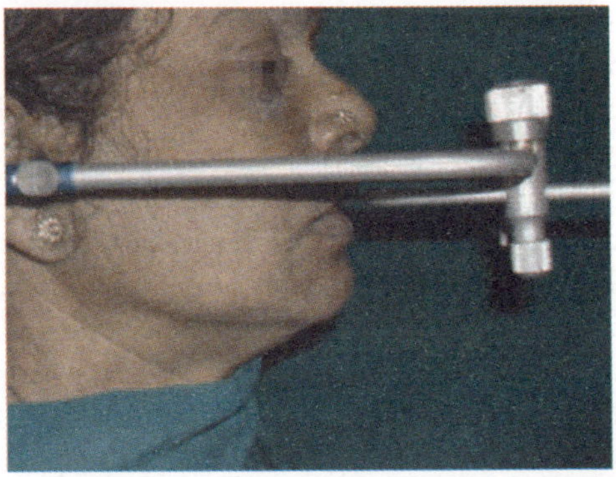

Fig. 13.5 Face bow is positioned in the auditory meatus and attached to the fork .Face bow and long portion of yoke are parallel

The method

1. Arbitrary hinge axis point is located on the patient's face, on the cantho meatal line, 13 mm anterior to the most posterior point of tragus (only for facia type face bow).
2. Place the maxillary occlusal rim on the cast. Warm the bite fork and place it 3 mm above the occlusal plane. The warm fork will find its way by melting the wax. The midline line marked on the fork should coincide with the central line of the occlusion rim. (fig 13.2 - 13.5)
3. Preset the face bow on the face and tighten the condylar rods on the arbitrary hinge axis. Note the scale readings and remove the face bow. On averaging the readings, the scales can be adjusted equally on both sides. In the ear piece face bow, the rods are placed in the auditory meatus. (fig 13.6)
4. Place the occlusion rim with the fork in the mouth and position the face bow on the fork, making sure that the readings on the rods are equal. The face bow and the yoke of the fork are made parallel. Then tighten the assembly.
5. Connect the third point reference (orbitale, nasion or the point specified by the model of the articulator). (fig 13.7 - 13.8)

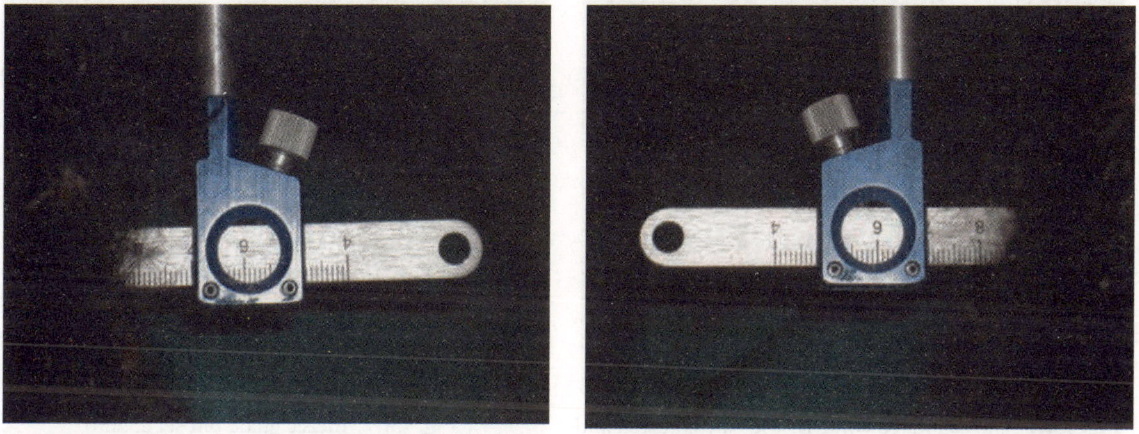

Fig. 13.6 a,b Equal scale readings on both the ear rods

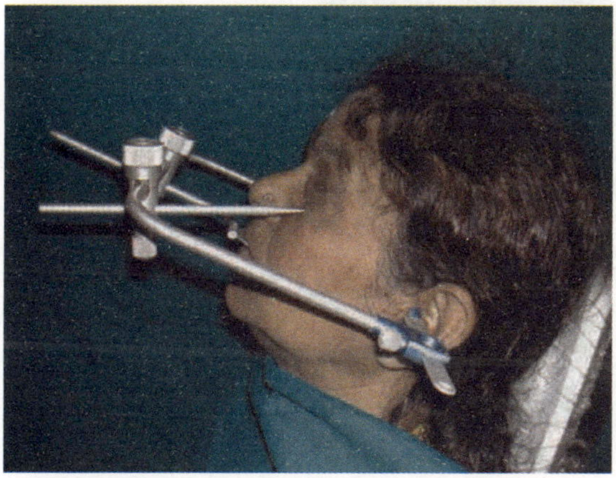

Fig. 13.7 Orbital pointer pin is attached

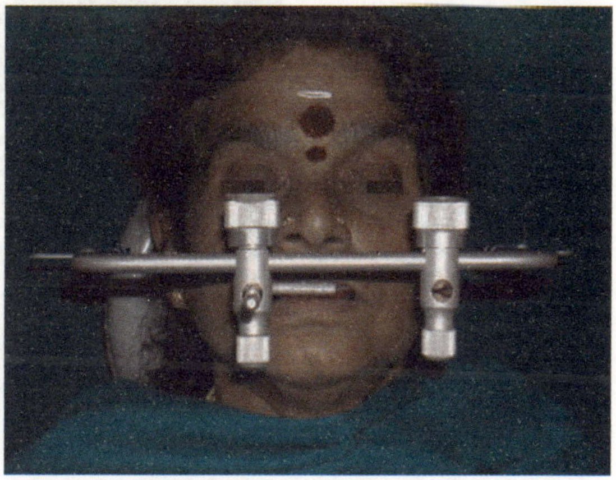

Fig. 13.8 Face bow and yolk are parallel

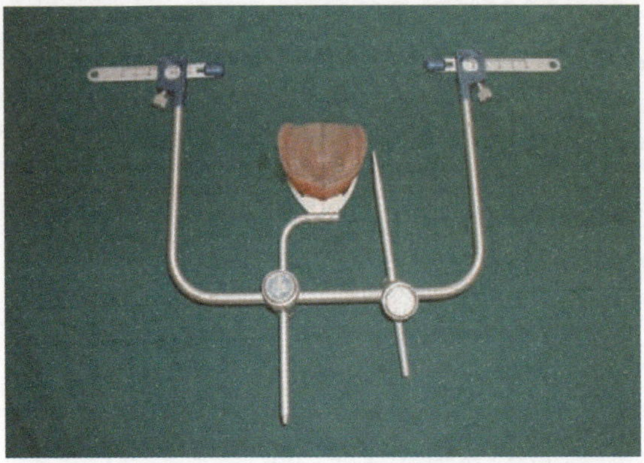

Fig. 13.9 Face bow assembly removed from the patient

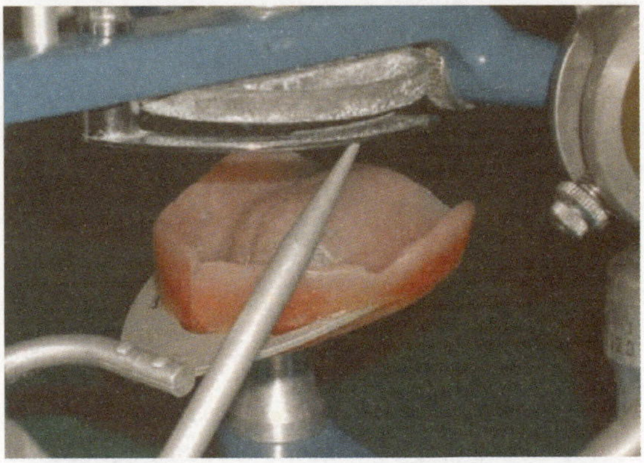

Fig. 13.10 Orbital pointer pin should touch the underside of the orbital axis plane indicator

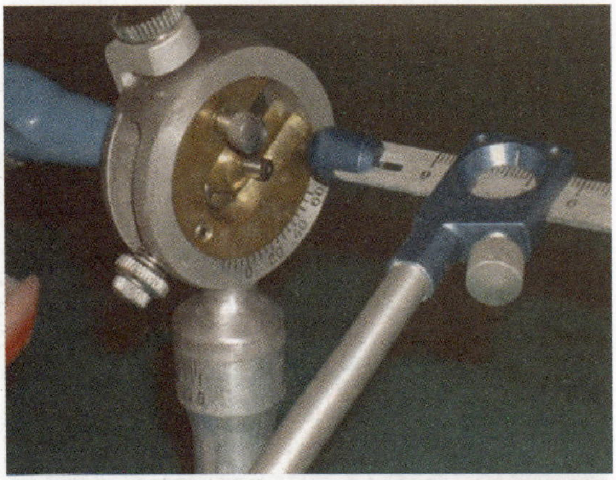

Fig. 13.11 The calibrated condylar rods are adjusted and locked at same readings on both the sides

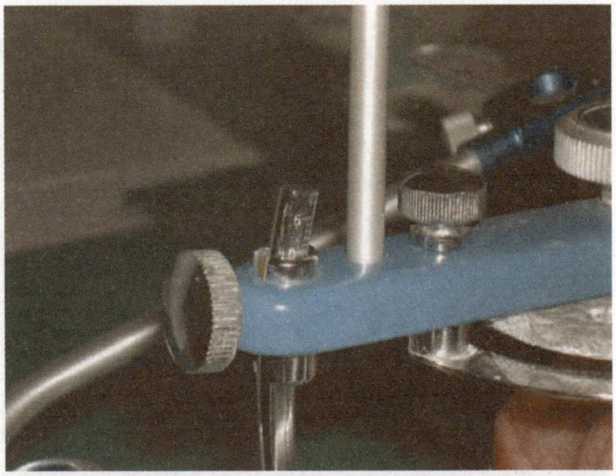

Fig. 13.12 Incisal guide pin set at zero

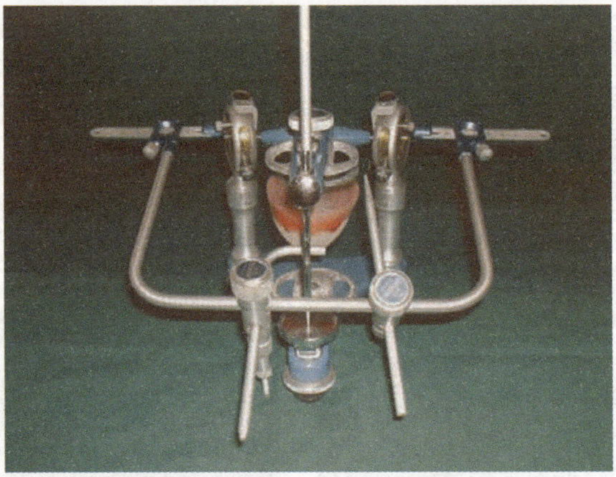

Fig. 13.13 Face bow relationship obtained in the patient is transferred to the articulator

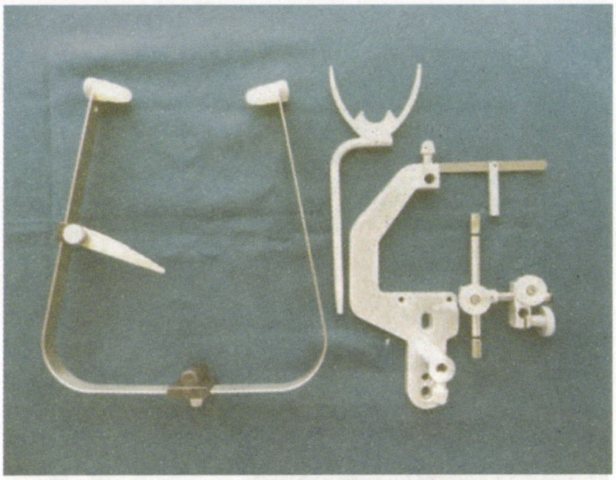

Fig. 13.14 Spring bow-Hanau

6. Loosen the condylar rods and remove the assembly from the face. (fig 13.9)
7. Position the maxillary cast in the base.
8. Place the condylar rods on the articulator hinge axis (for fascia type face bow) keeping the scale readings equal and adjusting the third point reference. (fig 13.10-13.13)

In Hanau and Dentatus classic articulators face bows can be connected with the cast assembly. In other models of Hanau transferring the relation is done through a jig. In wide vue articulators it is difficult to accommodate conventional face bows. Spring bows might even undergo permanent deformation. The use of jigs and spring bows have made the entire process simpler (fig. 13.14 - 13.20)

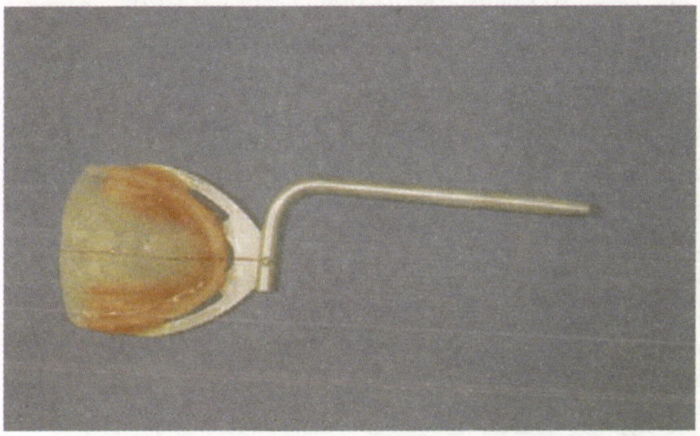

Fig. 13.15 Fork attached to the occlusal rim

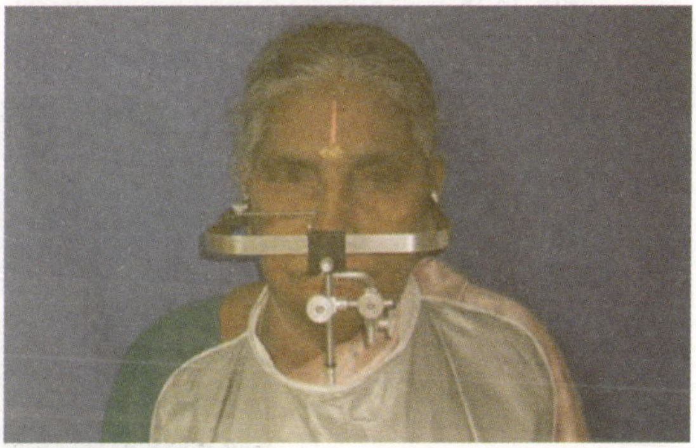

Fig. 13.16 Spring bow assembly

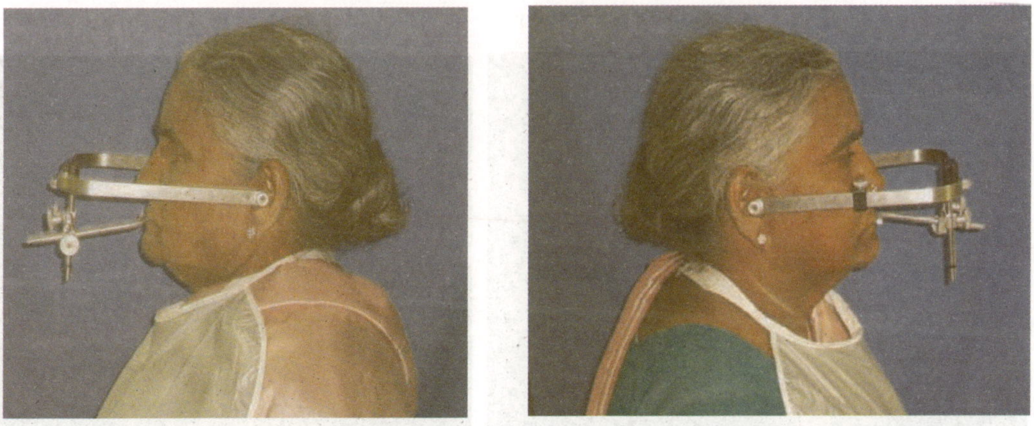

(a) (b)

Fig. 13.17 a,b Face bow is related to the FH plane

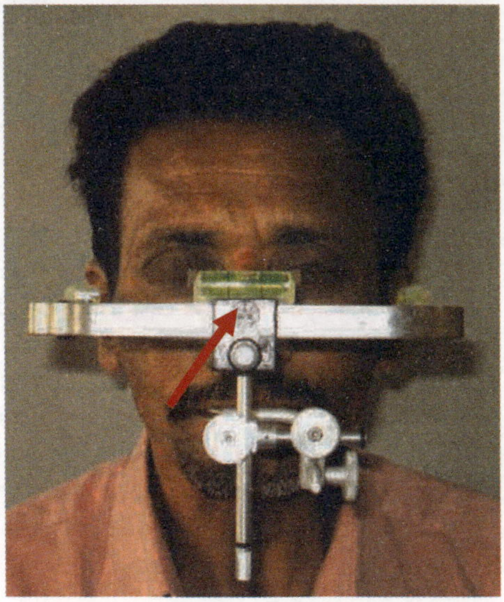

(a)

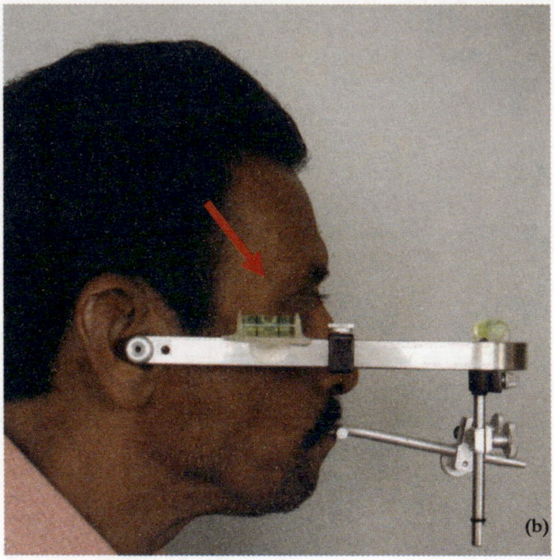

(b)

Fig. 13.18 a,b Spring bow modified by attaching spirit level to ensure horizontality while relating the bow to the fork

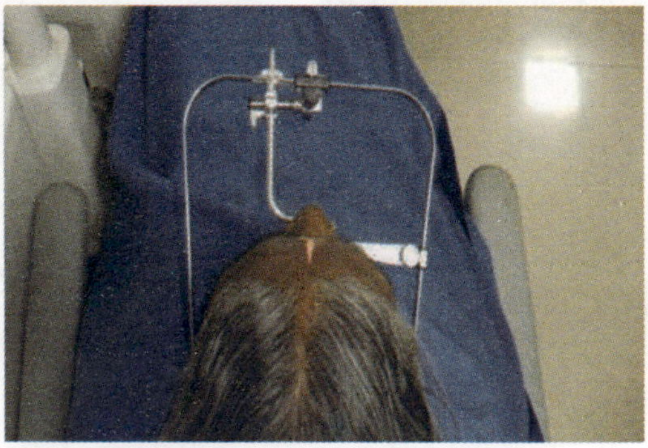

Fig. 13.19 Spring bow assembly viewed from top

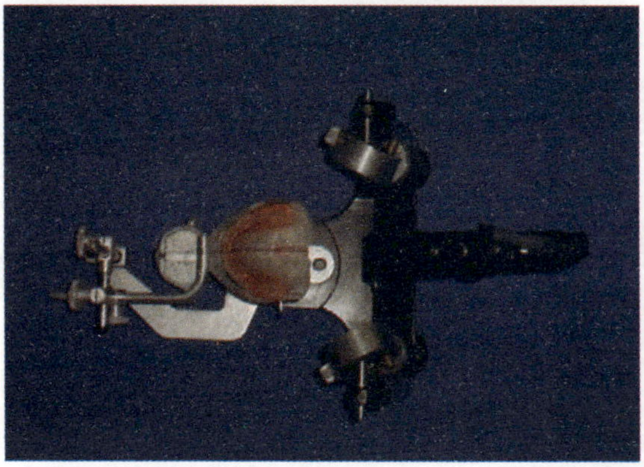

(a)

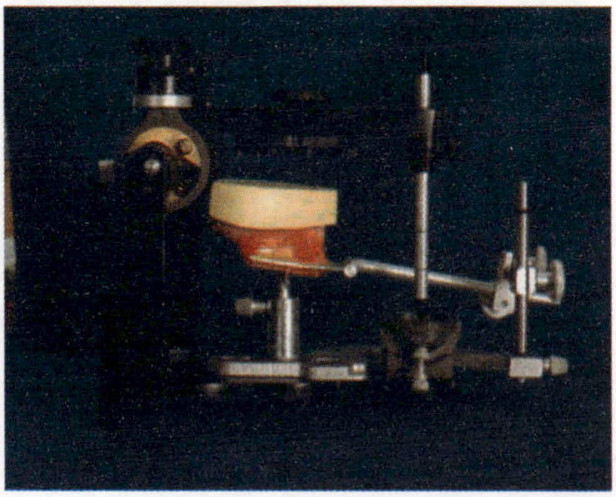

(b)

Fig. 13.20 a,b Face bow assembly transferred to the articulator with the transfer jig

By the process of face bow transfer, it can be ensured that the maxillary cast is placed in the articulator in an anatomically equivalent position of maxilla in relation to the skull. By this process of face bow transfer the static inter cuspal position designed in the articulator will match perfectly in the mouth because the opening arc is similar. The eccentric relations – balanced articulation - generated in the articulator will also match faithfully in the mouth. The cuspal slopes are designed in the articulator to obtain balanced articulation. Without the face bow transfer the above cannot be ensured.

Suggested Reading

1. Jerome M Schweitzer. *The Transograph and Transographics Articulation.* J Prosthet Dent 1957; 7 :595-621
2. Ulf Posselt. *Terminal Hinge Movement Of the Mandible.* J Prosthet Dent 1957;7:787-97
3. Christiansen.*Facebow In maxillary Cast Mounting* .J Prosthet Dent 1959;9:388-98
4. Lawrence.W.Weinberg .*An Evaluation Of Basic Articulators And Their Concepts :Part I –Basic Concepts.* J Prosthet Dent 1963;13:622- 44
5. Keki K Kotwal. *A need to use an arbitary facebow when remounting complete dentures with interocclusal records.* J Prosthet Dent 1979;42 :224
6. Carlo Ercoli, Gerald N. Graser, Ross H. Tallents Daniel Galindo *; Face-Bow Record Without A third Point of Reference, Theoritical Considerations and an Alternative technique*. J Prosthet Dent 1999; 82:237-41
7. Edgar N Starcke .*The History of Articulators : From Face-bows To The Gnathographs ,a Brief History of Early Devices Developed for Recording Condylar Movement: Part II.* JProsthodont 2002;11:53-62
8. William W Nagy, Thomas J Smithy and Carl G Wirth. *Accuracy Of A predetermined Transverse Horizontalmandibular axis point* .J Prosthet Dent 2002;87: 387-94
9. Olaf Bernhardt,Nina Kuppers ,Micheal Rosin and Greg Mayers .*Comparative Tests of Arbitary and Kinematic Transverse horizontal axis recordings of mandibular movements.* JProsthet Dent 2003;89:175-9
10. Jack D Preston .*A reassessment of the mandibular hinge axis theory.*JProsthet Dent 2004; 91: 505-12
11. Wilkie Noel, *The anterior point of reference,* J Prosthet Dent, 1979; 41(5); 488 – 96
12. Reddy L Chandrika, S Srividya, Nair Chandrasekharan , Shetty Jayakar, *A study on self centring of face bows,* J Indian Prosthodont Soc (July-Sept 2010) 10(3):165–167
13. KV Sadhvi, Nair Chandrasekharan, Shetty Jayakar, *Spirit level markers for face bow articulation,* Kerala Dental Journal, Apr 2009;32:65-6
14. Lauritzen G Arne, Wolford W Llyod, *Occlusal relationships: The split cast method for articulator techniques,* J Prosthet Dent, 1964;14(2): 256- 65

14

Gothic arch tracing

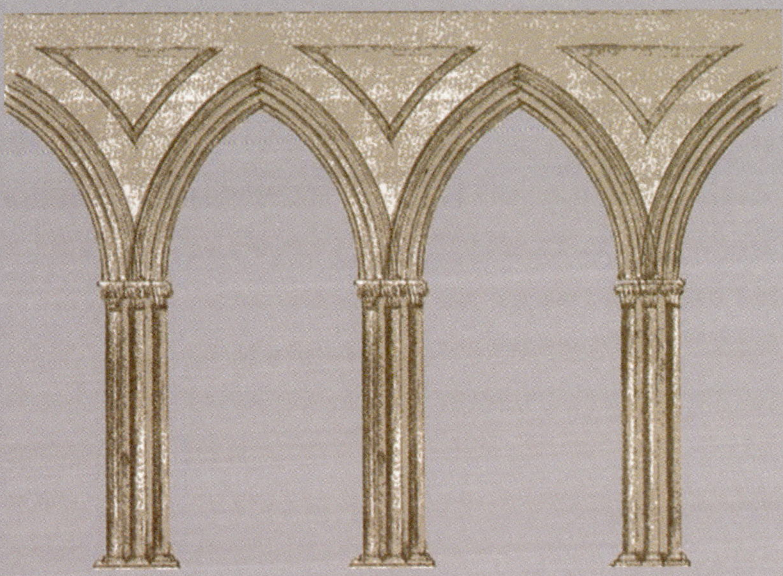

Graphic tracing method is mainly used to verify the check bite method of registering jaw relation. Both the methods are equally good.

Registration of centric relation is conventionally done by check bite method. This is further verified by graphic tracing method. For this purpose, the casts are mounted in a semi-adjustable articulator using check bite method and a tracing assembly is attached to the bite blocks. The tracing assembly is of two types - (a) intra oral and (b) extra oral. The tracing devices employ a stylus which could trace the path of jaw movement on a pigmented metallic plate.

In the intra oral method, the stylus is fixed to the mandibular arch and the tracing platform is fixed to the maxillary arch. The tracing platform is usually pigmented with colored wax. The vertical height is maintained by the stylus. A gap of 3mm (minimum) is provided between the upper and the lower occlusion rims usually made by reducing the lower occlusion rim.

In the extra oral device (Hight tracer) the stylus and the tracing table are positioned extra orally. The vertical height is maintained by a set of central bearing plates. The mandibular plate contains a spherical central bearing point and the maxillary plate provides a highly polished metallic surface. A gap has to be maintained between the plates as well as the occlusion rims. The central bearing plates are fixed mutually parallel. The extra oral tracing stylus is provided with a spring attachment which will allow the stylus to go up when the mandible is protruded and the gap between the occlusion rims gets diminished. (fig 14.1)

The occlusion-rim with the tracer assembly is placed in the patient's mouth and the patient is instructed to make eccentric movements namely protrusive, right lateral and left lateral. After making the eccentric movements, patient is instructed to bring back the mandible to centric position. The stylus will make a tracing which looks like an arrow (gothic arch). The arrow point designates the centric relation. The protrusive tracing is not always a straight line where as the lateral excursive movements will be seen as straight

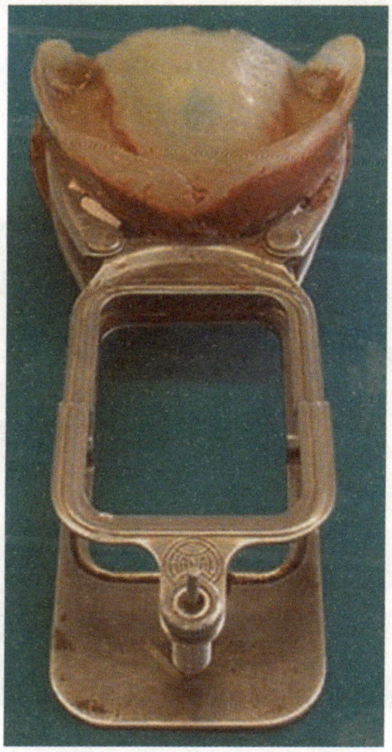

Fig. 14.1 Hight extra oral tracing assembly

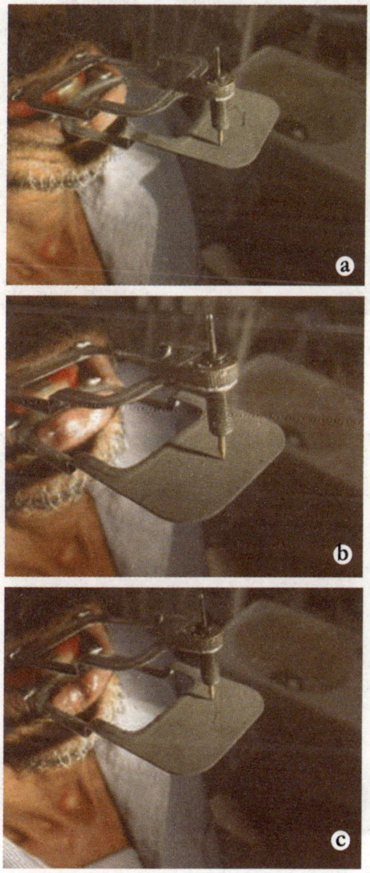

Fig. 14.2 a,b,c Tracing made on soot coated table

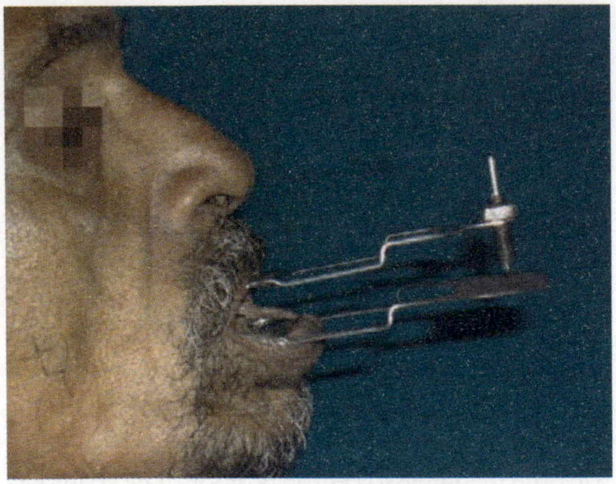

Fig. 14.3 Tracing assembly in the mouth

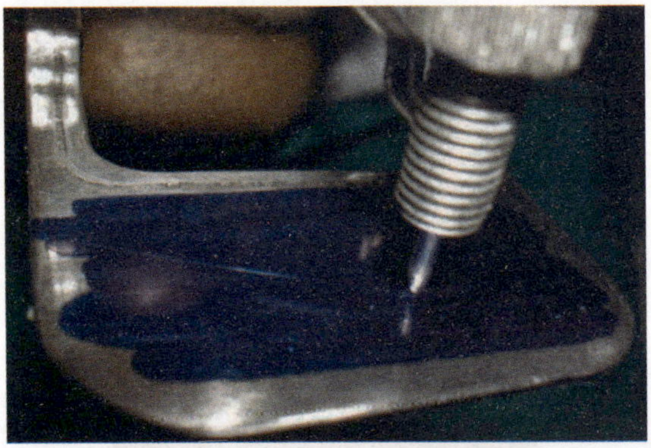

Fig. 14.4 Stylus making tracing over pigment coated table

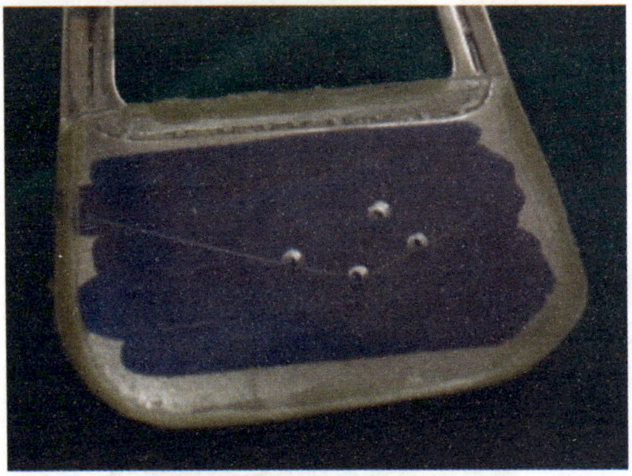

Fig. 14.5 Plastic sheet kept over the tracing and holes drilled

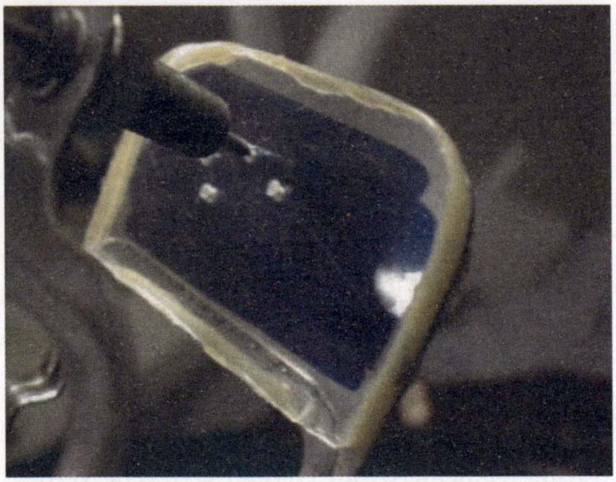

Fig. 14.6 Stylus held by the hole drilled in the plastic sheet

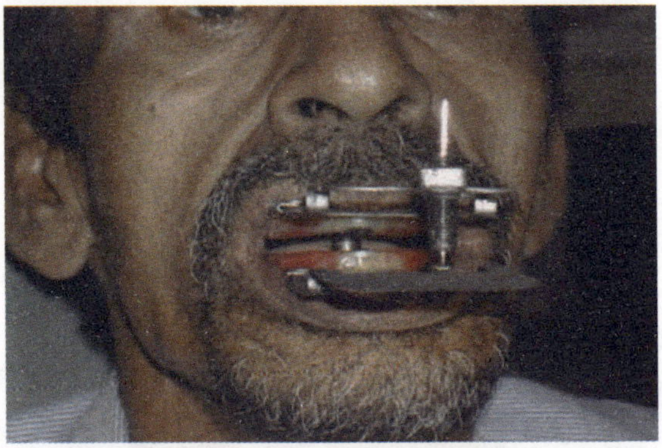

Fig. 14.7 Tracing assembly with interocclusal space for the plaster

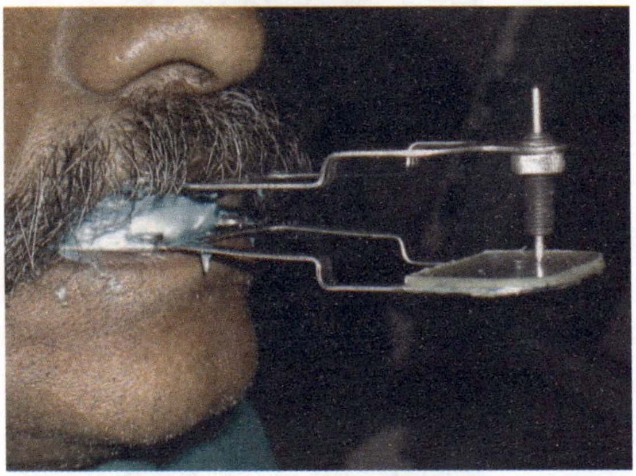

Fig. 14.8 Plaster injected between the rims to make the record

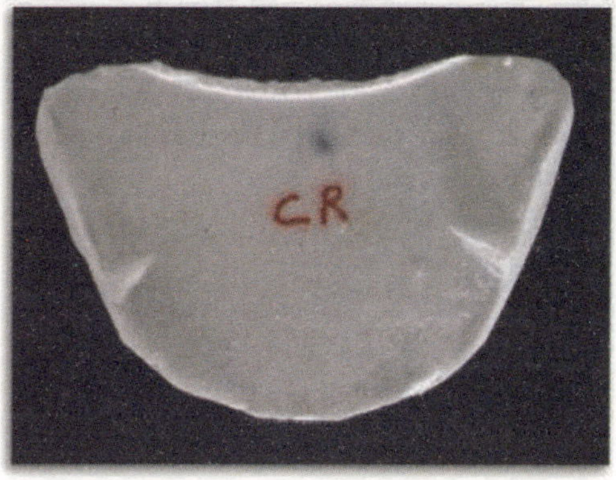

Fig. 14.9 Plaster record - Centric

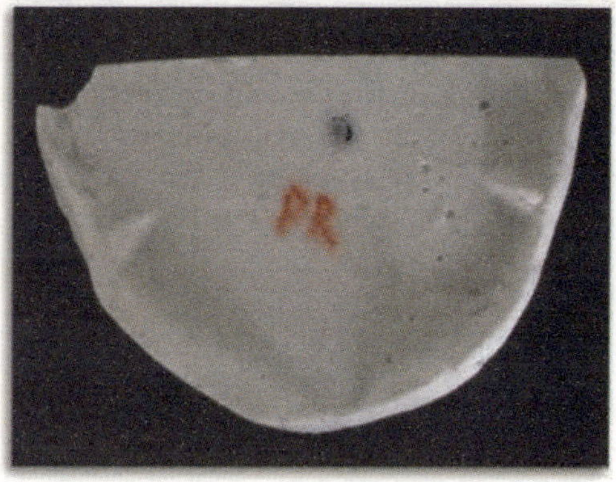

Fig. 14.10 Protrusive record - note the perforation

lines. These lines represent the border positioning of the mandible. Both in the intra and extra oral tracings, the arrow design can be obtained but the only difference will be in the direction of the arrow point. In the intraoral tracing, the arrow will be directed, towards the patient, where as in extra oral tracing the arrow point will be directed away from the patient. A patient with a reasonably good neuromuscular control can repeat the tracing with precision. Better results are obtained with training and guidance. (fig. 14.2 - 14.4)

The tracings are made to make inter occlusal records. Inter occlusal records are made in different positions namely- centric, protrusive, right lateral and left lateral. In eccentric positions records are not made at the extreme positions; instead it is made at a distance of 6mm away from the centric (arrow point). The number of records will depend on the type of articulator used. The reasons for making eccentric records at 6mm from the arrow point are the following:

The normal functions performed by an individual with the jaw will be with in 6mm.

Articulator will be optimally sensitive to be programmed for the horizontal angle and the Bennet angle only at 6mm distance or above.

Beyond 6mm the condyles will be positioned too anteriorly resulting in a reduction of the horizontal angle while programming the articulator

Once the tracing is completed, a transparent plastic sheet of 2mm thickness is fixed over the tracing and holes are drilled at the centric point and on the eccentric tracings at 6mm away from the centric. Holes are drilled to hold the stylus while the interocclusal records are prepared. Interocclusal records are usually made by injecting quick setting plaster between the metallic plates. Rigid materials are always preferred to make the records.

Programming the Articulator

Once all the records are made, the occlusal rims with the tracers are transferred to the articulator. The stylus of the extraoral tracer and the incisal guide pin of the articulator are raised from the respective table/ platform. The centric lock of the articulator is loosened and the condylar spheres are made free. The centric record is then placed between the upper and the lower occlusal rims. The cast and occlusal rims with the interocclusal record are firmly united with a stick and super glue or by fixing die pins and tying them with a thread. The split of the maxillary cast is loosened and it is allowed to approximate. When the cast assembly approximates without a gap, the condylar spheres are to be observed. If the spheres are in close proximity with the stops, it can be presumed that the centric relation registered using check bite method coincides with the centric identified through graphic tracing method. If there is a discrepancy, it is preferred to redo the entire clinical process from registering the jaw relation using check bite method. The protrusive record is then used to adjust the horizontal angle. When the split cast approximates closely while the interocclusal protrusive record is positioned, the condylar spheres sets the condylar angle automatically but care must be taken to keep the lock nuts properly loosened. The Benett angle is adjusted arbitrarily in the Hanau Articulator using the Hanau formula (L = H/8 + 12). Where as in Dentatus articulator the lateral records are used to programme the Bennett angle.

Evaluation of Gothic Arch Tracings

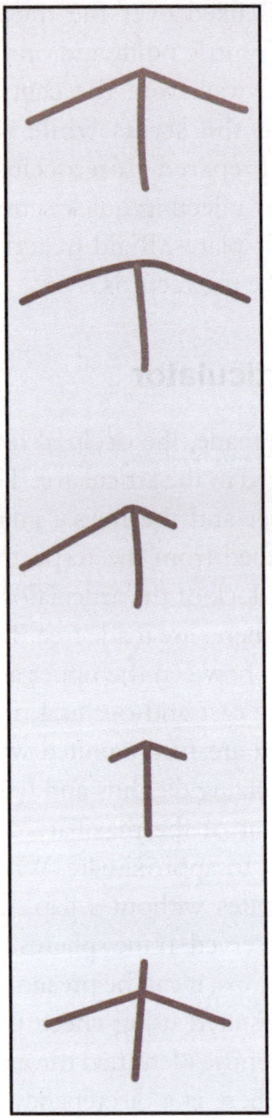

Classical, pointed form

The symmetry indicates an undisturbed movement sequence in the joints and uniform muscle guidance.

Classical flat form

The picture indicates distinct lateral movements of the condyles in the fossae.

Assymmetrical form

The tracing indicates a distinct inhibition of the forward movement in the right joint.

Miniature Gothic arch tracing

The tracing points to cramp-like movements, badly fitting and pain-causing record blocks, edentulous state of long standing with inhibited movement in the joints, badly constructed prosthetic appliances, etc.

Vertical line protrudes beyond the arrow point

This tracing was produced either by forcible retraction or pushing of the mandible. It is, however, possible that the Gothic arch was obtained with a protruded mandible. Too much stylus pressure can also cause this.

Suggested Reading

1. Payne AG.*Gothic arch tracing in the edentulous. Some properties of the apex point.*Br Dent J 1969;126(5):220-3.
2. Smith HF Jr.*A comparison of empirical centric relation records with location of terminal hinge axis and apex of the gothic arch tracing.* J Prosthet Dent. 1975;33(5):511-20.
3. Myers, M., Dziejma, R. and Goldberg, J. *Relation of gothic arch apex to dentist-assisted centric relation.* J Prosthet Dent 1980; 44:78-81.
4. el-Gheriani AS, Winstanley RB.*The Gothic arch (needle-point) tracing and condylar inclination.* J Prosthet Dent. 1987; 58(5):638-42.
5. el-Gheriani AS, Winstanley RB. *The value of the Gothic arch tracing in the positioning of denture teeth.*J Oral Rehabil. 1988;15(4):367-71.
6. el-Gheriani AS, Davies AL, Winstanley RB. *The gothic arch tracing and the upper canine teeth as guides in the positioning of upperposterior teeth.* J Oral Rehabil. 1989;16(5):481-90.
7. Obrez A, Stohler CS. *Jaw muscle pain and its effect on gothic arch tracings.* J Prosthet Dent.;75(4):393-8. Apr 1996
8. Raigrodski AJ, Sadan A, Carruth PL. *A technique to stabilize record bases for Gothic arch tracings in patients with implant retained complete dentures.* J Prosthodont. 1998;7(4):273-6
9. Watanabe Y.*Use of personal computers for Gothic arch tracing: analysis and evaluation of horizontal mandibular positions with edentulous prosthesis.*J Prosthet Dent. 1999;82(5):562-72.
10. Scott M.*Gothic arch tracing.* Br Dent J. 2002; 26;192(2):62
11. Keshvad A, Winstanley RB. *Comparison of the replicability of routinely used centric relation registration techniques.*J Prosthodont. Jun 2003;12(2):90-101
12. Watanabe Y.*Observation of horizontal mandibular positions in an edentulous patient using a digital gothic arch tracer: a clinical report.*J Prosthet Dent. Jan 2004;91(1):15-9
13. Williamson RA, Williamson AE, Bowley J, Toothaker R.*Maximizing mandibular prosthesis stability utilizing linear occlusion, occlusal plane selection, and centric recording.*J Prosthodont. Mar 2004;13(1):55-61
14. Rahman MD, Kohno S, Kobayashi H, Sawada K.*Influence of the inclination of the plate of an intra-oral tracing device on the condylar position registered by tapping movement.*J Oral Rehabil. Jun 2004 ;31(6):546-53.
15. Wojdyla SM, Wiederhold DM.*Using intraoral Gothic arch tracing to balance full dentures and determine centric relation and occlusal vertical dimension.*Dent Today Dec 2005;24(12):74-7
16. Villa Honorato, *Gothic arch tracing,* J Prosthet Dent 1959; 9(4):624-28

15

Programming the semiadjustable articulator

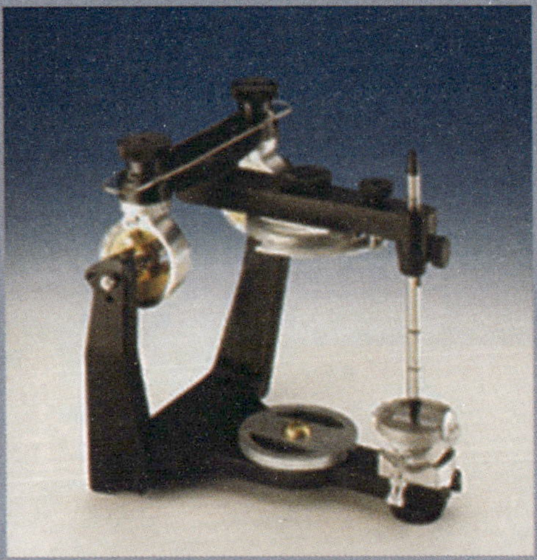

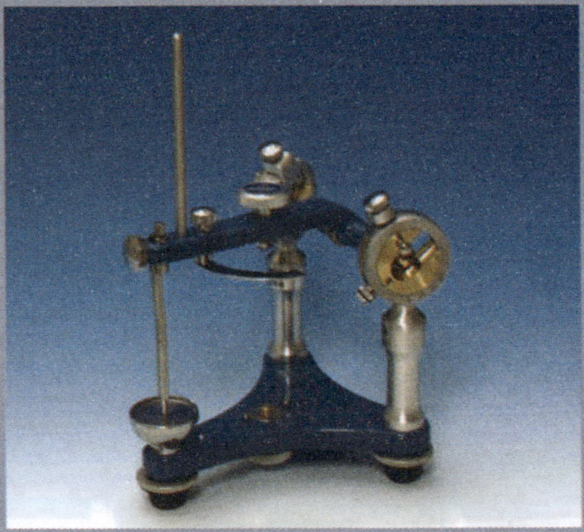

Articulator functions as a simulator of human jaws only when programmed

Maxillary cast is mounted to the upper member of the semi adjustable articulator using a face bow. A split cast is made (Fig 15.1). Tentative jaw relation is registered. Mandibular cast is mounted to the lower member of the articulator using tentative centric record (Fig 15.2). This is further verified using a graphic tracer. Extra oral tracer consists of central bearing point and plate. Tracer unit consists of stylus and table. The central bearing plate and central bearing point are attached to the occlusal rims in such a way that the height - the established vertical dimension is maintained and at the same time a uniform gap is provided (Fig 15.3, 15.4). The central bearing plate is submerged into the maxillary occlusal rim but the shape of which is kept unaltered (Fig 15. 5). Height of the mandibular occlusal rim is reduced by 4mm and is maintained parallel to the maxillary occlusal rim. The plate carrying the central bearing point is kept flush with the modified mandibular occlusal rim (Fig 15.6). The height of the central bearing point is adjusted to make a point contact with the central bearing plate attached to the maxillary occlusal rim. Central bearing point is positioned at the centre of the mandibular arch. The central bearing point is in the form of a sphere because, the central bearing point should maintain contact when the mandible protrudes; the condyles translate and the anterior portion of the occlusal rims get approximated. If the central bearing point is not a sphere this movement will not be accommodated. Next, testing is done in two phases. First testing is done in the articulator. The central bearing plate and points are attached and upper member is moved to simulate protrusive and lateral movements. Care should be taken that 3mm gap is maintained between heels of the bases. Now the bases are transferred to

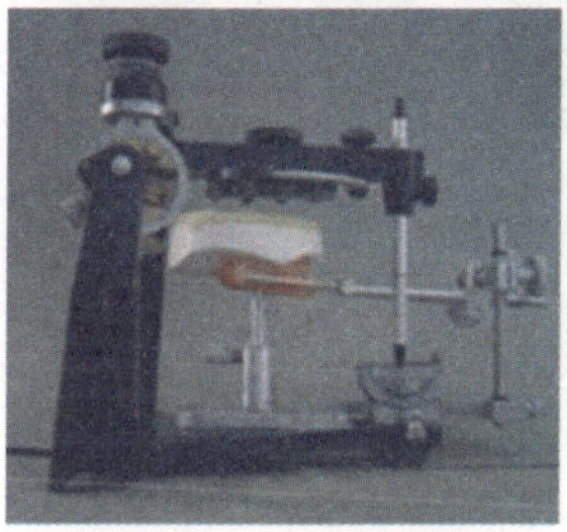

Fig. 15.1 Maxillary cast is mounted to the upper member of the semi adjustable articulator using a face bow with a split cast

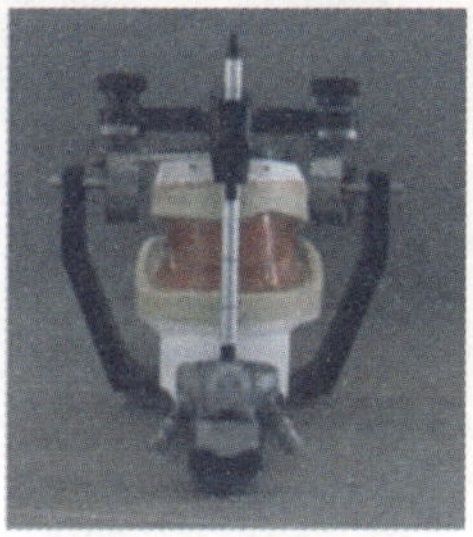

Fig. 15.2 Mandibular cast is mounted using tentative centric record

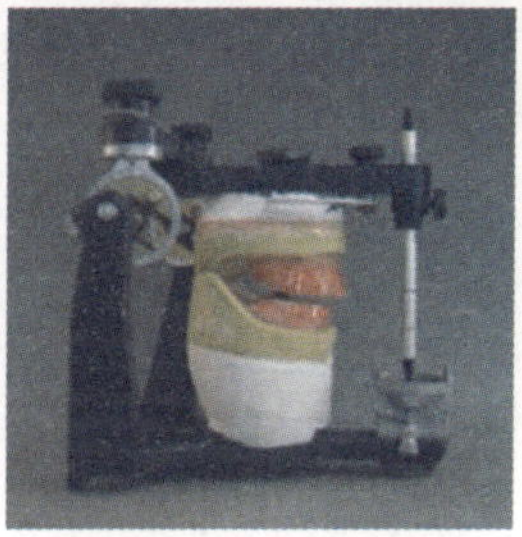

Fig. 15.3 The Central bearing plate and central bearing point are attached to the occlusal rims while maintaining established vertical dimension

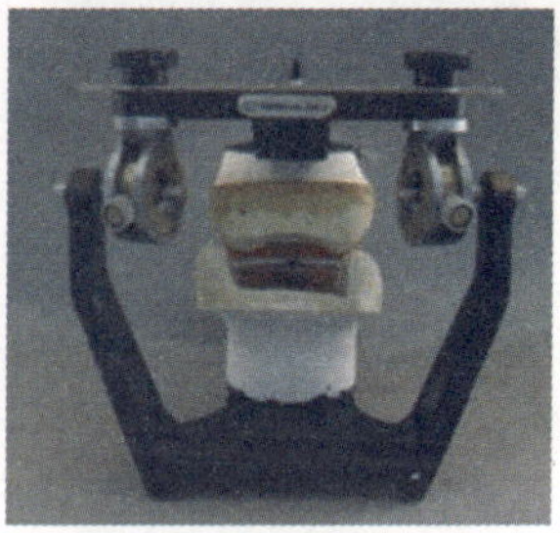

Fig. 15.4 Uniform gap provided between the maxillary and mandibular occlusal rims

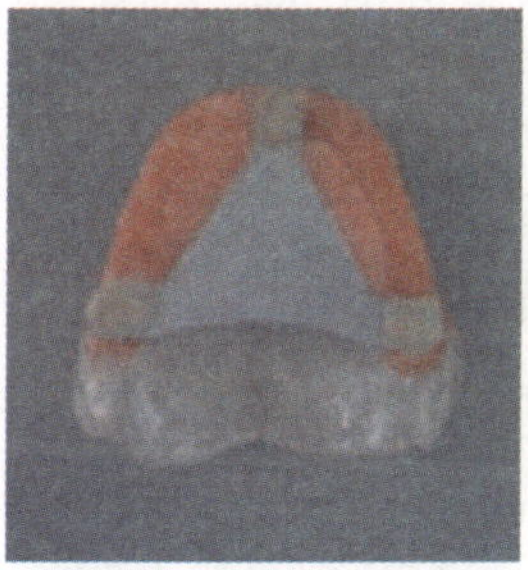

Fig. 15.5 The central bearing plate is submerged in to the maxillary occlusal rim

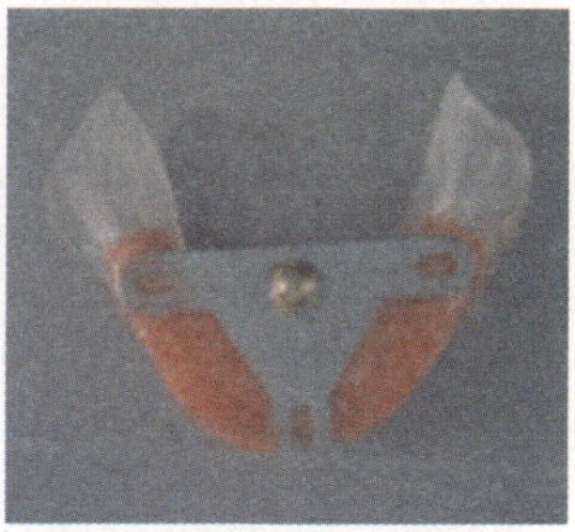

Fig. 15.6 The plate carrying the central bearing point is in flush with the modified mandibular occlusal rim

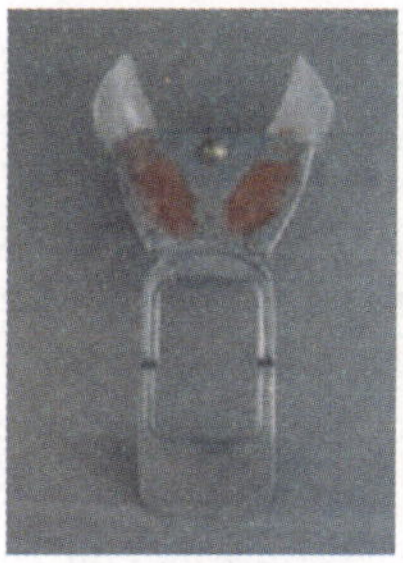

Fig.15.7 The tracing table is attached to the buccal surfaces of the mandibular occlusal rim

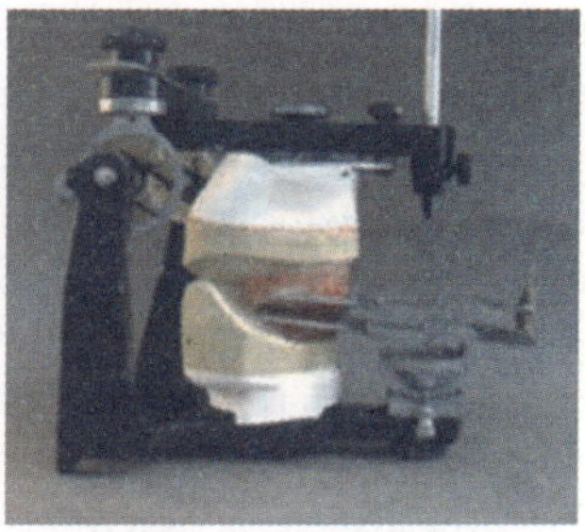

Fig. 15.8 The tracing table is attached such that it does not interfere with incisal guide table

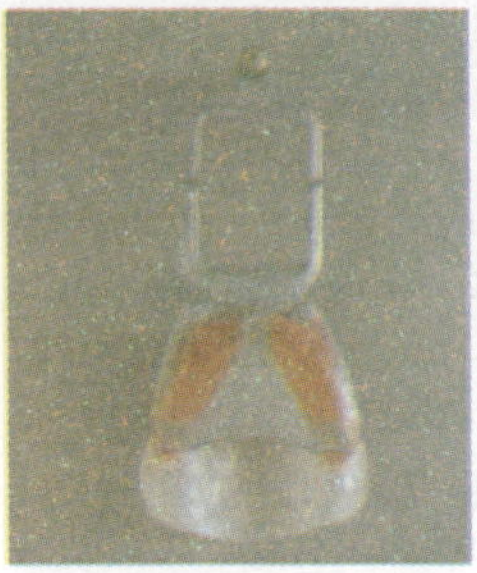

Fig. 15.9 Stylus unit is attached to the maxillary rim

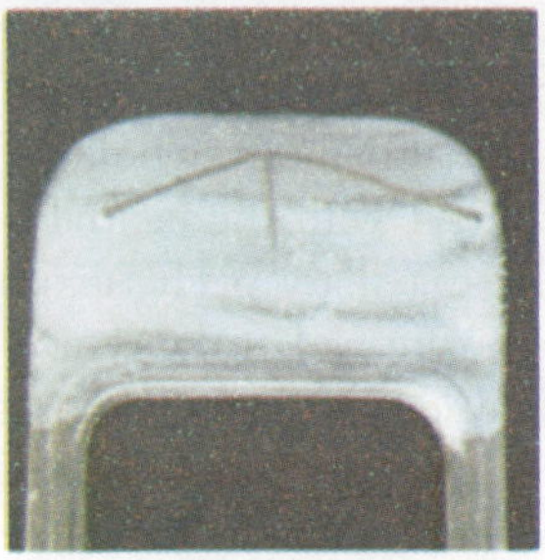

Fig. 15.10a Gothic arch tracing made by the patient on a mixture of zinc oxide and spirit

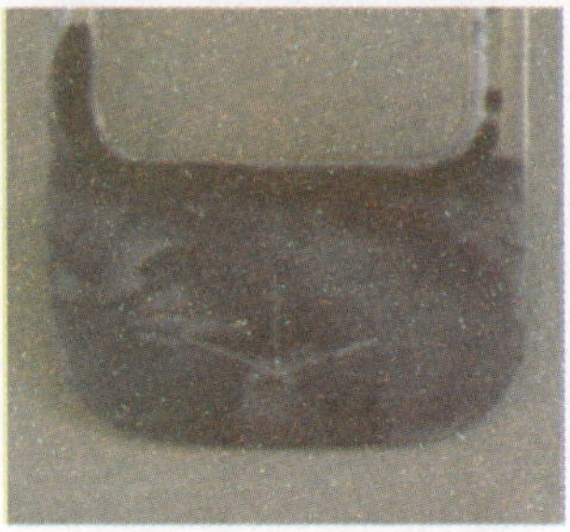

Fig. 15.10b Gothic arch tracing made by the patient on wax medium

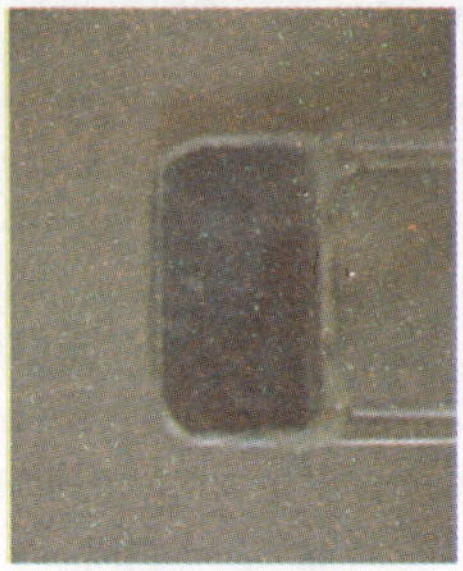

Fig. 15.11 Plastic template with hole made at centric and 6 mm protrusion

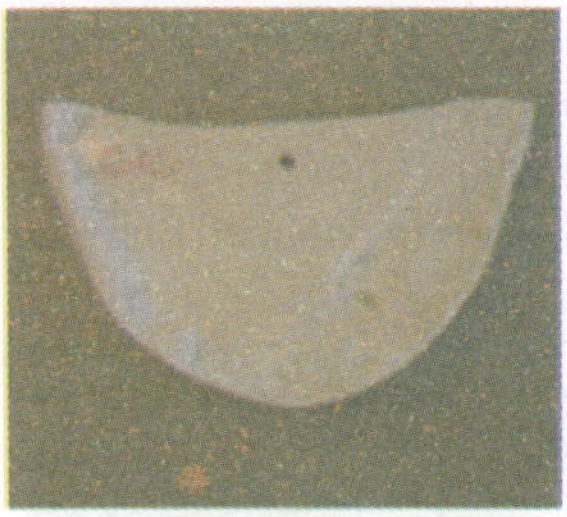

Fig. 15.12 Record obtained at centric

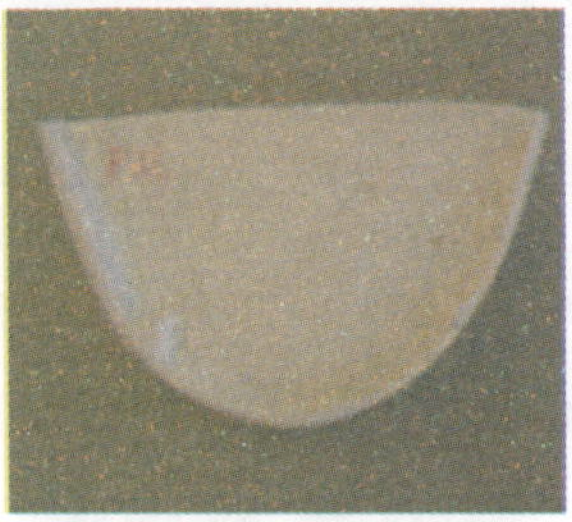

Fig. 15.13 Record obtained at 6mm protrusion

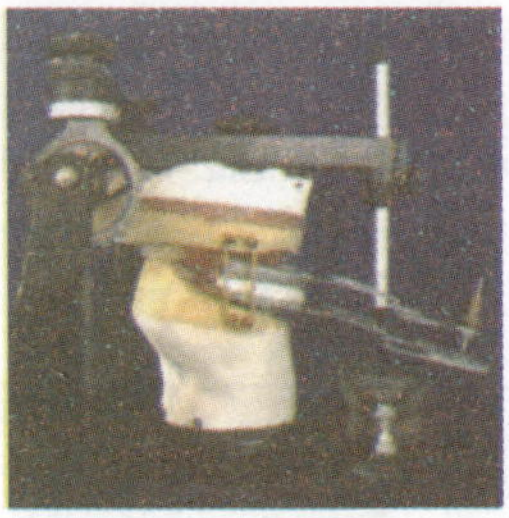

Fig. 15.14 Pins fixed onto the casts

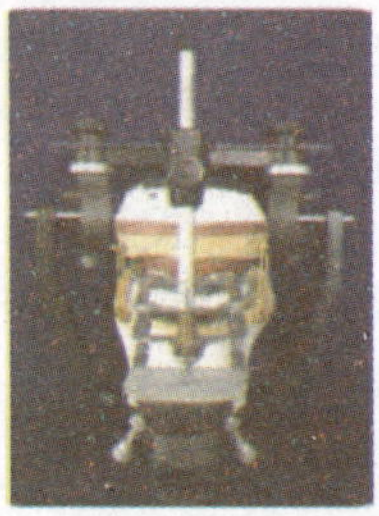

Fig. 15.15 Incisal guide pin and stylus raised up

the patient's mouth and movements are simulated. A minimum 3 mm of gap should be maintained in the posterior region. The next step is to attach the tracing unit. The tracing table is attached to the buccal surfaces of the mandibular occlusal rim such that it is parallel to the maxillary occlusal plane and will not interfere with the incisal guide table (Fig 15.7, 15.8). Stylus unit is attached to the maxillary rim (Fig 15.9). The stylus is provided with spring loading so that it can move in a vertical direction to accommodate the approximation of occlusal rims in the protrusive position. After the tracing unit is attached, the stylus movement is checked whether it is contained with in the table. Assembly is now transferred to the patient's mouth and patient is asked to make protrusive and retrusive movements only. Once consistency at centric relation point is obtained, the patient is asked to make excursive movements, one after the other. First the patient is asked to make right lateral and come back to centric then left lateral and back to centric. Patient if trained few times will be capable of making a tracing in a singular line. Then a thin layer of contrast medium using okelson spray, marker pen, wax or mixture of zinc oxide and spirit is applied on the tracing table and the patient is asked to perform the jaw movements.

By training, each edentulous individual will be able to make a gothic arch tracing. It has an arrow point that represents the centric relation (Fig 15.10a,b). The excursive movements – protrusive, right lateral and left lateral movements of the mandible will be represented by straight lines. However the tracing obtained from the protrusive movement need not always be a straight line because it is controlled by both the joints. With a caliper an arc is drawn on the tracing which will cut at 6 mm distance on all the lines from the centric point. The number of records to be obtained is based on the type of the articulator used. If Hanau wide vue articulator is used, two records are to be made, one at the centric and the second at the protrusive point which was marked before. Articulators like Dentatus require records made on the lateral tracings also. While making the record, the stylus has to be held at the desired points and for that a plastic template is used. A transparent plastic sheet is selected and trimmed according to the dimensions of the tracing table and it is fixed over the tracings made. The points at which the records are to be made are marked on the plastic plate and a fine hole is drilled. This hole will hold the stylus at the desired point, for example at centric and at 6 mm protrusion (Fig 15.11). Now the occlusion rims are to be modified by closing the gaps between the central bearing plates and the rim. On the wax rim, triangular locating notches extending to the buccal surfaces are prepared both on the maxilla and mandible. Petroleum jelly is smeared on the wax and metal surface to act as a separating medium between wax and plaster. Patient is asked to hold the stylus first at the centric position and an accelerated mix of plaster is injected between the upper and lower occlusal rims. Alternatively plaster mix can be spread first on the mandibular plate and then it can be inserted in to the mouth and the patient's mandible is guided to the required position. Excess material flowing out should be wiped. Once the plaster is set, the assembly can be removed and the record is carefully separated out. Record can be considered as accurate if the central bearing point makes clear perforation in the plaster record (Fig 15.12, 15.13). Similarly all records are obtained which will serve in programming the articulator.

Programming

First the centric record has to be placed and it has to be found out whether it matches with tentative centric relation. For this purpose the bases with the tracing assembly is brought back to the casts mounted in the articulator. After keeping the interocclusal record, the upper cast and the lower cast are to be secured and for that retentive pins have to be incorporated on both sides. Fine holes can be drilled on the casts and on each side 2 pins on the upper and 2 pins on the lower can be fixed. While fixing on the maxillary pins, care should be taken to drill the holes well below the split (Fig 15.14). Before securing the pins the split has to be separated. With a thread the lower cast, the lower base, the plaster record, the upper base and the upper cast should be secured in to a singular block. The incisal guide pin and the stylus have to be raised at this point and they need not make contact with the respective tables (Fig 15.15).

The upper member of the articulator with the upper split of the cast should now be approximated. At this point it is desirable to release the centric lock. When it is approximated, both the parts of the split cast must approximate closely. While it is closed, if the condylar spheres are making contact with the respective stops it can be considered that the tentative centric is matching with graphic tracing. If it is not matching it is desirable to go back to the check bite and re-register the tentative centric and repeat the entire process. If the centric matches the articulator can be programmed. Upto this stage the articulator simulated the patient in the opening and closing movement. The articulator has the capability to make translatory movements for which the horizontal condylar path has to be adjusted similar to the condylar path inclination present in the patient. For this purpose the protrusive record is used. In the place of the centric record, protrusive record is positioned and the casts are secured. The centric lock, as well as the thumbscrew present behind the condylar housing will be released so that both the condylar elements and the condylar paths can be moved. The upper member with the upper split cast is approximated. If there is a gap, the brass disc containing the condylar path can be moved so that the split completely gets obliterated. When it is obliterated, hold the upper member and the lower member of the articulator tight and note down the condylar path set by itself. The path is fixed at this point. The lateral condylar path in Hanau articulator is adjusted using the formula which will approximately be 15 degrees. From now onwards the articulator will function as a simulator of the patient's jaw with movement capability both in opening and in translation.

Suggested Reading

1. Nair K Chandrasekharan, *Programming the semiadjustable articulator,* Trends in prosthodontics and Dental Implantology, 2011;2(1):12-14

16

Facts about denture aesthetics

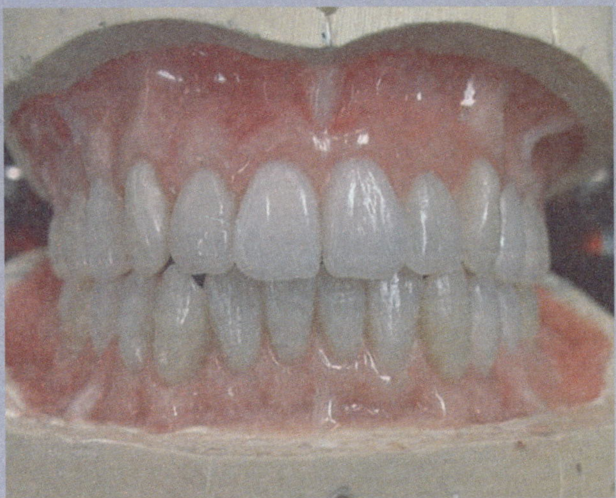

Aesthetics in complete dentures means creating a natural appearance harmonious with the face

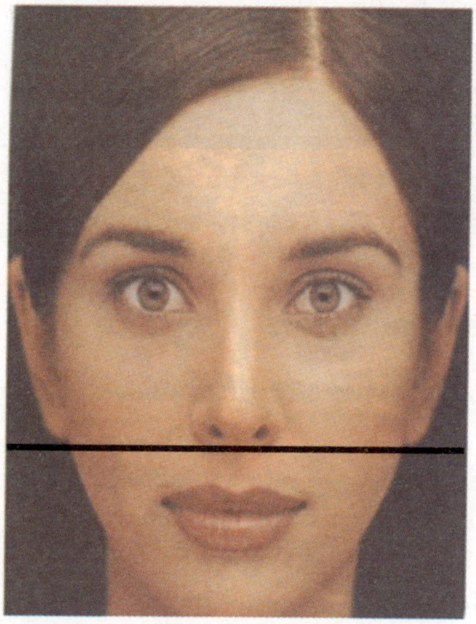

Fig. 16.1 Lower third of the face provides beauty

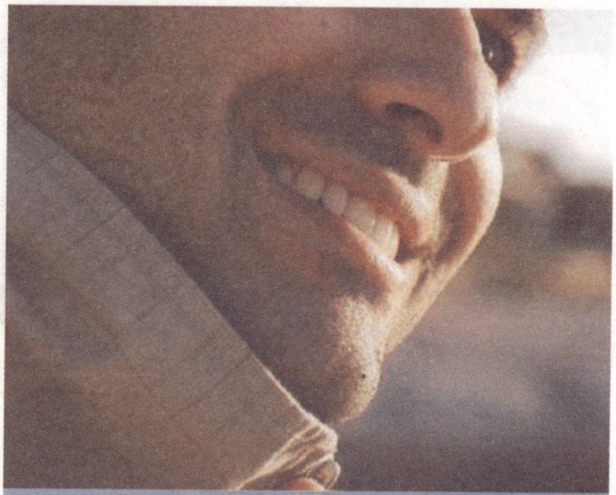

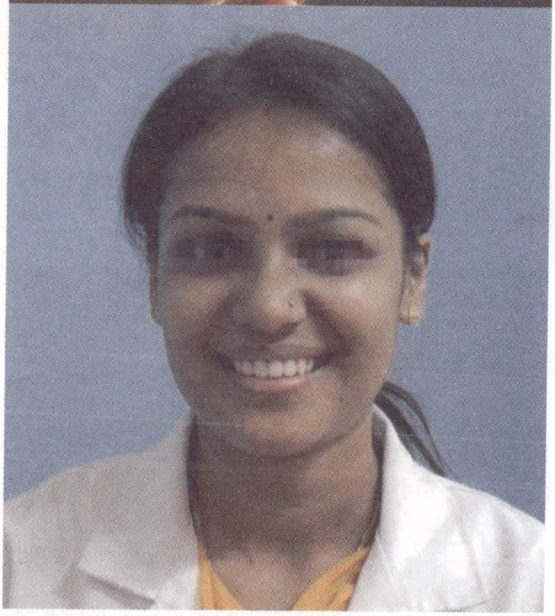

Fig. 16.2 Beautiful face always provide a good background for smile

History confirms that humanity has always been preoccupied with facial beauty. Aesthetic norms have changed with time and predictable success can be obtained only if we know the definitions of modern ideals which have considerable social acceptance. Lower third of the face provides significant beauty and that is mainly due to the presence of mouth (Fig. 16.1). When teeth are lost lips loose their shape and one cannot smile. Importance of smile has made the aesthetics of dentures a significant factor.

Aesthetics by definition is the science of beauty. It provides details so that an object becomes appealing to the onlooker and pleases him. Beautiful face always provides a good background for smile. (Fig.16.2) Pleasing smiles are related to the visual attention of teeth. When a person smiles, if too much attention is attracted by the teeth it is bad. Very white teeth on a dark skinned individual have this defect. If insufficient attention is drawn by the teeth, then the person will appear edentulous. The optimum nature of attention is very difficult to define but a dentist can train his eyes by looking at normal faces and derive his own optimum perception.

If artificial teeth resemble natural teeth it is generally considered as aesthetic. (Fig.16.3). But natural dentition need not be pleasing always. Incorporation of crowding, diastema and rotation have got questionable value in dentures. Diastema is closed with composites and teeth are derotated by orthodontic correction. If these things can happen in natural teeth, then how are we justified in incorporating them as aesthetic features in dentures.

Face can be divided into three equal parts viz trichion to nasion (upper third) fig.16.4. nasion to subnasale (middle third) subnasale to menton (lower third)

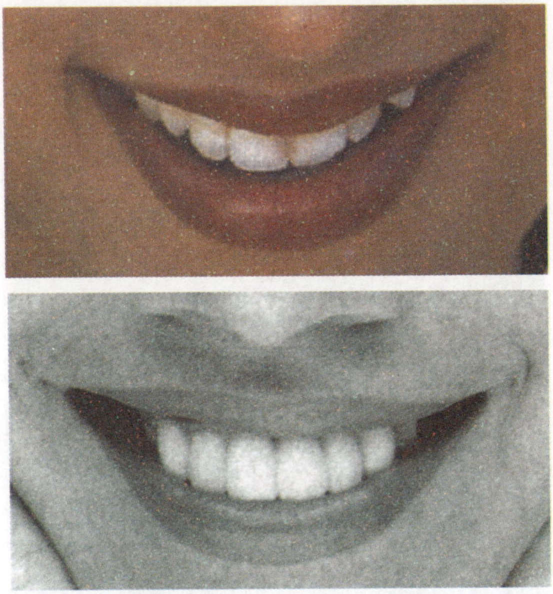

Fig. 16.3 If artificial teeth resemble natural teeth it is generally considered as aesthetic

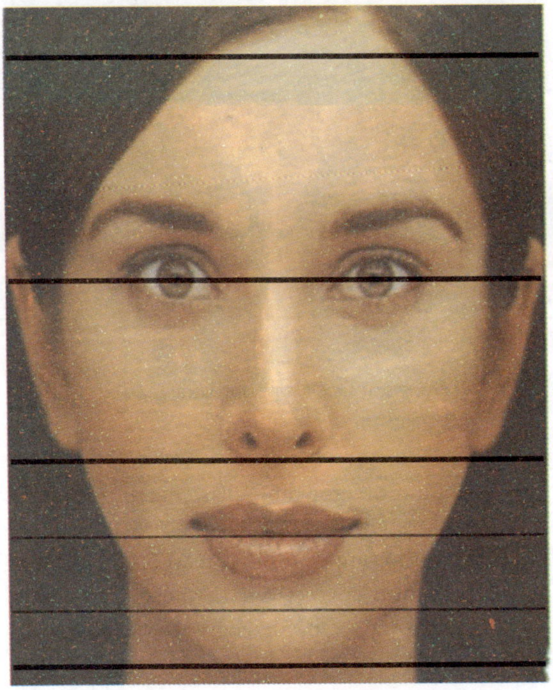

Fig. 16.4 Face can be divided into three parts: trichion-nasion-subnasale-menton. Lower third can further be divided into three. The incisal edges fall at the junction of the upper and middle thirds

Lower third can further be divided into three parts. The incisal edges of the maxillary anteriors fall at the junction of the upper and middle thirds.

Denture aesthetics is mainly related to maxillary anteriors. (Fig.16.5). Text book chapters are titled either selection of anteriors or denture aesthetics.

Shade of anteriors

Shade of teeth has no correlation with eye, hair or skin.

From anterior to posterior, the value of colour shifts to darker side Females have comparatively lighter shade.

Shade is first suggested by the dentist but mainly selected by the patient who will definitely opt for a lighter shade.

Shade contrasting to the skin colour should not be selected because it will make the teeth more conspicuous.

As age advances, the value of colour shifts towards darker side.

Shade guide-Vita 3 D master provides an appropriate distribution of shades according to the age. Groups 1and 2 for youngsters, 3 for middle aged and 4 and 5 for older individuals.

Cervical region of teeth is yellowish and incisal edge is gray.

Old dentures and natural teeth can act as a guide in the selection of shade.

Shape: Length, width and morphology

Mesio-distal dimension of anterior segment is usually between 48 to 52 mm. Above 52 it is considered as big. It can go as low as 39 mm.

Intercommissural width and anterior teeth are in golden proportion ie. 1:1.618.

Width of the philtrum and width of centrals almost match.

Width of central incisor is ¼ of the canine cusp to canine cusp distance.

Width of one central incisor is 1/16 th of bizygomatic width.

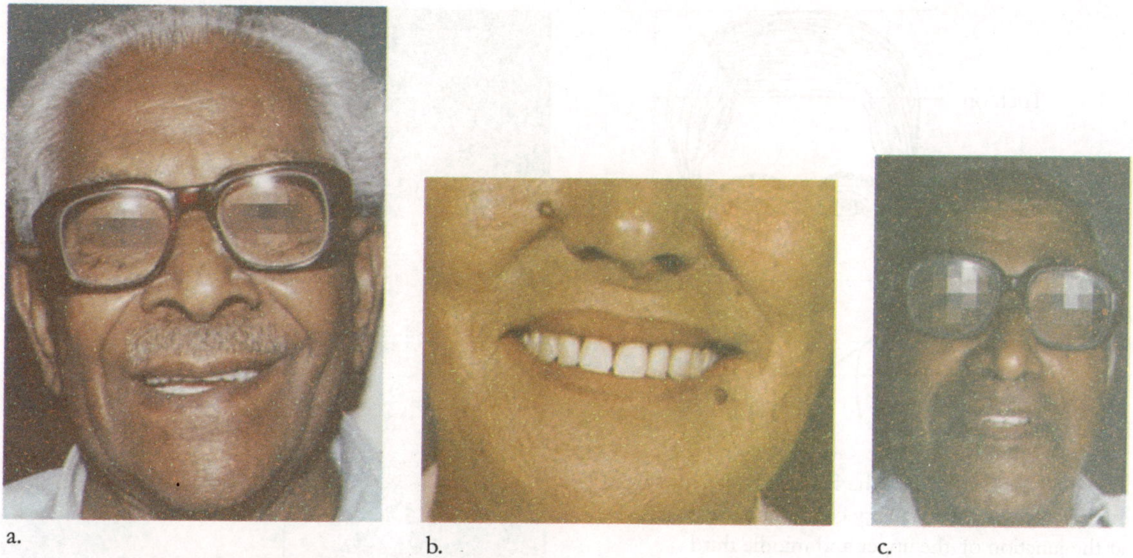

Fig. 16.5 Denture aesthetics is mainly related to maxillary anteriors. a) Anteriors not visible b) Anterior teeth more visible and midline error c) Adequate visibility

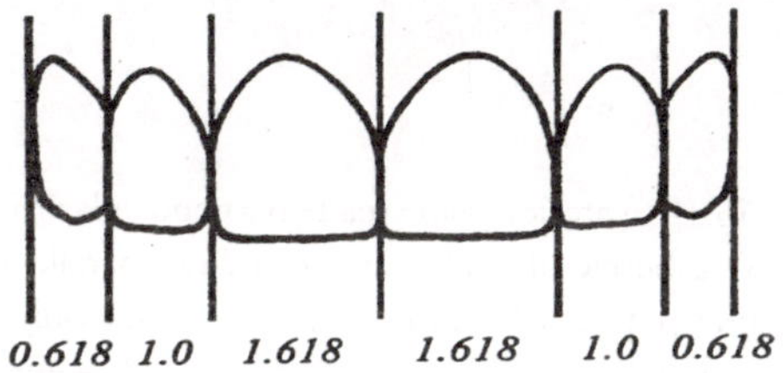

Fig. 16.6 Golden proportion can be maintained between central, lateral and canine 1.6 : 1 : O.6

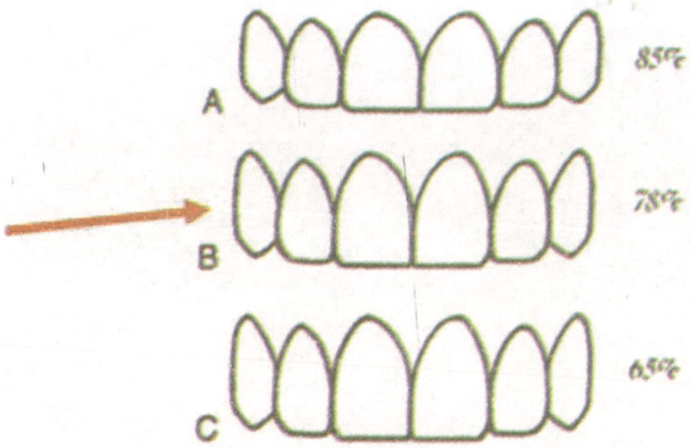

Fig. 16.7 Width of the central incisor if made 78% of the length, it will be pleasing. Golden proportion makes the centrals appear longer

Width of anterior segment is 1/3 of bizygomatic width.

Length of maxillary central incisor is 1/16 (1/20) of face length trichion to menton.

Golden proportion can be maintained between central, lateral and canine 1.6 : 1 : O.6. The reduction is at the rate of 62%. With this proportion anterior segment can be narrower. If it is felt so, the proportion can be enhanced to 70%. The reduction proportion should be maintained constantly. The proportion is designated on the visibility when viewed from the front and not on tooth size. (Fig. 16.6).

Width of the central incisor if made 78% of the length of the incisor, it will be pleasing. Golden proportion makes the centrals appear squarish. (Fig. 16.7, 16.8).

Arrangement of anterior teeth

All these statements are for maxillary central incisor

Lower third of the face is divided into three. Incisal

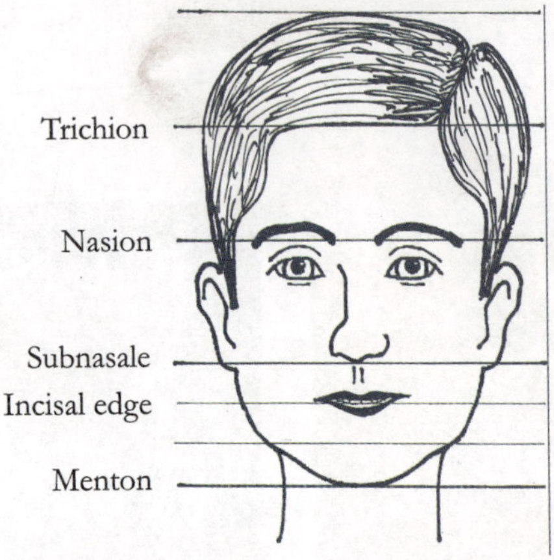

Fig. 16.9 Lower third of the face is divided into three. Incisal edge of the maxillary central incisor should fall at the junction of the upper and middle third

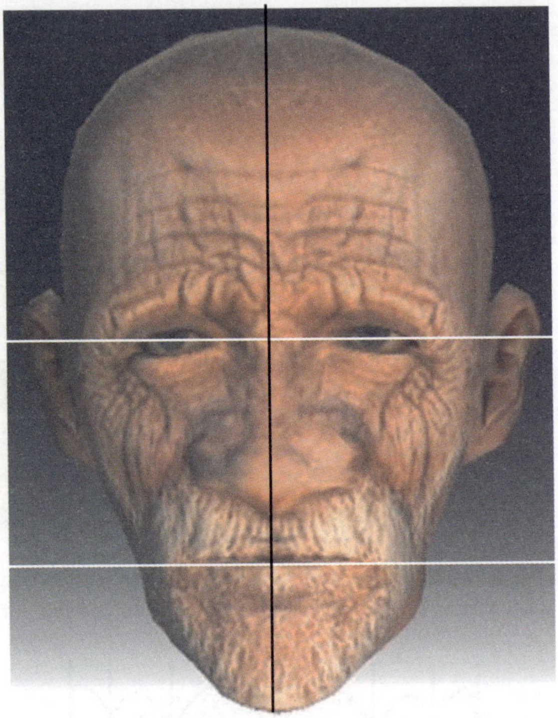

Fig. 16.11 Anterior plane made perpendicular to the nasion-tubercle of philtrum line and not parallel to the inter pupillary line. Plane selection done only after ensuring adequate lip support. Incisal 2/3 of incisor supports the lip

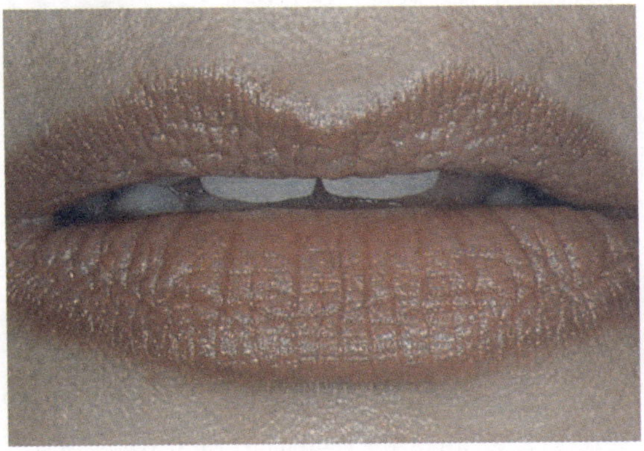

Fig. 16.10 At rest position of the lip-slightly parted-incisal edge of the central incisor should be visible 1 or 2 mm

edge of the maxillary central incisor should fall at the junction of the upper and middle third (Fig.16.9).

At rest position of the lip-slightly parted-incisal edge of the Central incisor should be visible 1 or 2 mm (Fig. 16.10).

Mesial angle of the central incisor is placed 8 mm anterior to the incisive papilla

While pronouncing F and V, incisal edge should meet the dry wet junction of the lower lip

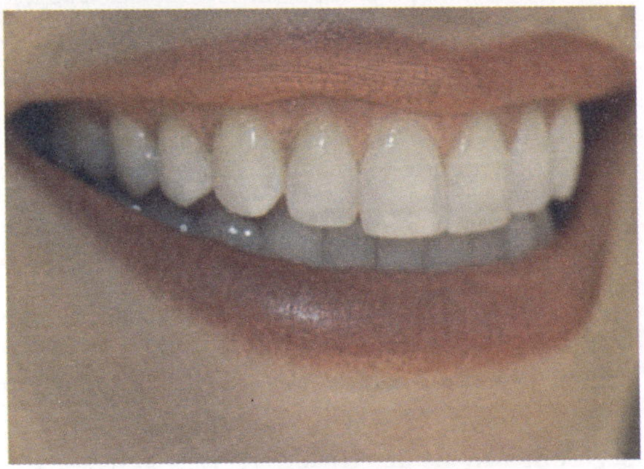

Fig. 16.12 Contact point raised in step ladder fashion. Perceived contact area between centrals, 50% of the length of the central, between central and lateral 40%, between lateral and canine 30% Distal angle is more rounded

Anterior plane is made perpendicular to the nasion-tubercle of philtrum line and not parallel to the inter pupillary line. (Fig.16.11).

Plane selection is done only after ensuring adequate lip support. Incisal 2/3 of the incisor supports the lip

Lateral incisor should be in golden proportion or the selected constant proportion to the central

Mesial angle is rotated forward in females

It is slightly depressed than the central in males

Contact points of the anteriors are raised in step ladder fashion. (Fig.16.12).

Perceived contact area between centrals 50% of the length of the central. Between central and lateral 40%. Between lateral and canine 30%

Distal angle is more rounded

Canine-papilla-canine line passes through the tip of canine

Canine is placed 10 mm away from the tip of the first rugae

Canine is placed slightly above lateral incisor

Axially rotated –distal half not seen from front in males

Cervical region is prominent

Never position canine with cusp jetting out labially

Labial ridge is prominent in males

Incisal embrasure between lateral and canine is triangular

Premolar visibility from front should be in golden proportion to Canine

Premolar should not be made more prominent than canine

Axes of all anteriors are mesially inclined to improve aesthetics. (Fig.16.13).

All the incisal edges form a curve smile curve along the upper border of the lower lip. (Fig.16.13).

Facial form and tooth form have no correlation. Harmony is the watch word

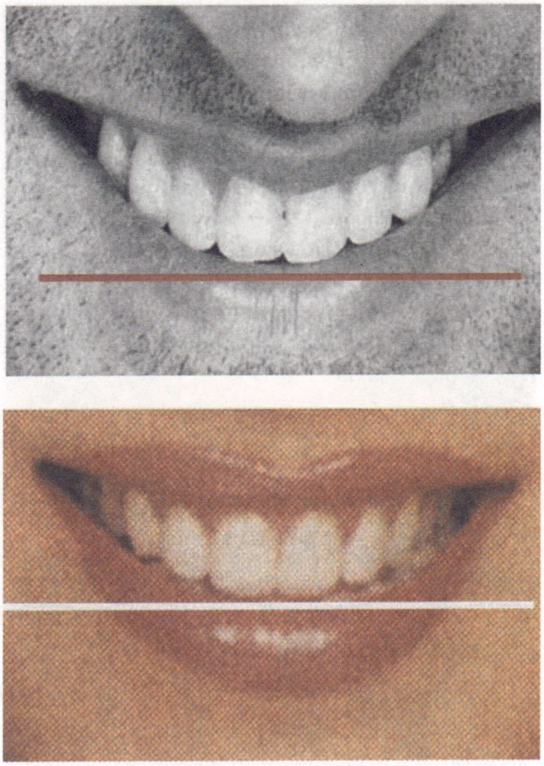

Fig. 16.13 a and b Axes of all anteriors are mesially inclined. All the incisal edges form a curve – smile curve along the upper border of the lower lip

SPA factor is not a reliable guide. Both the halves of dentition Sex, Personality, Age (SPA) may not express characteristic male/female features. Only one half will have the predominant sex feature. Inclusion of personality is a myth because personality is not a physical feature completely. Age changes if overtly incorporated will not be cherished by most of the individuals. Every one wants to appear young and hence incorporation of dark attritited teeth will not be appreciated. Visibility of incisors at rest position can be reduced as age advances. In youngsters it can be 2 mm in middle aged 1.5 mm and in old aged 1 mm or less

Preparation for denture aesthetics should start from impressions.

Thick and over extended borders made in the impression stages will make the lips over supported especially below the nose.

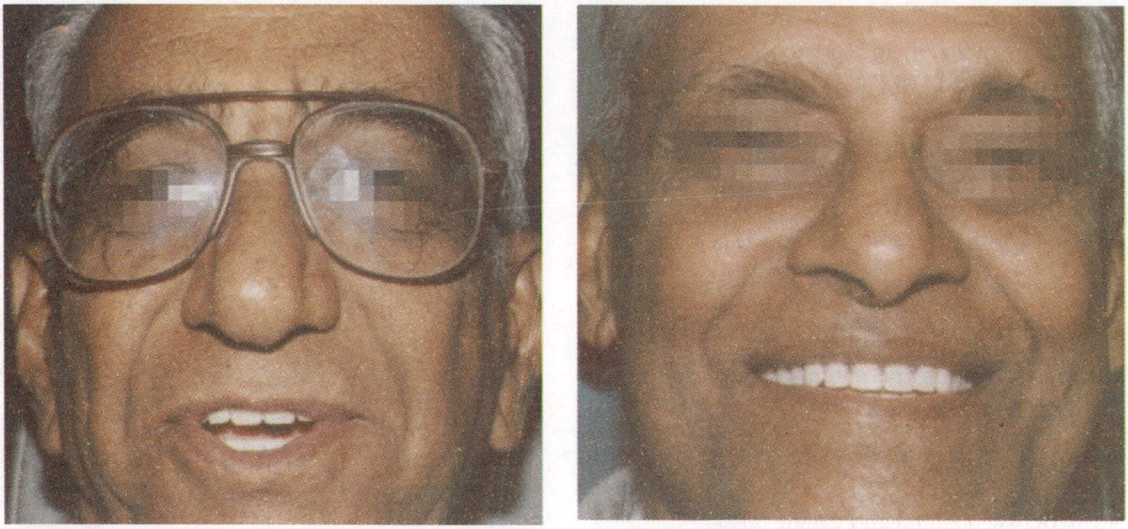

Fig. 16.14 Establishing correct vertical dimension is essential in positioning the perioral musculature

Normal shape of the philtrum should be retained during the impression stage

Establishing correct vertical dimension is essential in positioning the perioral musculature. Viewing the face from the front and from the side will guide the operator. If trial is not performed under correct soft tissue support, there is a possibility of change in visibility during denture insertion stage. (Fig.16.14).

Teeth should be arranged according to the factors mentioned already

During the try in check for midline, lip support, cuspid neck prominence, position of teeth, incisal and occlusal plane, visibility and phonetic relations

Digital images and Polaroid camera photos are to be used for patient evaluation. Mirror shows reverse images.

Like teeth, denture base also is important in providing aesthetics to the denture. While carving the gingival outline, the zenith is shifted to the distal in centrals and canines. In laterals it is kept at the centre.

Gingival border of the lateral incisor is kept at a lower level when compared to those of central and canine. Gingival border of the first premolar is at a lower level than that of canine.

In most cases tip of the papilla will be seen below the lip. Its relative length follows the contact placement.

Colour of the denture base resin should match that of mucosa.

Many of the resins available in India are too pink or too light.

Addition of umber colour to the monomer will compensate this.

Incorporation of stippling is better achieved with a slightly bent round bur and running it at a slow speed. Stippling should not be done in the free gingival region.

Interdental papilla if carved too deep will act as food traps

Denture base tinting is successful only limitedly. Tinting is mainly done to simulate melanin pigmentation.

Denture space impressions will confirm whether the teeth are within the biologic functional limit.

Aesthetics may not be appreciated always. Some people like the old looks even if it is bad. Do not try aesthetic modifications.

Suggested reading

1. Frush, J. P. and Fisher, R. D. *Introduction to dentinogeni-crestorations.* J Prosthet Dent 1955; 5 :586-595.
2. Frush, J. P., Fisher, R. D. *The dynesthetic interpretation on the dentogenic concept.* J Prosthet Dent 1958;8:558-581.
3. Lombardi, R. E. *The principles of visual perception and their clinical application to denture esthetics.* J Prosthet Dent 1973;29:358-382.
4. Pound, E. *Controlling anomalies of vertical dimension and speech.* J Prosthet Dent 1976;36:124-135.
5. Mathews, T. G. *The anatomy of a smile.* J Periodont Res 1978;39:128-134
6. Vig, R. G. and Brundo, G. C. *The kinetics of anterior tooth display.* J Prosthet Dent 1978; 39:502-504.
7. Levin, E. I. *Dental esthetics and the golden proportion.* JProsthet Dent 1978;40:244-252.
8. Tautin FS. *Denture esthetics is more than tooth selection.*J Prosthet Dent. Aug 1978;40(2):127-30.
9. Cade, R. E. *The role of the mandibular anterior teeth in complete denture esthetics.* J Prosthet Dent 1979;42:368-370.
10. Brisman, A. S. *Esthetics: A comparison of dentist's and patient's concepts.* J Am Dent Assoc 1980;100:345.
11. Mavroskovfis, F. and Ritchie, G. M. *The face-form as a guide for the selection of maxillary central incisors.* J Prosthet Dent 1980;43:501-505.
12. Lorton, L. and Whitback, P. *Esthetic parameters of mandibular anterior teeth.* J Prosthet Dent 1981;46:280-283.
13. Scandrett, F. R., Kerber, P. E. and Umrigar, Z. R. *A clinical evaluation of techniques to determine the combined width of the maxillary anterior teeth and the maxillary central incisor.* J Prosthet Dent 1982;48:15-22.
14. Tjan, A. H. L., Miller, E. D. and The, J. G. P. *Some esthetic factors in a smile.* J Prosthet Dent 1984;51:24-28.
15. Murrell GA.*Esthetics and the edentulous patient.*J Am Dent Assoc. Sep 1988;117(4):57E-63E.
16. Murrell GA. *Complete denture esthetics. Review.*Dent Clin North Am. Apr 1989;33(2):145-55.
17. Engelmeier RL.*Complete-denture esthetics.* Dent Clin North Am. 1996 Jan;40(1):71-84.
18. Devlin, Reddick. *Biological guides… Dental update* Dec 2001; 492- 5.

17

Arrangement of anterior teeth

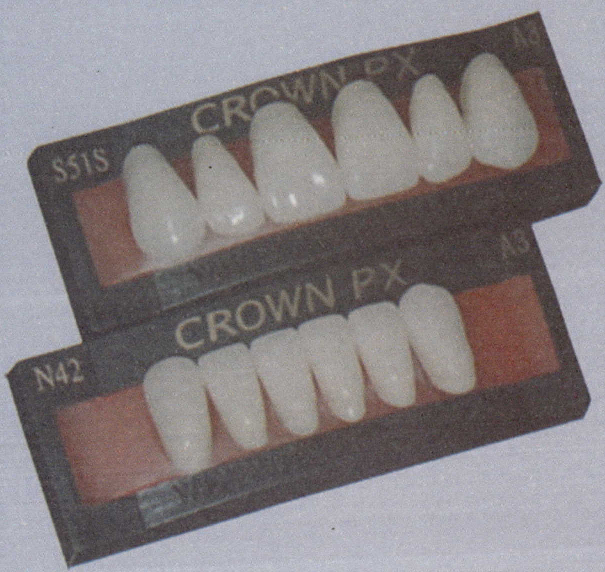

Success of complete denture treatment depends greatly on clear understanding of the possibilities and the limitations

Position of the maxillary and mandibular casts is fixed in the articulator and the appropriate teeth set is selected. Now the teeth have to be arranged in the available space between the maxillary and mandibular ridges. It would be desirable to have an inter ridge space of 15 to 20mm but in all the cases it is not obtained. The space must be ascertained first by removing the bases with the occlusal rims and by measuring it. First the anterior teeth are arranged. For this the operator requires the orientation of midline, canine line and the occlusal plane which are present in the occlusion rim. While arranging the teeth, the wax rim will be removed and there is every possibility that the markings made on the wax rim will be lost. Hence these markings are extended on the land of the cast with a pencil. The occlusal

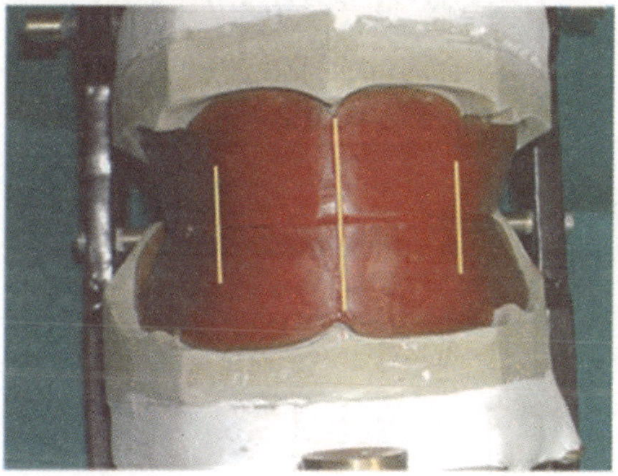

Fig. 17.1 Occlusal rims with central and canine lines marked

plane can be marked as a horizontal line drawn at a known distance away from the occlusal plane and the distance must be noted on the land. (Fig. 17.1)

Once the space available for the anterior teeth is known, appropriate teeth can be selected. (Fig. 17.2-17.3) Teeth are available in different shapes, sizes and shades. Tapering, square and ovoid shapes are generally seen. Human face is also seen in these forms. A tapered outline of the tooth will harmonise very well with a tapered face. Size of the anterior teeth is selected by two parameters. The width of the anterior segment will be roughly one third the bizygomatic width of the face. Width of the

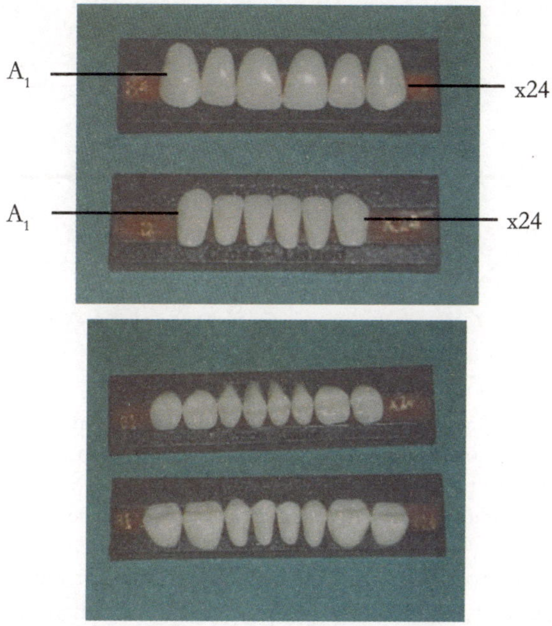

Fig. 17.2, 17.3 Anterior and posterior teeth set. Markings on the left side indicate the mould and right side indicate shade.For anteriors the mould indicate the shape where as in the posteriors it indicates the combined mesio-distal dimension of two premolars and two molars.

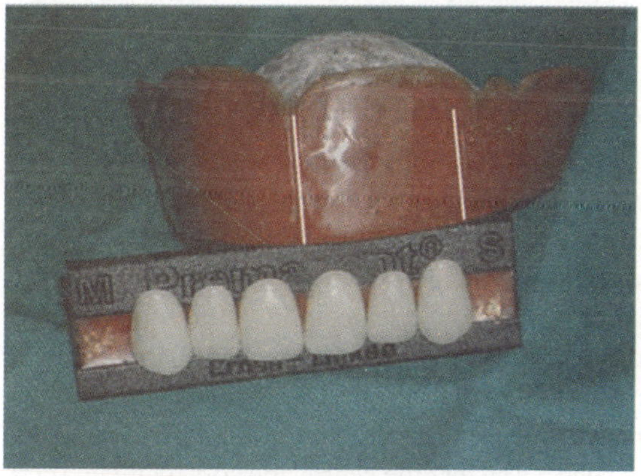

Fig. 17.4 Comparision of the distance between the central and canine lines and the tooth size.

maxillary central incisor will be one sixteenth of the bizygomatic width of the face. (Fig. 17.4) Length to width proportion is usually done based on golden proportion. If length is 1, the width will be 0.6. In

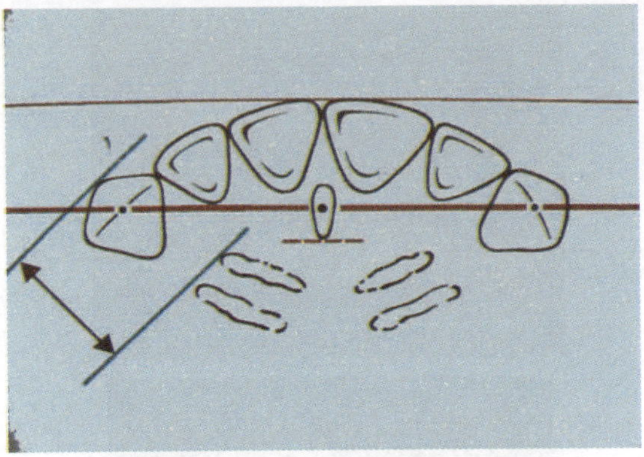

Fig. 17.5 Mesial angle of the maxillary central incisor is positioned 8mm anterior to the midpoint of the incisive papilla. Cusp tips of canines and the centre of the papilla fall in a line called canine papilla canine line.

other words width is 60% of the length. For more realistic aesthetics this proportion can be enhanced to 78%. Position of the central incisor is of critical importance especially for aesthetics. It is positioned generally 8 mm anterior to the mid point of the incisive papilla. (Fig. 17.5) This anthropometric measurement need be considered only as a guideline and not as a rule. Aesthetic perception of the operator and the approval of the patient will have a more important say in the finalization of the central incisor position. Shade of the teeth is selected so that there is no contrast for the teeth from the face.

Acrylic teeth supplied by the manufacturer will have considerable bulk at the neck region and hence it may not be possible to accommodate the same without trimming. It is always desirable to grind the binding surface in order to improve the bond between the denture base and the acrylic teeth. Modifications made on the acrylic teeth should be well suited to the patients' facial features. Anterior teeth are arranged in such a way that the central incisors maintain their axis vertical and parallel. The lateral incisors are tilted so that the mesial angle moves medially. Canines are arranged in a vertical axis. For esthetic reasons it can also be tilted mesially. Incisors are generally proclined labially by about 15 degrees from the vertical plane so that it can provide adequate support to the lips and the teeth will be adequately visible during smile.

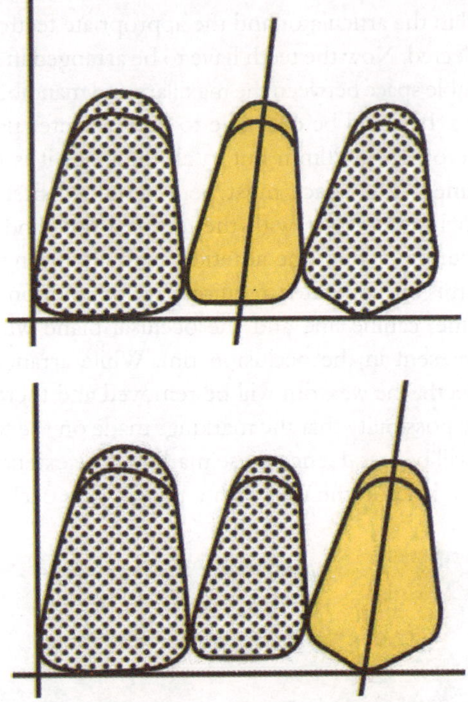

Fig. 17.6 Lateral incisor is slightly raised from the occlusal plane in middle aged individuals and in old aged both central and lateral are arranged at the same level.In certain individuals cervical region of the canine is pushed distally as an acceptable variation

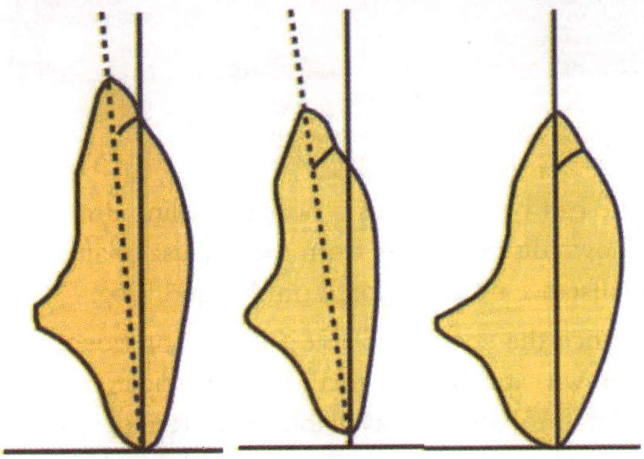

Fig. 17.7 Both central and lateral incisors are tipped labially by approximately 15^0. This tipping is achieved by depressing the cervical region. Axis of the canine is vertical in contrast to that of the incisors.

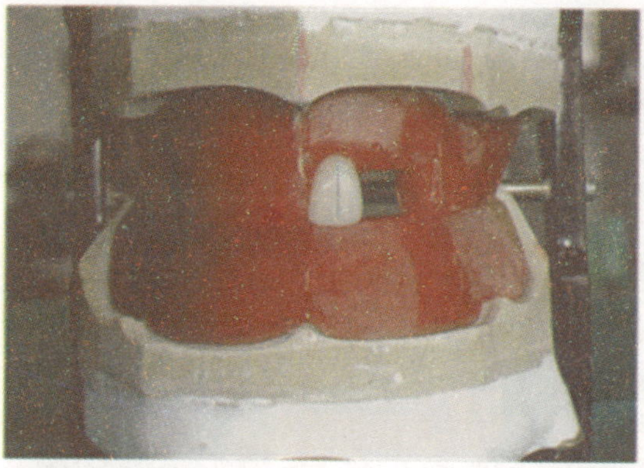

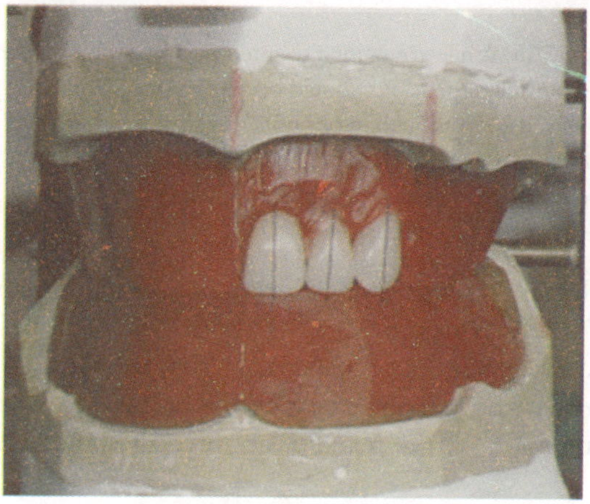

Fig. 17.8, 17.9 Before arranging the anterior teeth the occlusion rim representing the tooth portion is completely removed. Central incisor and canine are arranged vertically when viewed labially. However,axis of lateral incisor is tilted.This tilt is achieved by tilting cervical region distally.

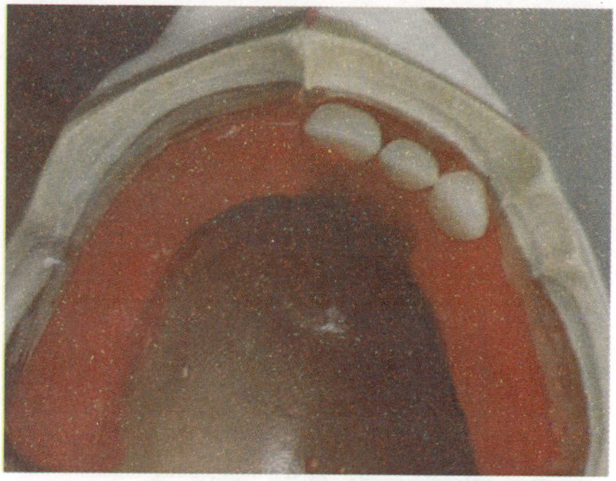

Fig. 17.10 Anterior teeth when viewed incisally form an arch. The arch is incorporated by rotating the lateral and canine in an axial direction. Lateral incisor is depressed in males where as in females it slightly overlaps the distal angle of the central.

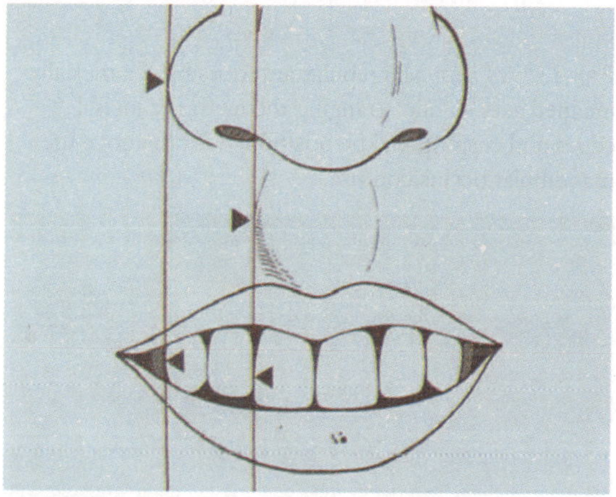

Fig. 17.11 A drop line passing through the lateral borders of the philtrum generally coincides with the distal border of the central incisor. Drop line passing through the ala of the nose passes through the distal slope of the canine. The line should be drawn when patient smiles.

(Fig. 17.6, 17.7), The above rules need be considered as a guide line but an operator can take the liberty to arrange the teeth in an aesthetic and acceptable form. (Fig. 17.8, 17.9, 17.10) The ultimate aim in teeth arrangement is that, they should harmonize with the facial features otherwise the teeth will stand out and attract the attention of the onlooker. (Fig. 17.11) After positioning the maxillary anteriors, mandibular anteriors can be arranged.

Mandibular incisors are slender teeth and at the same time long. If particular care is not taken the mandibular incisors will look like a singular block after processing. While arranging the mandibular anteriors the labial surfaces should be positioned in such a way that they do not cross the mid point of the labial sulcus in the labio lingual direction. If these teeth are placed further labially, they will exert pressure on the lips which in turn will dislodge the mandibular denture. Many a time this restriction

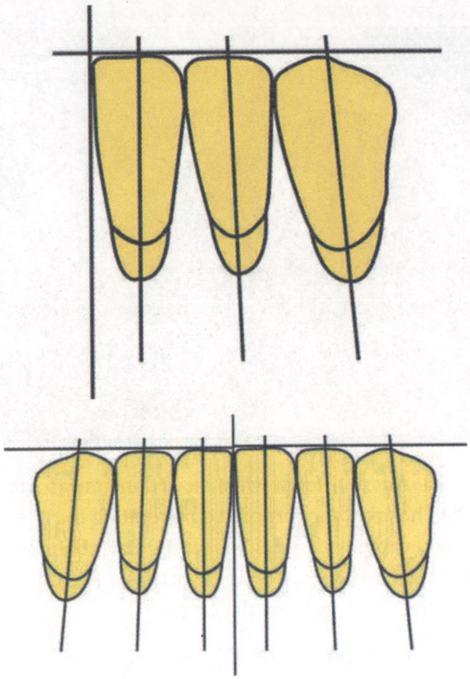

Fig. 17.12, 17.13 Mandibular anteriors have a mesially inclined axes. While arranging the teeth the incisal edges and cusp tip will be positioned 2mm above the mandibular occlusaion rim

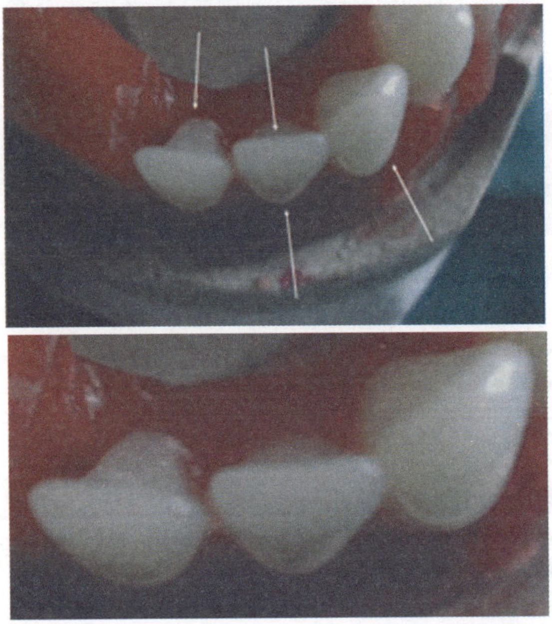

Fig. 17.14, 17.15 In order to obtain naturality mandibular central incisor is tipped labially,lateral positioned straight and canine tipped lingually

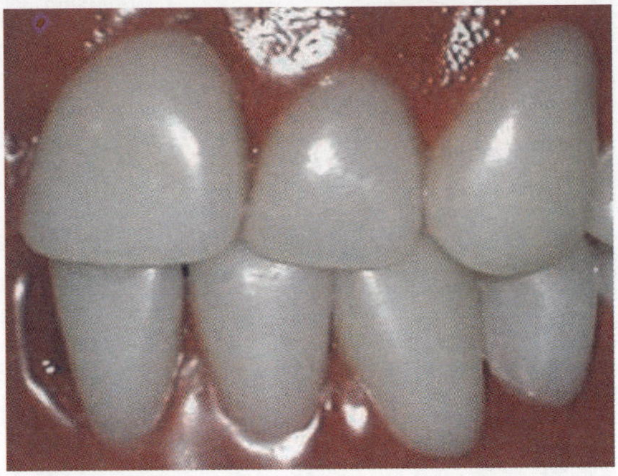

Fig. 17.16 While arranging the anteriors,proportion of the mesio distal dimensions should be adhered to. Mandibular canine cusp tip should be positioned against the maxillary embrasure between the lateral and the canine. The distal border of the mandibular canine should fall in line with the maxillary canine cusp.

will make the operator provide a horizontal overlap of more than 2 mm. Once the horizontal overlap is increased the vertical overlap has also to be increased, so that the patient can incise. The mesio distal dimension of the mandibular anteriors should be

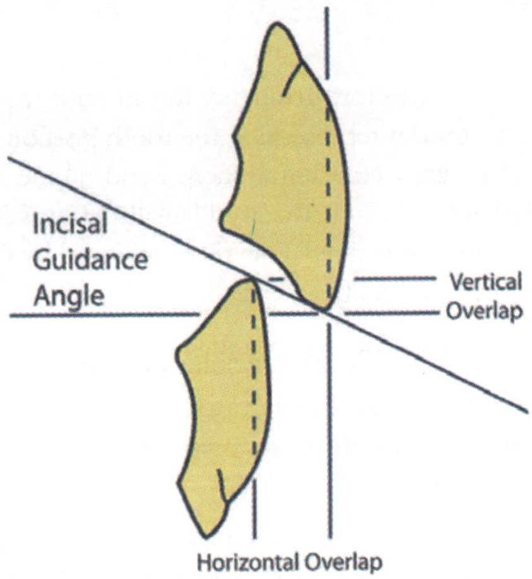

Fig. 17.17 Incisal guidance angle

restricted within the cusps of maxillary canines. The axis of mandibular anteriors are in general mesially oriented. (Fig. 17.12, 17.13) While the central incisors are labially tilted, the laterals are positioned straight.

This will make a distinction between centrals and laterals. Canines are lingually tilted. (Fig. 17.14, 17.15, 17.16) Care should be taken, not to give very close contacts between the anteriors. When the anteriors are arranged, the upper member of the articulator can be pushed backwards to simulate a protrusive movement and an act of incision. Upper and lower incisors are normally arranged to get an inter incisal contact during protrusion and which would help to perform the act of incision. (Fig. 17.17) At this stage the patient can be called back and a trial insertion can be performed. Changes in the arrangement can be done at this stage. It is always desirable to make the midline of the dental arch coincide with the midline of the face.

Note: While the incisal edges of the maxillary anteriors almost coincide with the occlusal surface of the rim, the incisal edges of the mandibular incisors are 2 mm above the occlusal surface of the lower rim. It is desirable to conduct clinical trial separately for the anteriors and posteriors.

Suggested Reading

1. Mavroskoufis F, Ritchie GM.*The face-form as a guide for the selection of maxillary central incisors.*J Prosthet Dent. 1980 May;43(5):501-5.
2. Lang BR, Razzoog ME.*A practical approach to restoring occlusion for edentulous patients. Part I: Guiding principles of tooth selection.*J Prosthet Dent. 1983 Oct;50(4):455-8.
3. Hoffman W Jr, Bomberg TJ, Hatch RA.*Interalar width as a guide in denture tooth selection.*J Prosthet Dent. 1986 Feb;55(2):219-21.
4. Young L Jr, Glaros AG, Moore DJ, Collins JF.*Assessing shade differences in acrylic resin denture and natural teeth.*J Prosthet Dent. 1994 Jun;71(6):575-80.
5. Sellen PN, Jagger DC, Harrison A.*Methods used to select artificial anterior teeth for the edentulous patient: a historical overview.*Int J Prosthodont. 1999 Jan-Feb;12(1):51-8.
6. Bissasu M.*Use of lingual frenum in determining the original vertical position of mandibular anterior teeth.*J Prosthet Dent. 1999 Aug;82(2):177-81
7. McCord JF, Grant AA.*Registration: stage III--selection of teeth.*Br Dent J. 2000 Jun 24;188(12):660-6.
8. Sellen PN, Jagger DC, Harrison A.*An assessment of the ability of dental undergraduates to choose artificial teeth which are appropriate for the age and sex of the denture wearer: a pilot study.*J Oral Rehabil. 2001 Oct;28(10):958-61.
9. Al Wazzan KA.*The relationship between intercanthal dimension and the widths of maxillary anterior teeth.*J Prosthet Dent. 2001 Dec;86(6):608-12.
10. Sellen PN, Jagger DC, Harrison A.*The selection of anterior teeth appropriate for the age and sex of the individual. How variable are dental staff in their choice?*J Oral Rehabil. 2002 Sep;29(9):853-7
11. Varjalo FM, Nogueira SS.*Intercommissural width in 4 racial groups as a guide for the selection of maxillary anterior teeth in complete dentures.*Int J Prosthodont. 2005 Nov-Dec;18(6):513-5.
12. Varjalo FM, Nogueira SS.*Nasal width as a guide for the selection of maxillary complete denture anterior teeth in four racial groups.*J Prosthodont. 2006 Nov-Dec;15(6):353-8.
13. Gomes VL, Gonsalves LC, do Prado CJ, Junior IL, de Lima Lucas B.*Correlation between facial measurements and the mesiodistal width of the maxillary anterior teeth.*J Esthet Restor Dent. 2006;18(4):196-205
14. Varjalo FM, Nogueira SS, Filho JN.*The center of the incisive papilla for the selection of complete denture maxillary anterior teeth in 4 racial groups.* Quintessence Int. 2008 Nov;39(10):841-5.
15. Guldag MU, Sentut F, Ceylan G.*Relationship between pterygomaxillary notches and maxillary anterior teeth.* J Prosthodont. 2010 Apr;19(3):231-4

18

Occlusion in complete dentures

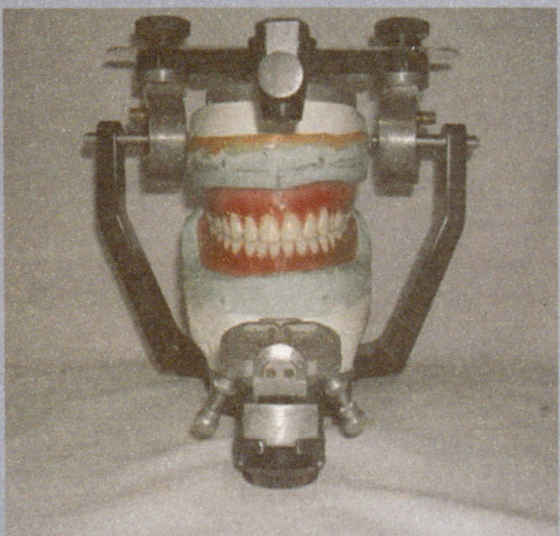

Opposing teeth contacts in static and dynamic positions ensures stability and success of dentures

When an individual chews food with natural teeth a force is generated and it will be transmitted through the teeth, finally producing a tensile force in the surrounding alveolar bone. Tensile forces stimulate bone growth and that is how the jaw bones are maintained when natural teeth are present. When one becomes completely edentulous, the above mentioned loading becomes impossible and by providing a denture an attempt is made to transmit forces to the bone. However, there is a difference in the direction and quality of the force generated by the denture. The force generated is mainly compressive in nature and which will restrict the blood supply to the jaw bones provided through the periosteum. The restriction in blood supply can cause resorption. The difference in the nature of forces so far described is due to the loss of periodontal ligament and the loss of a well developed mechanism of proprioception. The periodontal ligament area is calculated to be 45 sq. cm. whereas the residual ridge area is only 22 sq. cm for the maxillary and 12 sq.cm for the mandibular residual ridges. The masticatory load generated is the same; whereas the supporting tissue, present both in maxilla and mandible differ in their area. This will result in a greater concentration of force on the mandibular ridge and which will result in its greater resorption. The above factors should be considered while we generate an occlusion for the dentures.

When an individual has natural teeth the stable intercuspal position which is otherwise called as occlusion does not usually match with the centric relation position of the mandible. But there will be no discrepancy felt by an individual and that is because of the well developed proprioception. When the mandible moves to the eccentric positions like protrusion and lateral excursion, contact between the upper and the lower teeth are mostly restricted to either incisors or the canines. In other words during eccentric positions of mandible, a gap will be present between the upper and lower posterior teeth. When we generate an occlusion for complete dentures we cannot simulate an occlusal system similar to this. For a denture wearer both the centric relation and the inter cuspal positions will be made to coincide. This is because in an edentulous individual the proprioception is highly restricted and hence it is difficult to achieve desired mandibular positions precisely. This is the reason for generating the occlusion at the centric relation position. An individual can bring the mandible to this position repeatedly. It is also presumed that all eccentric movements get started from this position and also terminate in it. As in the natural dentition, dentures cannot provide a gap between the posterior teeth when the anteriors make a contact because artificial teeth function as two units and which are not well anchored to the jaw bone as the natural teeth. For example, in a denture wearer, if a gap appears between the upper and lower posterior teeth while trying to bite on an object the dentures will get destabilised and denture will fall off. In order to prevent this, occlusion in dentures is designed in such a way that simultaneous contacts are present anteroposteriorly and bilaterally in any eccentric position or articulation. This will ensure stability for the denture. This particular system is otherwise known as the so called balanced occlusion or precisely balanced articulation.

Occlusion in dentures is dependant upon different factors. For any movement of the mandible the condyles have to glide through a path provided by the glenoid fossa. The condylar position in centric relation and the condylar position during an eccentric movement are different. If these two positions are connected through a straight line and if it is related to a horizontal plane it will produce an angle. If this angulation can be determined and if the articulator has a facility to incorporate it, the occlusion generated in the articulator will be faithful in the patient's mouth also. This factor is designated as the condylar guidance.

When a dentulous individual protrudes the mandible, the mandibular incisors make a continuous contact with the palatal surface of the maxillary anteriors. This is known as the incisal guidance. In the case of dentures, such a continuous incisal guidance is not provided. That is because of the difficulty in providing balancing contacts during the entire act of protrusion. Moreover for that purpose greater cusp heights are to be used which is not preferred in dentures for fear of generating horizontally directed forces which would destabilize them. However in dentures, anteriors are arranged in such a way that when the maxillary and mandibular incisors contact as in the action of incision, there will be simultaneous bilateral posterior contacts. In order to achieve this, the vertical overlap is limited to aesthetic and phonation requirements and an equal amount of horizontal overlap is also provided. Maxillary and mandibular anteriors are arranged to suit the requirements of the individual and the incisal guide table of the articulator is adjusted in such a way that when the anterior teeth meet as in the action of incision, the incisal guide pin should make contact with the guide table. However, it is desirable to keep the vertical overlap to the minimum.

Positioning of the occlusal plane appropriately between the maxillary and mandibular residual ridges is of importance because it helps in getting synchronous occlusal movements matching that of the condyles. Usually it is placed midway between the upper and the lower ridges so that when masticatory load is applied it will directly be transmitted through the middle of the ridges without generating any destabilizing forces. However, in long standing edentulism the occlusal plane happens to be positioned considerably away from the mandibular ridge in comparison to that of the maxillary ridge. On most of the occasions the operator is at a loss and hc will be forced to keep the occlusal plane closer to the mandibular ridge to enhance stability but the vertical dimension gets reduced. The judgement however requires considerable clinical experience.

While describing the difference between the natural and complete denture occlusions, the inability of the operator to simulate the natural occlusal contact was mentioned. To be specific, when an individual protrudes the mandible a gap appears between the posterior teeth.

Christensens phenomenon which if copied in the denture will be detrimental to the stability. So in complete denture occlusion, especially in eccentric positions the gap in the posterior region is eliminated and a contact is ensured (balanced articulation). In order to achieve this, the posterior teeth are positioned in an antero posterior curve and a lateral curve the radii of which are controlled by the requirements of that patient. This is done in the articulator which is programmed according to the records obtained from the patient. The articulator has a programmed condylar path copied from the patient through interocclusal records. Programming of incisal guidance is done by the operator according to the position of anterior teeth, the overlap and an occlusal plane oriented in the middle of the inter arch space. Now the posterior teeth are positioned according to the two curves running anteroposteriorly and laterally. By a trial and error method the positions of teeth are found out so that in eccentric movements anterior and posterior teeth will make simultaneous contact i.e., balanced articulation. The curve on which the posterior teeth are arranged is known as compensating curve because it compensates the limitations of the natural teeth curve that provides the gap between the posterior teeth in articulation or eccentric positions.

Height of the cusp helps in mastication because of the sharp eminences they provide which pass through the food material very easily. Initially the young natural teeth have sharp cusps. Though these cusp tips are efficient, it limits the movement of the mandible in the horizontal plane. As age advances the cusp height reduces and the chewing activity becomes more horizontal in nature. In complete dentures thc cusp height is always limited in order to facilitate a reduction in interfering contacts when the mandible makes eccentric movements. The design of the teeth especially the occlusal morphology is heavily modified to facilitate a smooth glide from intercuspal position to an eccentric position. Some of the clinicians prefer to grind off the transverse ridges present on the occlusal surfaces of the posterior teeth. However, the vertical height must be maintained by the holding cusps and at the same time they should not interfere with the movements. The holding cusps should be successful in transmitting the load directly over to the residual ridges. The

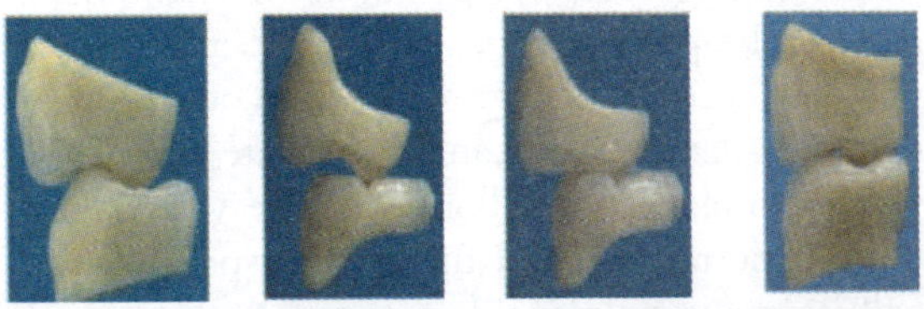

Fig.18.1a Teeth in different occlusal schemes

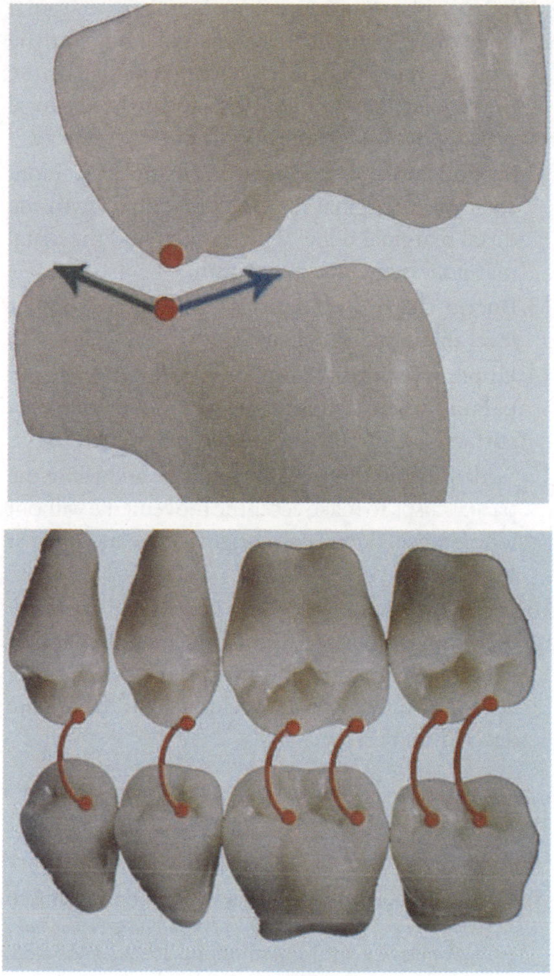

Fig. 18.1b Lingualised occlusion

mandibular arch is comparatively wider than the maxillary arch. Hence in order to direct the forces through the ridges, maxillary posteriors are tilted and placed buccally. The mandibular posteriors are placed lingually tilted. In order to eliminate the interfering contacts during the excursive movements, the mandibular and maxillary buccal cusps are reshaped. The maxillary cusps are least modified to retain the normal shape of the teeth.

While considering the occlusion generated in complete dentures, any one is easily confused because of the multiplicity of concepts evolved in the past half a century. In the recent past however there was a disinterest on the part of clinicians and teachers presuming that there is a considerable reduction in the number of patients demanding complete dentures. But in reality the adult population is going to increase. Hence, a policy statement on occlusion is made.

1. Occlusion refers to the static relationship where mandible is in centric relation position and maximum intercuspation is intended. Articulation refers to the contact between the upper and lower teeth when the mandible is in eccentric positions viz. protrusive and lateral.
2. Four occlusal concepts can be identified viz. balanced articulation, non balanced articulation, monoplane articulation and lingualised articulation (while describing the concepts both occlusion and articulation are used without much distinction)
3. In order to develop a particular occlusal concept, anatomic, semi anatomic, zero degree teeth or specially developed teeth (for lingualised articulation) can be used. Mostly 30° teeth are used in clinical practice. Next in popularity is zero degree posteriors opted for compromised ridge conditions. Teeth exclusively developed for lingualised occlusion is also available.
4. The resorptive pattern observed in edentulous individuals confirm the fact that mandibular residual ridge becomes wider than the maxillary ridge compelling the operator to arrange the posterior teeth in such a way that maxillary posteriors are buccally tilted and the mandibular posteriors are lingually tilted. The occlusal plane is curved antero - posteriorly and laterally. Considering all these facts, lingualised articulation can be considered as the choice occlusal concept.
5. Lingualised articulation is preferred by the patients because of the improved chewing ability. Operators consider it superior because lateral interferences are minimum even in due course of wearing. Dentures will be stable, ridges will be less prone to trauma and discomfort will be less.
6. While observing this scheme it is desirable to observe the following:
   - At centric relation position maximum intercuspation should occur

- Deflective or interfering contacts must be eliminated
- Teeth should be arranged in such a way that cusp height should permit occlusal reshaping to avoid interferences
- Aesthetics should be achieved with tooth arrangement

7. Arrange anterior teeth for aesthetic and functional requirements. On protrusion anteriors must come into contact, enabling the patient to incise.
8. Angle of the mouth at occlusal position and a point 2mm below the upper border of the retro molar pad will initially decide the height of the occlusal plane.
9. The lingual surfaces of the lower posteriors should fall in the triangle formed by connecting the cusp of the canine, lingual and buccal border of the retromolar pad and centre of the retromolar pad.
10. Arrange the lower premolars perpendicular to the occlusal plane with buccal cusps at a higher level limiting the tilt to 5 degrees to form the lateral curve.
11. First molar is arranged with mesial marginal ridge on par with the distal marginal ridge of the second premolar. The distal marginal ridge of the first molar is raised by 1mm from the occlusal plane. This will ensure antero posterior curve.
12. Second molar is arranged in a similar fashion. Its mesial marginal ridge will be on par with the distal marginal ridge of first molar and the distal marginal ridge raised by 1 mm.
13. Buccal cusps of the molars will be at a higher level than the lingual cusps.
14. Upper posterior teeth are arranged with the palatal cusps holding the opposing occlusal surface – central fossa or marginal ridge.
15. Widen the holding area by grinding and allow the palatal cusps to make eccentric movements without interference. Buccal cusp height can be modified at the end.
16. If the space is not adequate, number of posterior teeth can be reduced. Substitute mandibular first premolar with a second premolar from another set to ensure sufficient occlusal area. Eliminate second molars.

Suggested Reading

1. Payne S.H. *A comparative study of posterior occlusion.* J Prosthet Dent 1952; 2:661-667,
2. Ortman HR. *Complete Denture Occlusion,* Dent Clin North Am. 1977;21(2):299-320
3. Clough H.E., Knodle J.M., Leeper H.L., Pudwill M.L. and Taylor D.T. *A comparison of lingualized occlusion and monoplane occlusion in complete dentures.* J Prosthet Dent 1983;50:176-79.
4. Applebaum M. *Plans of occlusion.* Dent Cli N Am: symposium on removable prosthodontics. W.B.Saunders,1984, Philadelphia. Pp 273-285.
5. Owen C.P. *The prophylactic reduction of cusps: is it desirable?* J Oral Rehabil, 1986;13:39-48.
6. Lang B.R. *Complete denture occlusion.* In: Dent Cli N Am Complete Dentures, 1996, Engelmeier R.L W.B.Saunders, Philadelphia. Pp 85-101
7. Parr G.R. and Ivanhoe J.R *Lingualised occlusion: an occlusion for all reasons.* In: Dent Cli N Am, Complete Dentures Engelmeier R.L. W.B.Saunders, Philadelphia, pp 103-112.
8. Ohguri T., Kawano F., Ichikawa T., and Matsumoto N. *Influence of occlusal scheme on the pressure distribution under a complete denture.* Int J Prosthodont. 1999;12:353-358.
9. Williamson RA, Williamson AE, Bowley J, Toothaker R. *Maximizing mandibular prosthesis stability utilizing linear occlusion, occlusal plane selection, and centric recording.* J Prosthodont. Mar 2004;13(1):55-61.
10. Nimmo.A. and Frank J. Kratochvil, *Balancing ramps in nonanatomic complete denture occlusion,* J Prosthet Dent 1985;53:431-433
11. S.Davies and R. M. J. Gray, *What is occlusion?* Br Dent J 2001;191(5):236-245
12. S. J. Davies, R. M. J. Gray and J. F. McCord, *Good occlusal practice in removable prosthodontics,* Br Dent J 2001;191(9):491-502
13. Ash M. *Occlusion: Reflections on science and clinical reality.* J Prosthet Dent 2003; 90: 373-84.
14. Levin Bernard, *A reevaluation of Hanau's Laws of articulation and the Hanau quint* J Prosthet Dent 1978; 39(3): 254- 58

19

Arrangement of posterior teeth

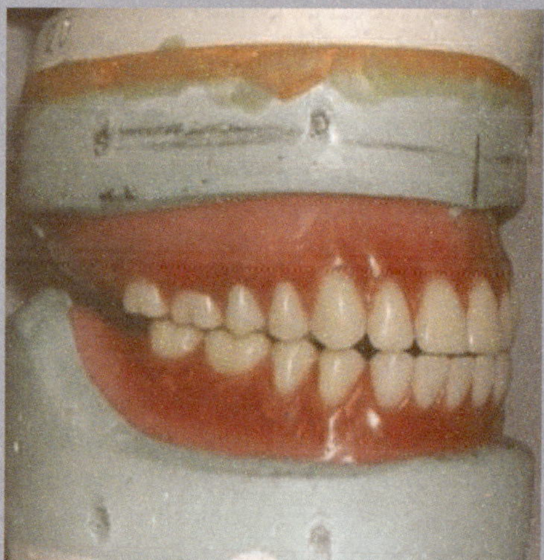

Masticatory process with dentures mainly depends on the correct positioning of posterior teeth

Once the anterior teeth are arranged the operator can decide on the mesiodistal dimension of the posteriors comprising of two premolars and two molars in each quadrant. The distance from the distal border of the canine to the anterior border of the retromolar pad is generally considered as the space available for the posterior teeth. If the posterior part of the ridge ascends in an angular fashion, that region should also be avoided for positioning the teeth. Manufacturer usually proportions the buccolingual width of the teeth according to the mesio distal dimension. However teeth broader than the width of the ridge, should not be selected because it will increase the forces applied on the residual ridge during mastication. Smaller teeth can pierce through the food easily and thereby the load is reduced. Posterior tooth selection is always dictated by the space constraints of the mandibular ridge. The mesio-distal dimension of the four posterior teeth is usually printed on the tooth pad in millimeter and designated as the mould size.

Operators usually prefer to arrange the maxillary posteriors first and then the mandibular posteriors. The mandibular teeth are arranged directly over the ridge. This is described in the chapter of occlusion in complete dentures. If these precautions are taken, on mastication the forces will be directed towards well supported area of the residual ridge. In order to get equal distribution of load on all sides of the ridge it is better to make the central fossae coincide with the crest of the ridge. This can very well be appreciated in lingualized occlusion. On arranging the posterior teeth, maximum intercuspation is to be achieved in the centric relation position. In eccentric positions such as protrusion and lateral excursions simultaneous tooth contact is desired in the anterior and the posterior regions so that the denture will be stable during function. During the act of protrusion maxillary and mandibular incisors and posterior teeth should maintain contact on both sides. On lateral excursions, anterior contact should be present on incisors and posterior contact should be present on both sides. In order to generate such a contact system and to obtain stability during function a semiadjustable articulator is to be used. In such an articulator the condylar path can be adjusted similar to that of the patient. The incisal guide table of the articulator is adjusted in an angle so that on protrusion the upper and lower incisors make a contact.

Once the articulator is programmed operator can arrange the posterior teeth in such a way that posterior teeth on both sides maintain a contact in all eccentric positions. To find out the position of the posteriors in the vertical direction first the maxillary and the mandibular molars are fixed in an arbitrary position on both sides. Then the protrusion is performed by pushing back the upper member of the articulator. When the incisors meet each other the molars should be checked to find out whether they are in contact. If not the molar can be rearranged in an upward or downward direction till a contact is achieved on protrusive movement. Once this is done the premolars can be set in the plane connecting the canine to the molar (fig. 19.1). In a fixed path articulator also the same technique can be employed. Once all the posteriors are set, that would successfully establish a curve. This curve would compensate for the disoclusion exhibited

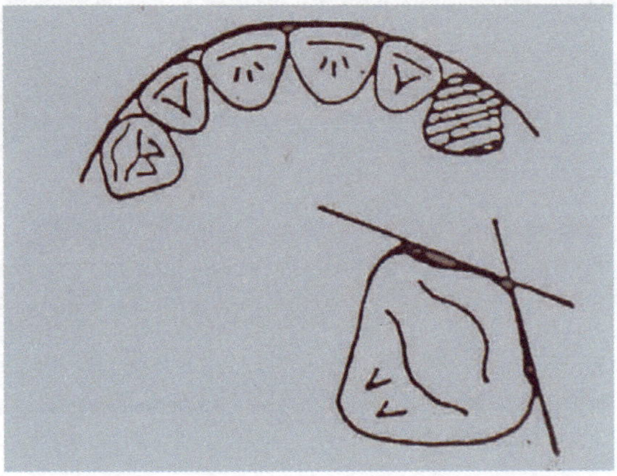

Fig. 19.1 Canine plays a significant role in determining the arch width. The mesial half of the canine in included in the anterior segment where as the distal half is included in the posterior segment.Axial rotation of the canine mesially will widen the arch whereas a distal rotation will narrow the arch.

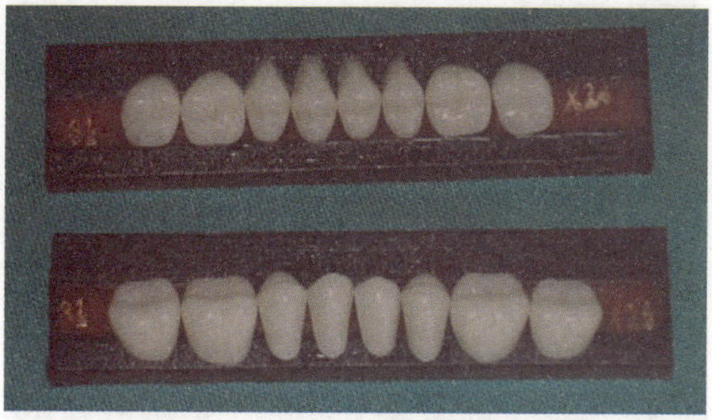

Fig. 19.2 Posterior teeth set. Markings on the left side indicate the mould and right side indicate shade. For anteriors the mould indicate the shape where as in the posteriors it indicates the combined mesio-distal dimension of two premolars and two molars.

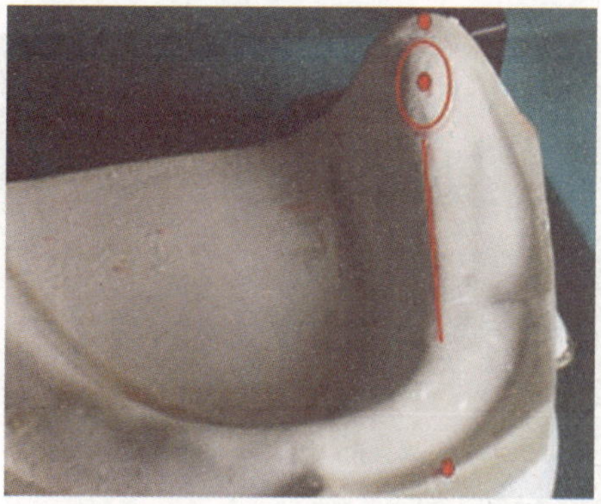

Fig. 19.3 Midpoint of the retromolar pad is marked and the direction of the posterior ridge is marked and projected on the land area

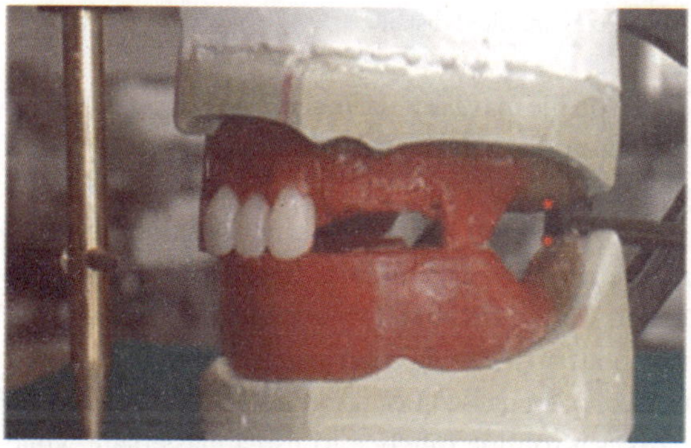

Fig. 19.4 Above the marking of retromolar pad a mark is made on the maxillary transfer base. Wax rim is partially removed from the premolar and molar space. The posterior most portion of the occlusal rim retained as a pedestal

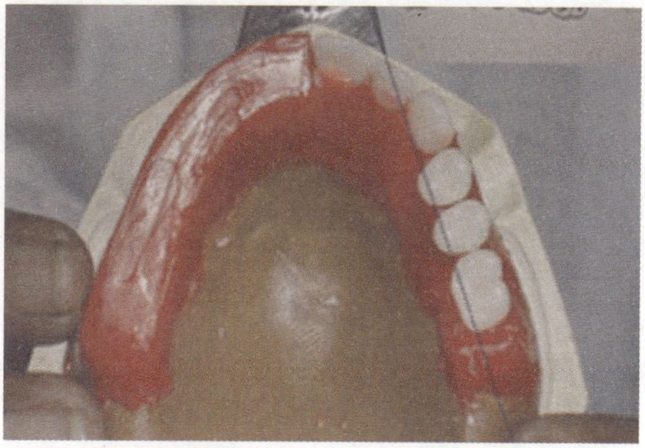

Fig. 19.5 Premolar and 1st molar are arranged in such a way that the palatal cusps fall into the line connecting mid point of the lateral incisor and the marking made against the retromolar pad

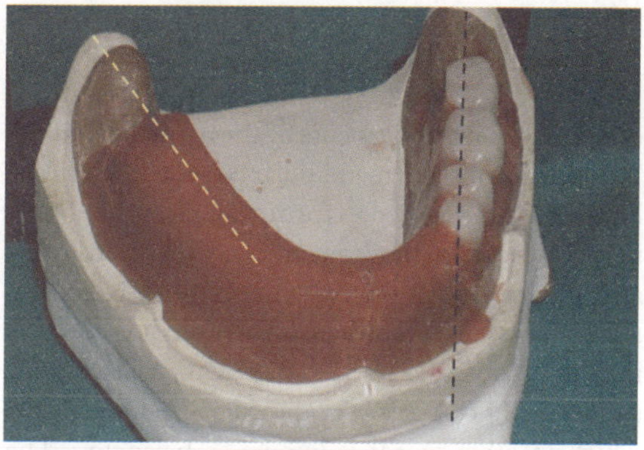

Fig. 19.6 Mandibular posterior teeth are arranged against the maxillary posteriors.The central fossae fall on the crest of the ridge

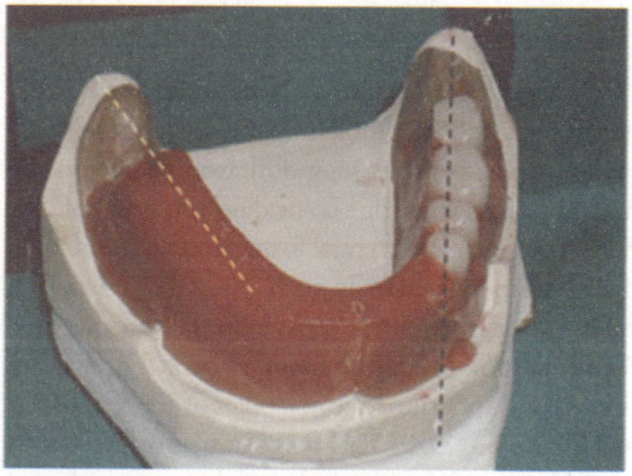

Fig. 19.7 Central fossae of mandibular posterior teeth and cusp tip of the canine fall a straight line

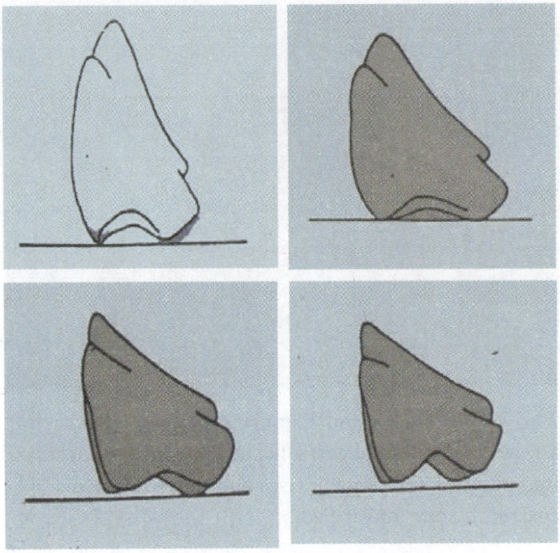

Fig. 19.8 Relationship of posterior teeth to occlusal plane

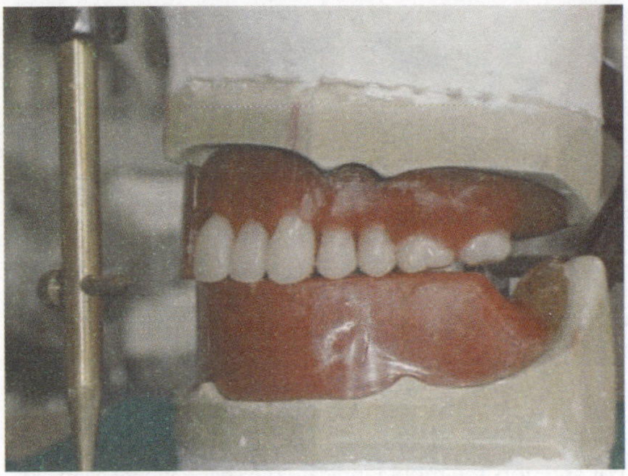

Fig. 19.9 Buccal cusps of the posterior make a curve and this is achieved by a buccal tilt given to the molars

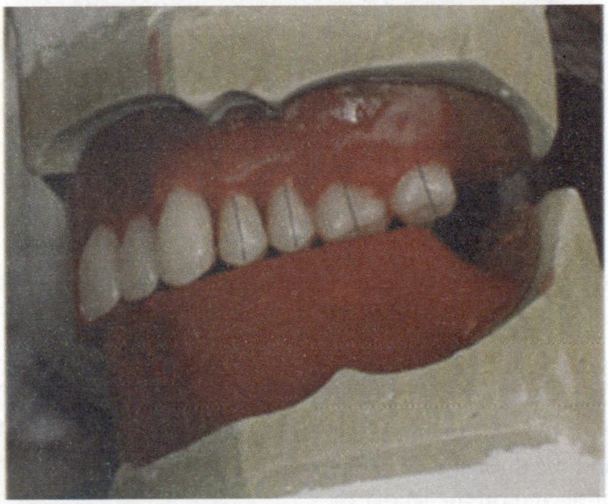

Fig. 19.10 The vertical axes of the premolars and molars. Molar axes are tilted distally

during excursive movements by the natural dentition. While arranging the mandibular posterior teeth, the buccal cusps are raised to form a lateral curve so that in lateral excursive movements simultaneous contacts are obtained both on the working and balancing sides. Curves that are successful in providing contacts in protrusive and lateral movements will provide simultaneous contacts in all the excursive movements which in other words is known as balancing. The occlusal plane thus established should behave faithfully in the mouth provided the horizontal angle set in the articulator is similar to that in the patient. However minor discrepancies will be adjusted by the resilient nature of the soft tissues.

Arranging the maxillary posteriors in the correct position may pose a problem to the novice. (Fig. 19.2) Hence some operators suggest drawing a line on the mandibular occlusal rim coinciding the crest of the ridge representing the central fossae, and then arranging the maxillary posteriors in such a way that the palatal cusps of the mandibular posteriors fall on this line. Some operators locate a posterior point on the maxillary occlusal rim opposite to the mid point of the retromolar pad. (Fig. 19.3, 19.4) This point is then connected to the mid point of the incisal edge of the maxillary lateral incisor. (Fig. 19.5). A line connecting these two points is drawn on the maxillary occlusal rim and while arranging the posterior teeth the palatal cusps are placed to fall on this line. (Fig. 19.6 - 19.7) Both the lines mentioned above will almost fall on the same position. In cases where the maxillary arch is broad posteriorly, the molars can be arranged towards the mid sagittal plane in contrast to the straight line arrangement. This pattern is used in lingualised occlusion also.

It is a routine practice to use a glass plate while arranging the maxillary teeth. As a guide line it can be followed in the preclinical situations and in the early stages of clinical training. When a glass plate is used it must be fixed on to the mandibular occlusal rim after reducing the height of the occlusal rim to accommodate the glass plate. It is generally advised to make all the cusps of the premolars contact the glass plate. The first molars are tilted buccally and distally so that only the mesiopalatal cusps contact the glass plate. The position of the second molar is similar to that of the first molar but it is placed at a higher plane so that no cusp touches the glass plate. (Fig. 19.8, 19.9, 19.10).

By this arrangement an anterioposterior curve can be developed and which can be appreciated, when viewed buccally. It must be noticed that all the techniques need not be utilized simultaneously. An operator has the freedom to take recourse to a technique of his choice and convenience so that he achieves the desired result of balancing. Once the operator gains experience, the relevance of glass plate becomes minimum. The compensating curve should be found out by trial and error method and by changing the position of the posterior teeth.

Simultaneous contacts in the anterior and posterior region is not always achieved just by positioning the posterior teeth. After arranging all the posterior teeth when the upper member of the articulator is pushed to an eccentric position the incisal guide pin gets lifted. While achieving simultaneous contacts on eccentric movements, it is mandatory that the incisal guide pin should maintain contact with the table. In order to achieve this, teeth may have to be ground selectively. Usually the lingual slopes of maxillary buccal cusps are modified. By this, a smooth glide can be achieved on most of the occasions and at the same time the centric holding can be left undisturbed. The exact point of grinding can be located by placing an articulating paper between the upper and lower teeth and pushing the upper member of the articulator. At the end of this modification, if loss of vertical height has occured, it can be verified for by loosening the incisal guide pin in the closed position of the articulator. If the modification has affected the centric holding, the upper member will move towards the lower member collapsing the vertical dimension and this can be measured by observing the incisal guide pin position. At any cost the final modification should not cause a reduction in the vertical dimension.

Suggested Reading

1. Frush IT, Fisher RD. *Dentogenics: its practical application,* J Prosthet Dent 1959; 9:914-921.
2. Jones PM *The monoplane occlusion for complete dentures,* J Prosthet Dent 1972; 85:94 100.
3. Lang B.R. and Razzoog M.E. *A practical approach to restoring occlusion for edentulous patients. Part I: guiding principles of tooth selection.* J Prosthet Dent 1983;50:599-606
4. Lang B.R. and Razzoog M.E. *A practical approach to restoring occlusion for edentulous patients. Part II: arranging the functional and rational mold combination.* J Prosthet Dent 1983;50:455-458.
5. Clough HE, Knodle 1M, Leeper SH et al. *A comparison of lingualized occlusion and monoplane occlusion in complete dentures,* J Prosthet Dent 1983; 50:176-179.
6. LaVere AM, Marcrof KR, Smith RC et al. *Denture tooth selection: size matching of natural anterior tooth width with artificial denture teeth,* J Prosthet Dent 1994;72:381-384.
7. Lang BR7. *Complete denture occlusion,* Dent Clin N A 1996;40:85-101.
8. Davies SJ, Gray RMJ, McCord JF, *Good occlusal practice in removable prosthodontics,* Br Dent J 2001;191:491-502

20

Trial insertion

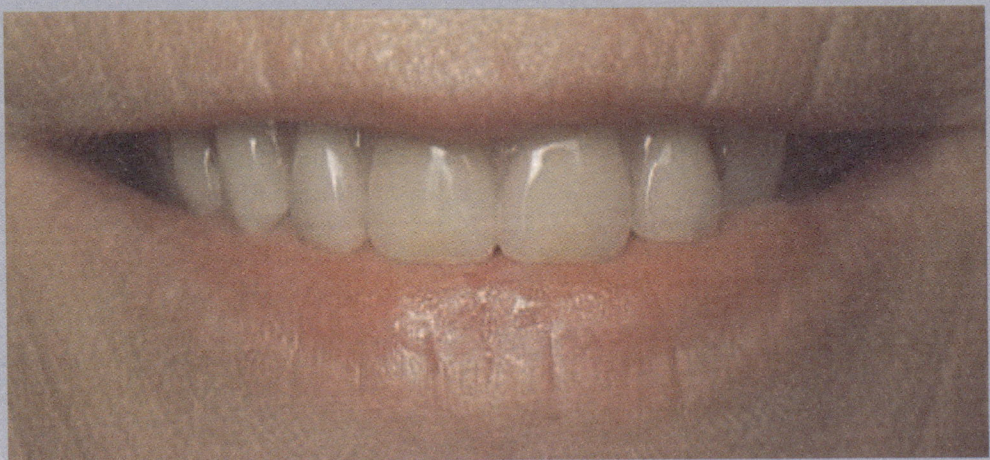

Trial gives an insight in to the future things that may happen

Even though dentist provides all information to the patient on the complete denture treatment, patients get the real experience of it only when they reach the stage of trial insertion. The trial denture should be fully extended and should provide adequate support to the soft tissues. Tooth visibility should be determined by adequate carving and once approved by the patient major changes should not be made. The trial denture is inserted and initially checked for stability. After that centric relation should be verified. i.e. when the patient is asked to close at centric relation position, there must be maximum intercuspation without disturbance to the stability. In complete dentures, occlusal relationship is generated at centric relation, and there should not be any discrepancy. If there is a discrepancy, re-registration of the jaw relation is to be done. For that the posterior teeth are removed, the occlusal rims remade and the centric relation is reregistered.

Once the centric relation is verified, vertical dimension is to be checked. Patient is asked to sit upright without head support. Patient is instructed to take deep breath twice or thrice so that the mandible attains a relaxed position. In the relaxed position lips must be competent. Observe the face from the front and the side. Once the operator is convinced of the relaxed position, instruct the patient to close or bite. During this act an upward movement of the mandible should be observable if sufficient freeway space is present. This is tried twice and if the operator is convinced of the presence of free way space, he can proceed further with the verification of closest speaking space. In case of doubt, vertical dimension can be ascertained by fixing dots on the nose and the chin and by measuring the distance. Closest speaking space is ascertained by asking the patient to say 'S' repeatedly. During this act, if the maxillary and mandibular teeth are contacting heavily it can be presumed that closest speaking space is not available. In such a condition it is desirable to increase the free way space. For this purpose establishment of vertical dimension should be repeated. Desirable closest speaking space is 1mm between the posterior teeth. Position of the maxillary anteriors is verified next. Patient is instructed to pronounce 'F'. During this act, the lower lip comes closer to the edge of the maxillary incisors and makes a contact at the dry wet junction. When the patient is instructed to pronounce 'V', first the maxillary incisors make a contact at the dry wet junction of the lip and then the lip moves away from the teeth. If both the upper and lower lips are making a contact, before the lower lip contacts the incisors while pronouncing 'F', it can be presumed that the incisors are not properly positioned, and the 'F' might sound 'Ep'

The mid line is to be verified next. It is always desirable to coincide the midline of the dental arch with the mid sagittal plane of the face. Patient is then asked to smile and observe for the adequacy of the visibility of teeth. Unless specifically requested for, denture base exposure is not desired. A triangular space present between the posterior teeth and the cheek (buccal corridor) is to be observed during smile. During a broad smile, the posterior teeth appear to vanish in buccal corridor space. This vanishing effect adds to the three dimensional effect especially in broad squarish arches. The operator should satisfy himself of the esthetic harmony first, then only he need proceed to show the trial denture to the patient. On most of the occasions the operator will be a better judge than the patient. No trial denture should be approved just because that patient has given the approval. After all, dentist is the creator who has to get himself satisfied. Patients are handicapped in appreciating his own image because most of the time they are given a mirror to judge. Mirror provides the facial image in a restricted and reverse manner. The comments made by the patient can be appreciated only if the operator also looks at the mirror by standing behind the patient. Use of a Polaroid camera, a digital camera or a computer imaging system is desirable where the patient can see his own image as the other individuals view it. Once the patient approves, after looking at the image for some time it is advisable to show the dentures to immediate relatives. However they should be asked to refrain from making any comments directly to the patient rather they should make it privately to the dentist. Most of the time the relatives and friends may not have a realistic perception but these negative comments have a long lasting impact on the patient. It must always be borne in mind that approval of the spouse in the Indian context is highly essential. A trial insertion phase should have a duration of 30 to 60 minutes. It is better to sign consent at this time.

Different Stages of trial

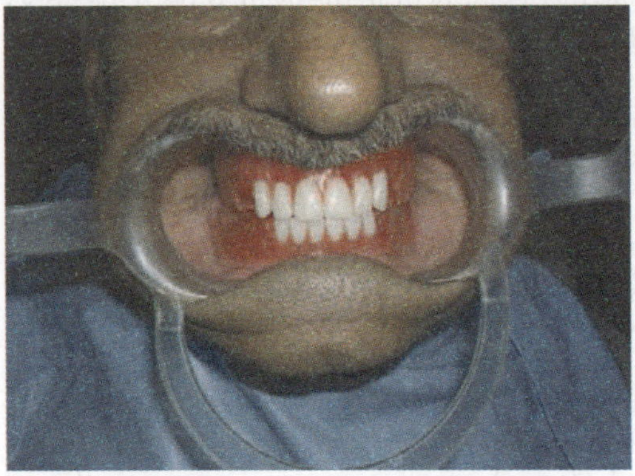

Fig. 20.1 Anterior trial - centric

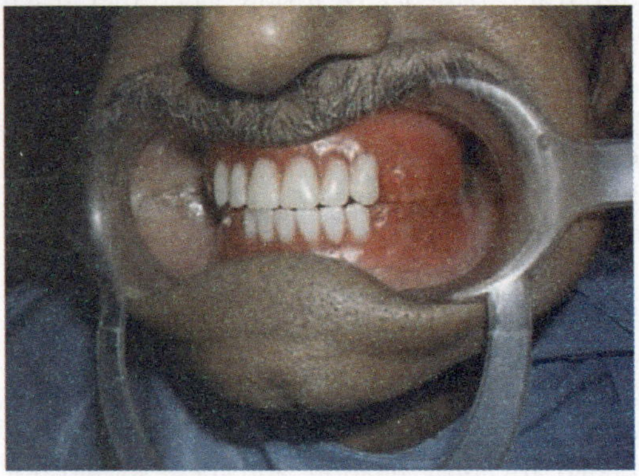

Fig. 20.4 Anterior trial – Left lateral

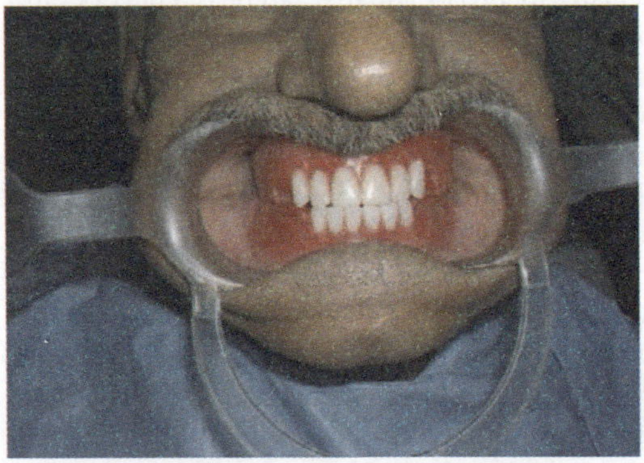

Fig. 20.2 Anterior trial - protrusive

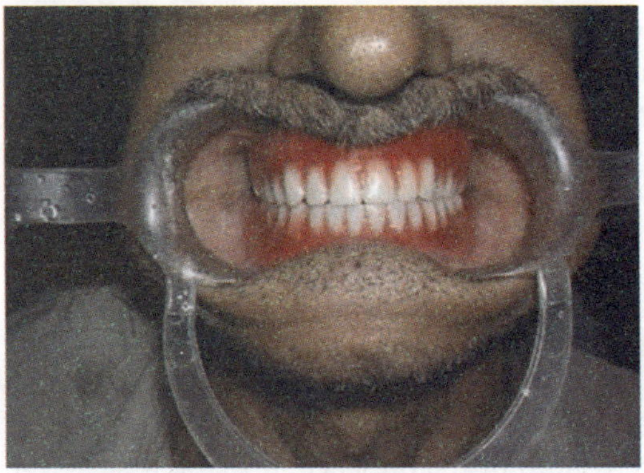

Fig. 20.5 Posterior trial – centric – frontal view

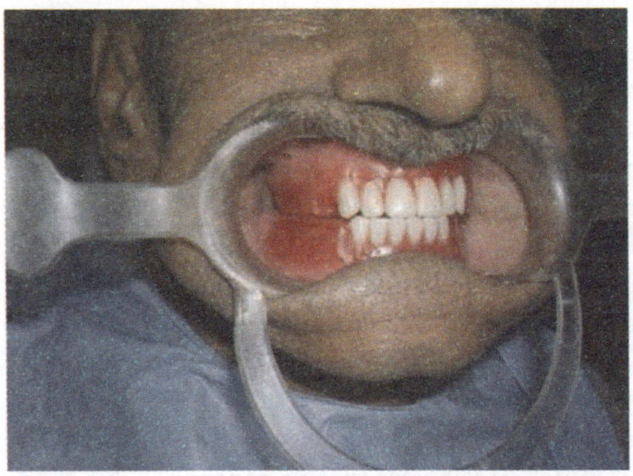

Fig. 20.3 Anterior trial – Right lateral

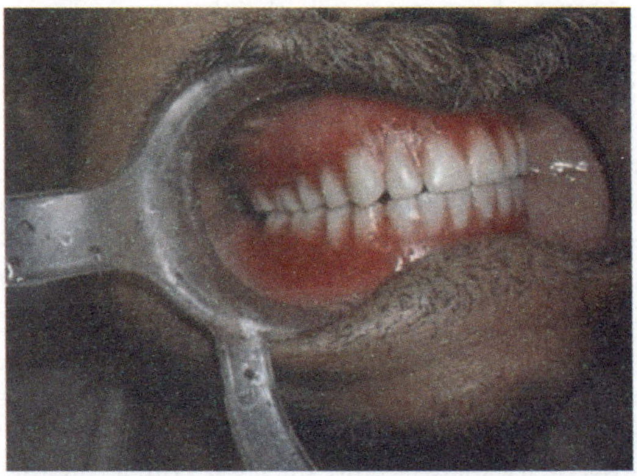

Fig. 20.6 Posterior trial – centric – right lateral view

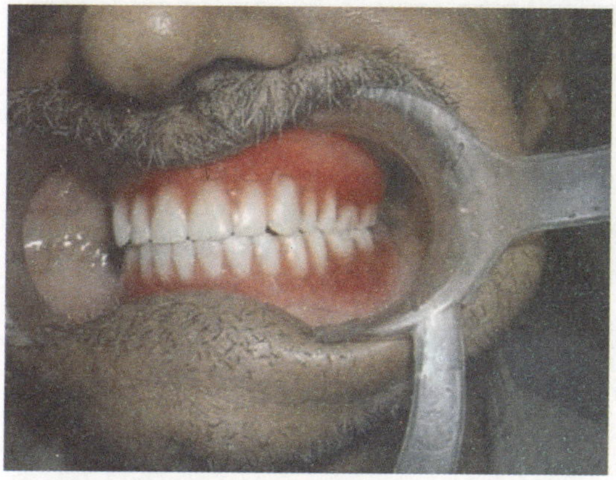

Fig. 20.7 Posterior trial – centric – left lateral view

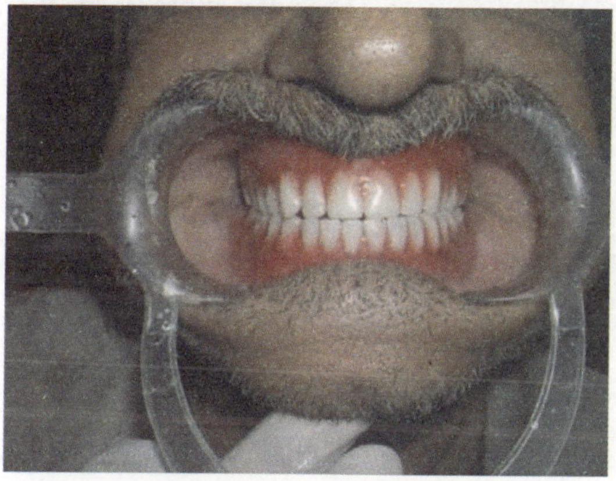

Fig. 20.8 Posterior trial–protrusive–frontal view

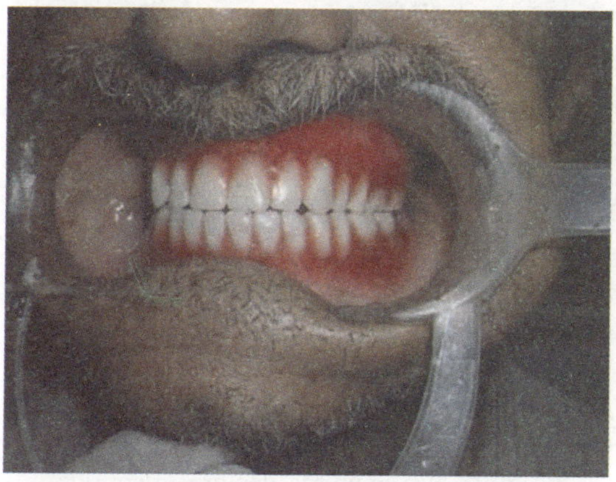

Fig. 20.9 Posterior trial–protrusive–left lateral view

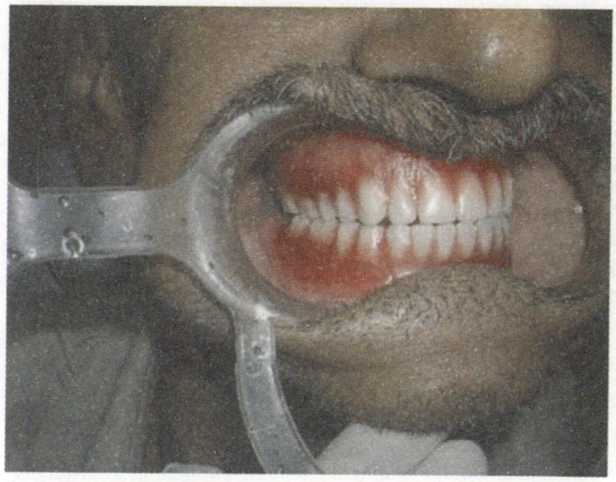

Fig. 20.10 Posterior trial – protrusive – right lateral view

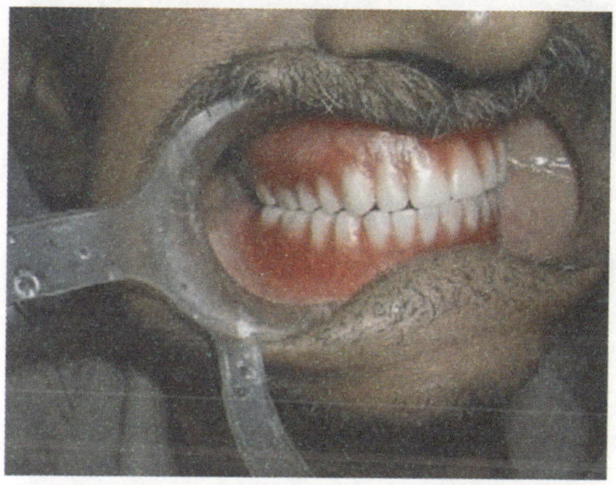

Fig. 20.11 Posterior trial – right lateral – working side

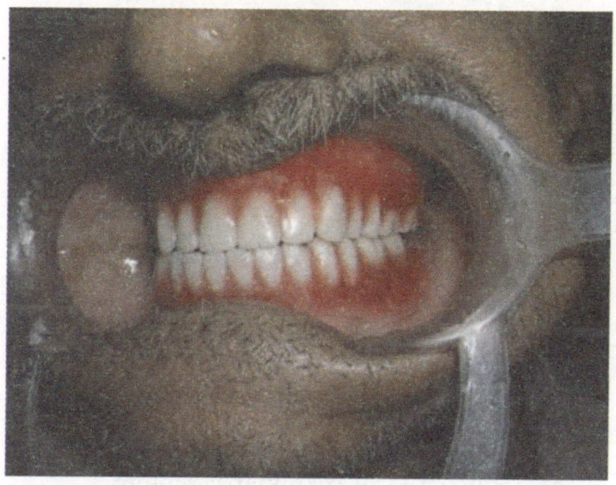

Fig. 20.12 Posterior trial – right lateral – balancing side

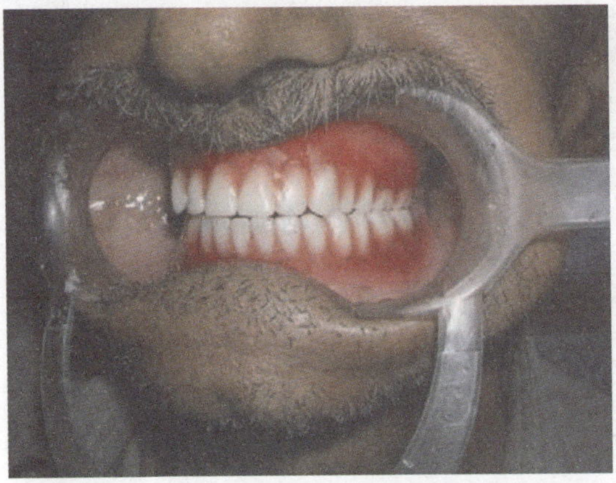

Fig. 20.13 Posterior trial – left lateral – working side

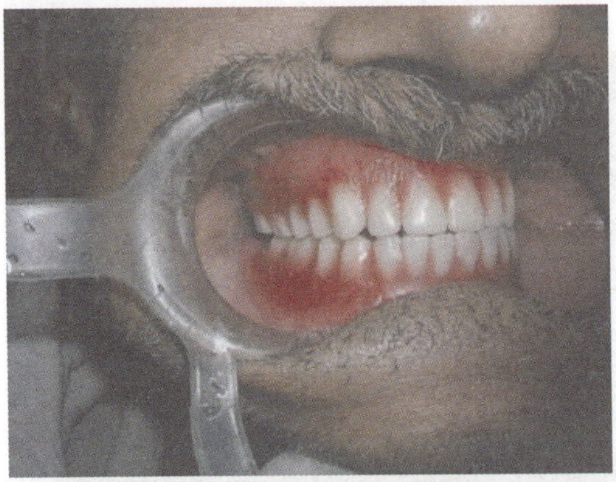

Fig. 20.14 Posterior trial – left lateral – balancing side

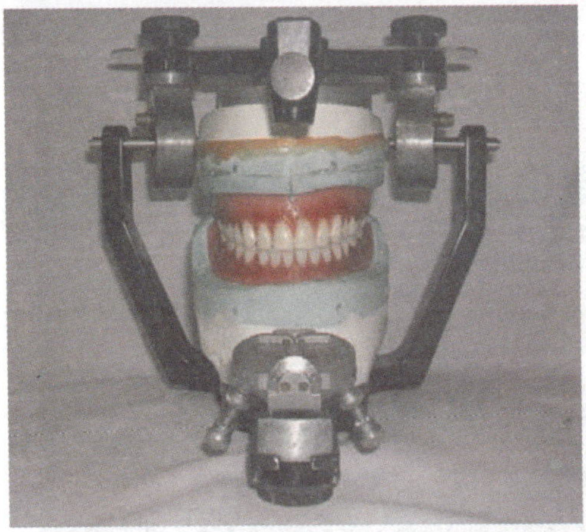

Fig. 20.15 Waxed-up trial denture

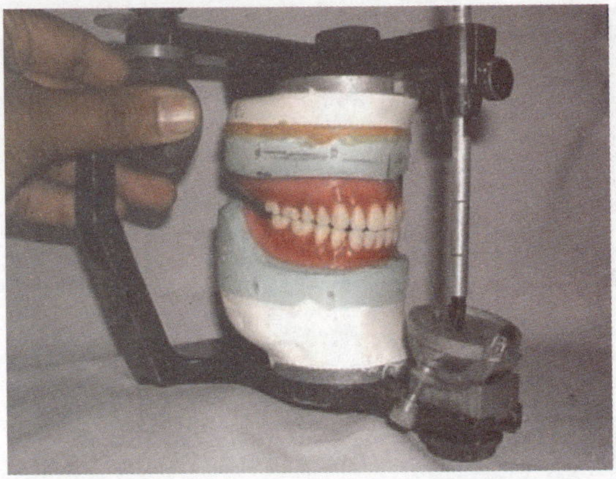

Fig. 20.16 Waxed-up trial denture – right lateral view in protrusive

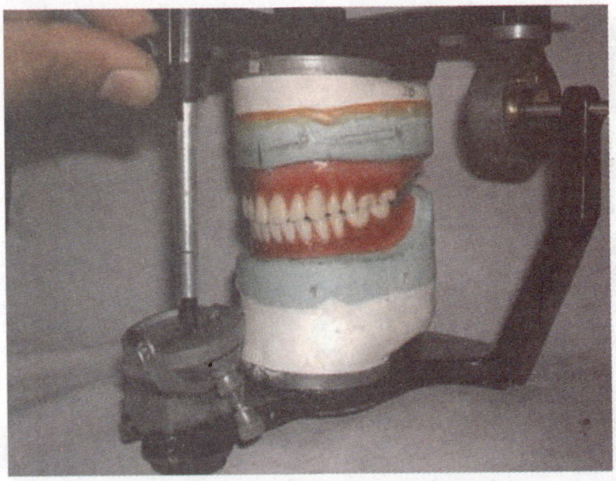

Fig. 20.17 Waxed-up trial denture – left lateral view in protrusive

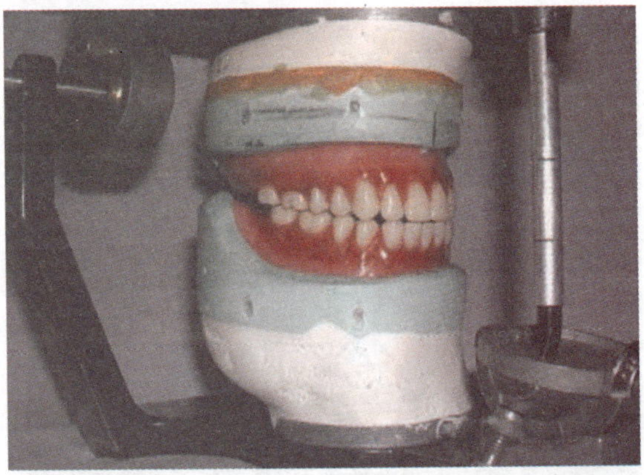

Fig. 20.18 Waxed-up trial denture – right side balancing

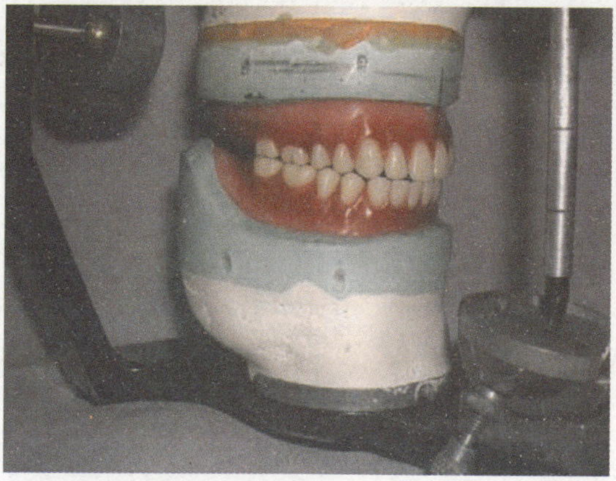

Fig. 20.19 Waxed-up trial denture – right side working

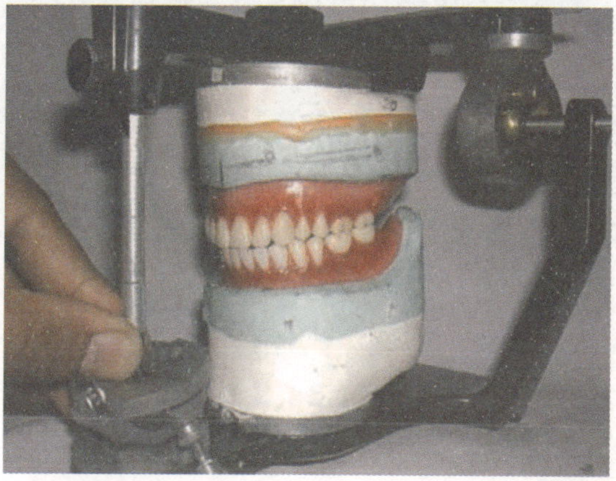

Fig. 20.20 Waxed-up trial denture – left side working

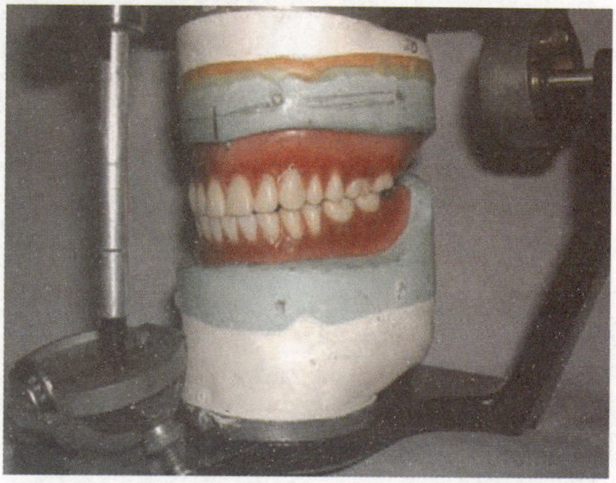

Fig. 20.21 Waxed-up trial denture – left side balancing

Suggested Reading

1. Desjardins RP. *Clinical evaluation of the wax trial denture.* J Am Dent Assoc. 1982 Feb;104(2):184-90.

21

Denture processing

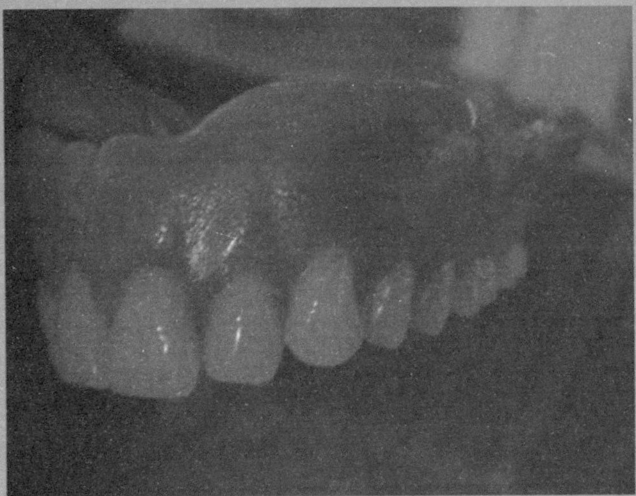

The most accurate trial denture can be made a failure if the processing is not done with precision

Once the teeth are arranged , waxing is done. Waxing is the process of adding wax on to the teeth covering the cervical portion of teeth labially and lingually. Labially the wax should cover the teeth by atleast 1 mm in the cervical region and lingually by 2mm. After completion of wax up procedure, the carving procedure is initiated. While carving, the dentures are held such that the flanges of denture face the palm of the hand and carving is directed towards teeth. After carving is completed, waxed up denture is polished and trial is done. (Fig. 21.1, 21.2, 21.3) Once the trial dentures are approved by the patient and the dentist, they are processed to obtain the final dentures. Denture processing involves replacing the trial base and wax with denture resin material which is usually the heat activated acrylic resin. There are basically two methods of processing heat activated acrylic resin dentures viz. compression molding technique and injection molding technique.

Compression molding technique involves creating a mold in a denture flask, placing the acrylic resin mixture in the dough consistency in the mold space previously occupied by the trial base and the wax holding the acrylic teeth and finally by applying heat and constant pressure the acrylic resin is polymerized. The advantages of this technique are ease of manipulation and is economical. The main disadvantage is polymerization shrinkage. The steps involved in compression molding technique are flasking, dewaxing, packing, bench curing, polymerization, bench cooling and deflasking.

The basic armamentarium required for compression molding technique are dental flask and clamp. The dental flask has three parts viz. base (drag), ring (cope) and lid (cap). The base has three lugs and ring has corresponding notches to accommodate these lugs. The denture flask should first be evaluated for ease of fit without resistance to closure. The base of the denture flask should be flat, if not the cast may break. The clamp has to be evaluated for free rotation of the central disc and the thread for any resistance to move upward or downward.

1. Preparation of denture for flasking: After the trial denture has been waxed up, carved and polished, the master cast is separated from the mounting plaster. In case of maxillary trial denture, the trial base in the palatal area is trimmed and removed and replaced with two layers of wax. In the palatal area, the acrylic that is used for temporary record base tends to lift away from the palate during polymerization. If processed directly with this record base, the denture will be too thick in the palatal area. The master cast is placed in the lower half of the denture flask and checked for 5 mm space all around between the cast and the rim of the denture flask (Fig 21.4a,b). Then the wax trial denture is sealed to the cast. The trial denture sealed to the cast is placed in the lower portion of denture flask and checked if adequate space is present between the occlusal surfaces of the teeth and the upper border of the ring of the denture flask. A minimum of 6mm space should be present. (Fig. 21.5)

2. Flasking/investing: The investing procedure is the placing of the waxed denture bases and teeth in suitable investing media in preparation for wax elimination and packing of acrylic resin in its place. Petrolatum jelly is applied on the inner surface of the dental flask so as to ensure ease of separation of mold from the flask while deflasking. The lower portion of denture flask is filled with freshly mixed dental stone and the master cast is placed in to this mixture and pressed to the bottom of the flask. The excess dental stone that is displaced is contoured when it is partially set so that it slopes towards the rim of the denture flask. This is done to facilitate wax elimination, packing, and deflasking procedures. Particular care should be taken while flasking mandibular cast such that no undercut is present in the posterior lingual region of the cast as well as the heels of the cast is adequately supported with stone (Fig 21.6). Separating medium is painted on the investing stone and on the land areas of the cast with a paint brush. Application of separating medium at this stage ensures easy separation of the different parts of the mold. Once the trial denture sealed to the cast is secured to the base or lower portion of the flask, the rest of flasking procedure

is completed by using either the two pour, three pour or stone core technique.

In the two pour technique, the ring of the denture flask is positioned atop the base of the flask, filled with investing stone. The lid is placed and secured tightly with clamps.

In the three pour technique, the ring is placed and filled with investing stone upto the occlusal/incisal edges. After the investing stone sets, apply separating medium, and fill the rest of the ring with stone and place the lid and secure tightly with clamps.

In stone core technique, the teeth portion of the trial denture is painted with dental stone. The stone core is around 2-4 mm thick and ends 2-3 mm below the occlusal /incisal surfaces of teeth. (Fig. 21.7, 21.8)

3. Dewaxing: After the investing stone is completely set, the denture flask is immersed in boiling water for 5 minutes for the melting of wax. The flask is lifted from the hot water bath and the segments are separated. The record base and the softened wax are eliminated with hot water flush. The teeth which remain firmly embedded in the investing stone are also cleaned (Fig 21.9, 21.10). The mold cavity is cleaned with a mild detergent solution and again rinsed with boiling water.

4. Packing: The placement and compression moulding of the resin into the mold cavity is termed packing. The alginate based separating medium is painted with a brush on to the exposed surfaces of the warm, clean mould. (Fig. 21.11, 21.12) The separating medium is carefully guided in to the interdental regions. If the separating medium has contacted the acrylic resin teeth , it has to be removed with a brush dipped in monomer. The purpose of applying separating medium at this stage is to prevent direct contact between the denture base resin and the mold surface. This is done so as to prevent diffusion of water from the mold surface in to the denture base resin, as it may affect polymerization rate. Also free monomer may enter the stone mold and affect the physical properties of the final dentures. The mold sections are then positioned such that pooling of the separating medium is prevented. Acrylic polymer and monomer are dispensed in to a mixing jar in the ratio of 3:1 by volume, mixed and allowed to reach dough consistency. Usually about 10 minutes is required to reach the dough consistency and remains so in this stage for at least 5 minutes. Within this time, the resin mixture has to be 'packed' in to the mold cavity. The resin is removed from the mixing jar in the dough stage, rolled in to the shape of rope and placed in the mould over the teeth (Fig 21.13). Two moistened and swelled cellophane sheets are placed over the resin, each covering two third portions of the resin. The cellophane sheets dipped in water for at least 30 minutes will prevent the resin from sticking to the sheet. The flask assembly is then placed in to a specially designed press and pressure is applied incrementally. Slow application of pressure ensures resin dough to flow evenly through out the mold space. Excess material comes out as flash. The application of pressure is continued until the metal rims of the flask make firm contact. The mould is separated and the cellophane sheets are removed. The flash found on the land area of the mould is removed using a sharp blade.(Fig 21.14). Fresh cellophane sheet is placed and process is repeated again until no flash appears. This procedure is called as trial closure. Final closure is accomplished without intervening cellophane sheet. The flask is then transferred to a flask carrier which maintains the pressure during processing. The packed denture base resin is kept as such for half an hour. This is called as bench curing.

5. Polymerization: The denture flask is placed in an acryliser and the polymerizing or curing cycle is programmed. The long curing cycle involves processing the denture base resin in constant temperature water bath at 74° C for 8 hour or longer with no terminal boiling treatment. In short curing cycle, the resin is processed at 74° C for 2 hours and at 100° C for 1 hour. Either of the two curing cycles can be followed.

6. Bench cooling: After the curing is complete, the denture flask is cooled slowly to room temperature. Rapid cooling results in warping of the denture base because of the differences in thermal contraction

of resin and investing stone. The flask is removed from the acryliser and bench cooled for half hour and then immersed in cool tap water for 15 minutes.

7. Deflasking: The denture flask is pried open gently with a knife at the junction of the base and ring . The mold along with the denture is retrieved from the flask by gently tapping on the sides of the flask using a resin hammer. Using a saw, cut through the stone mold in three areas viz in the middle of the mold opposite the central incisors and two on either side of tuberosity region in maxilla or retromolar area in the mandible. A knife is placed in these saw cuts and investing stone surrounding the denture is pried away. The denture is then retrieved systematically from the cast by making several saw cuts on the base of the cast and separating each stone piece from the denture.

8. Finishing and polishing: The stone adhering to the tissue surface is removed using shell blaster. The denture is trimmed with series of three grits of acrylic trimming carbide burs viz – black (extra coarse), followed by green and then red at 15,000 rpm. The frenal attachment areas are relieved using a No.558 or No.701 bur. Using silicone carbide paper mounted on mandrel in low speed handpiece, polish the palatal surfaces and flange areas of denture, using rag wheel polish with a mixture of pumice slurry mixed with water followed by rouge. Final gloss can be obtained with universal polishing paste. (Fig. 21.15)

The polished denture is stored in water until insertion.

Denture repair

The fractured segments of denture are aligned with cyanoacrylate resin.(Fig 21.16, 21.17) A cast is made out of denture using silicone putty impression material. (Fig 21.18, 21.19). The advantage is that the silicone material is flexible so that the denture need not be relieved in the undercut areas. Denture segments are separated from the cast (Fig 21.20,21.21). The fractured areas of the denture segments are ground to create space for the repair resin. Retentive grooves are made on either side of the fractured area(Fig 21.22). These grooves can end in a dovetail in the resin. Fractured denture is realigned in the cast (Fig 21.23). The polymer and monomer of the repair resin are dispensed and mixed. It is poured in to the area that is to be paired and ensured that the resin flows in to the space created as well as in to the grooves. The resin is allowed to complete polymerization. (Fig. 21.24) Then the repaired denture is removed from the putty cast.The fitting surface in the area of repair is examined for any porosities. To enhance the strength the denture can be splinted in plaster and subjected to pressure pot curing. The denture is finally polished and inserted in the patient's mouth. (Fig. 21.25)

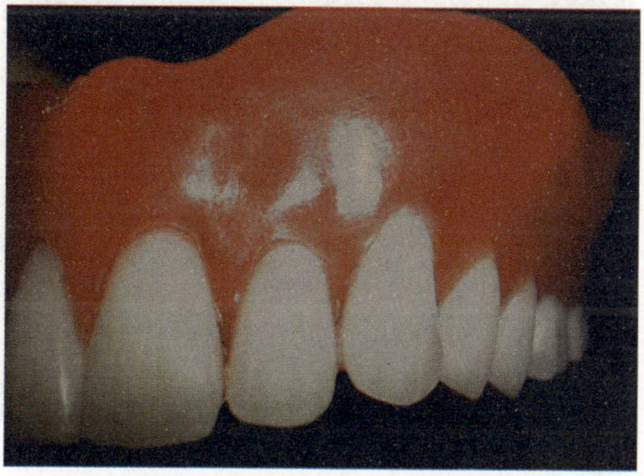

Fig. 21.1 Waxing up of trial denture

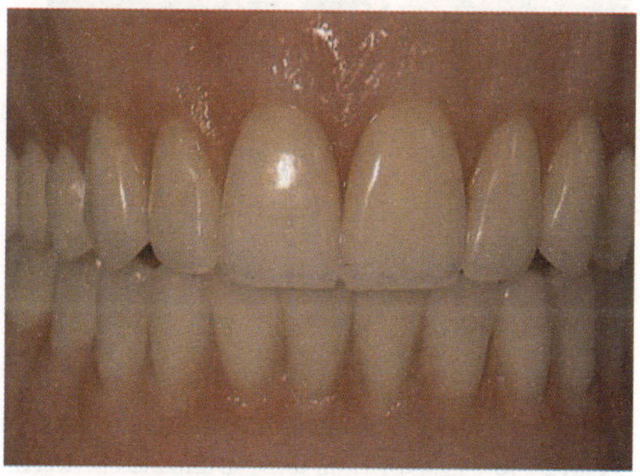

Fig. 21.2 Completed carving

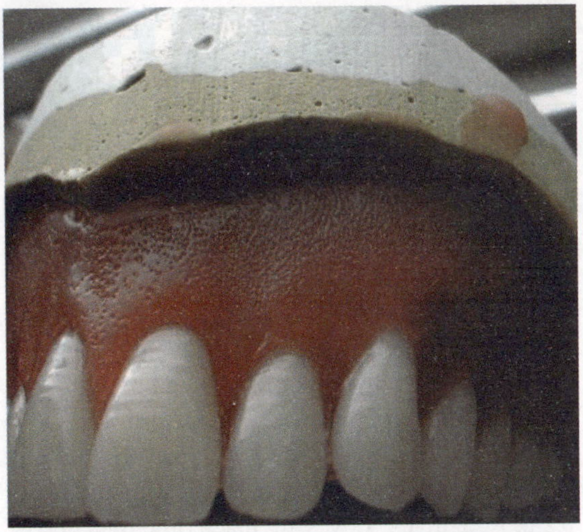

Fig. 21.3 Stippling incorporated

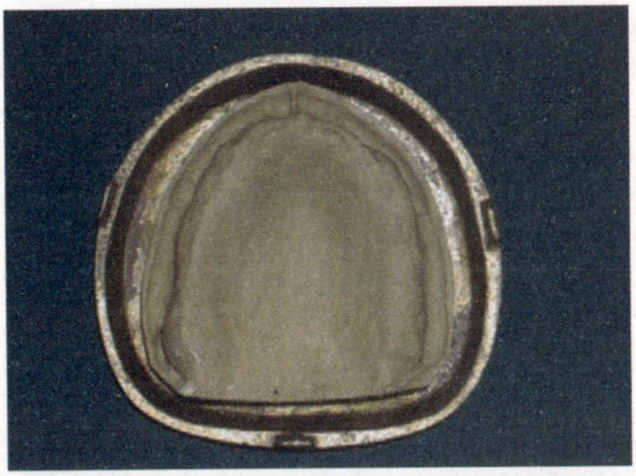

Fig. 21.4a A gap of 5mm to be maintained between the cast

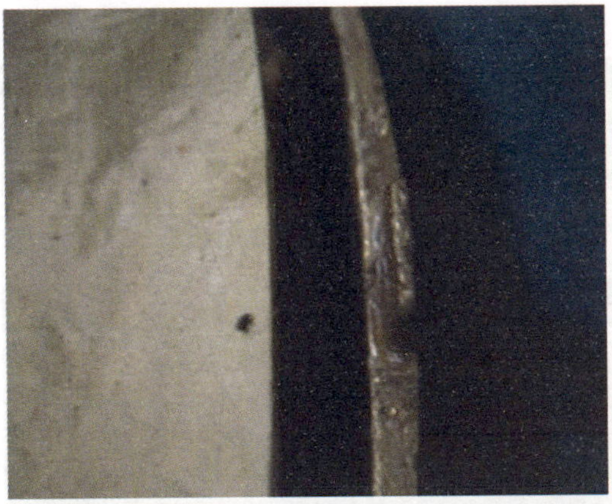

Fig. 21.4b A gap of 5mm to be maintained between the cast

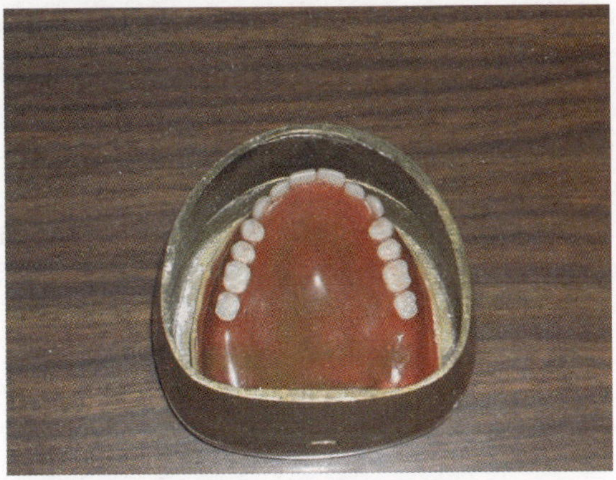

Fig. 21.5 Maxillary incisors of the waxed up trial denture should be 6mm below the upper border of the ring of the denture flask

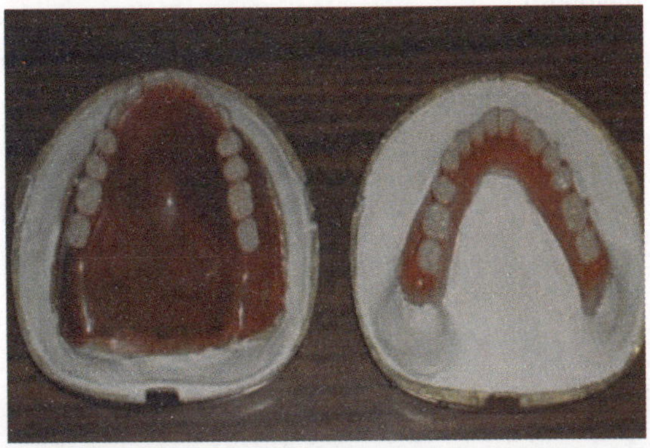

Fig. 21.6 Trial denture with the cast fixed to the base using investing plaster

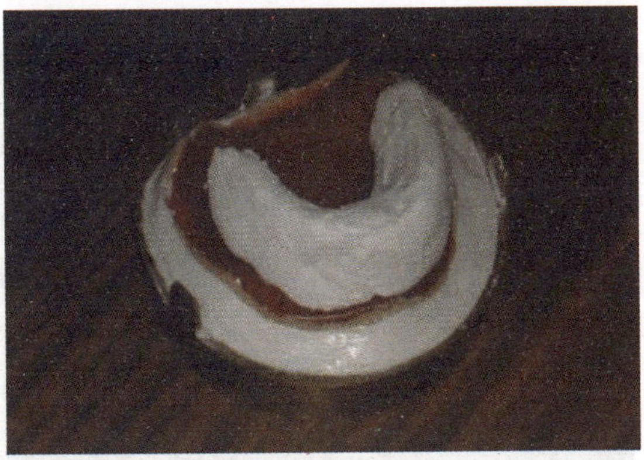

Fig. 21.7 The teeth portion painted with dental stoneto serve as a splint

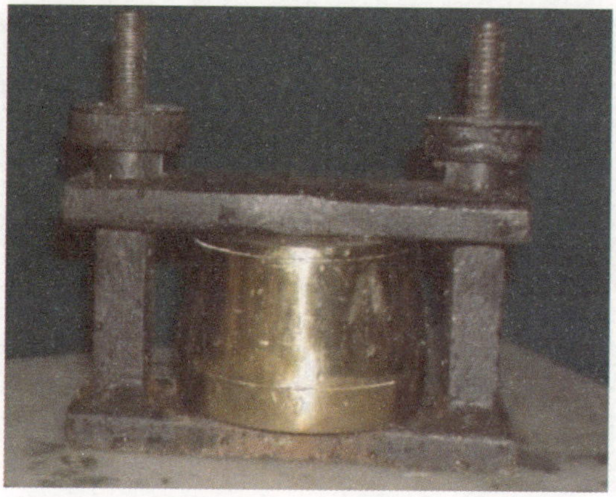

Fig. 21.8 Ring portion is filled with investing plaster and is secured tightly with clamps

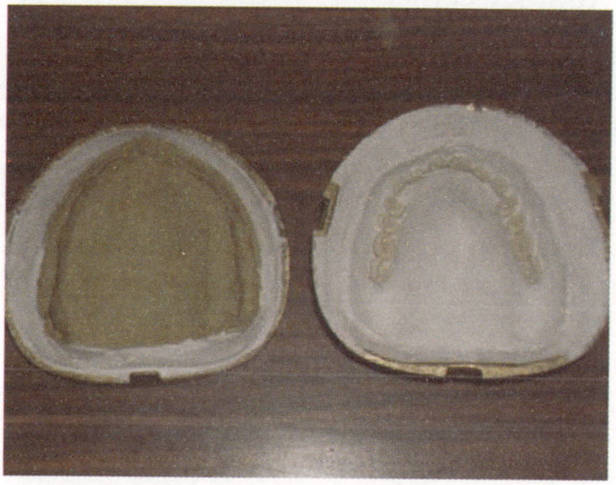

Fig. 21.9 Maxillary mould after dewaxing

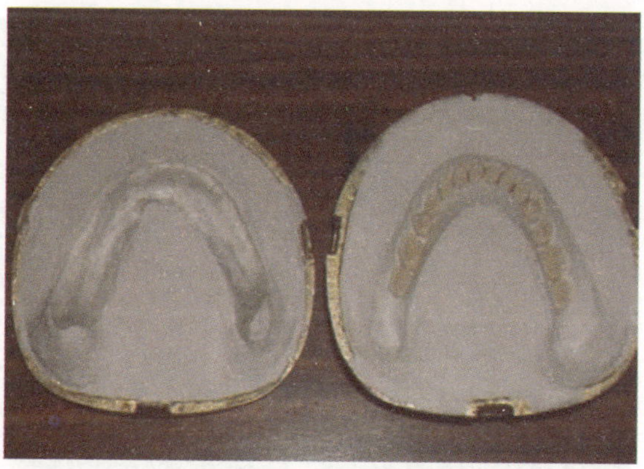

Fig. 21.10 Mandibular mould after dewaxing

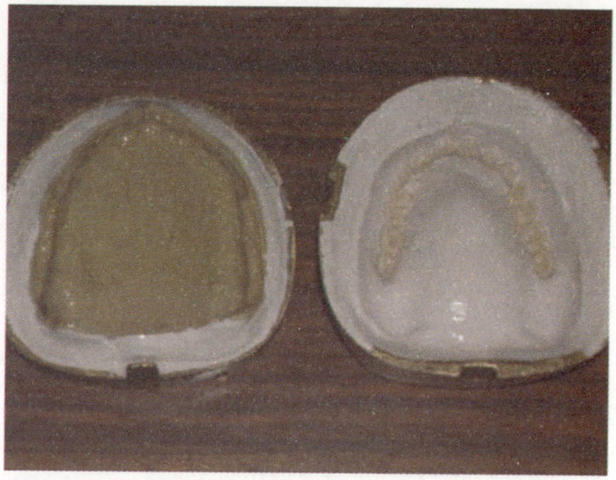

Fig. 21.11 Maxillary mould is painted with alginate separating medium

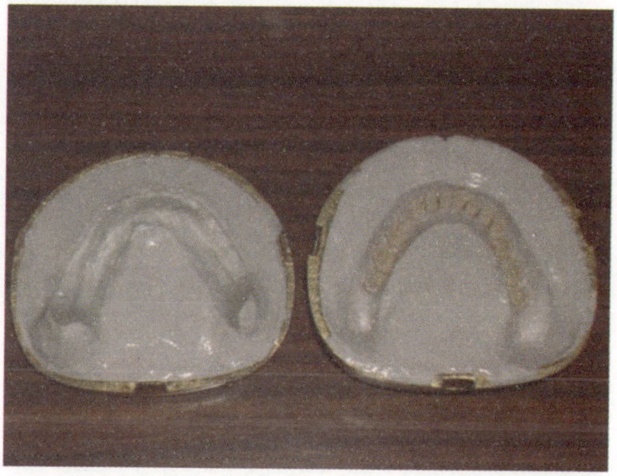

Fig. 21.12 Mandibular mould is painted with alginate separating medium

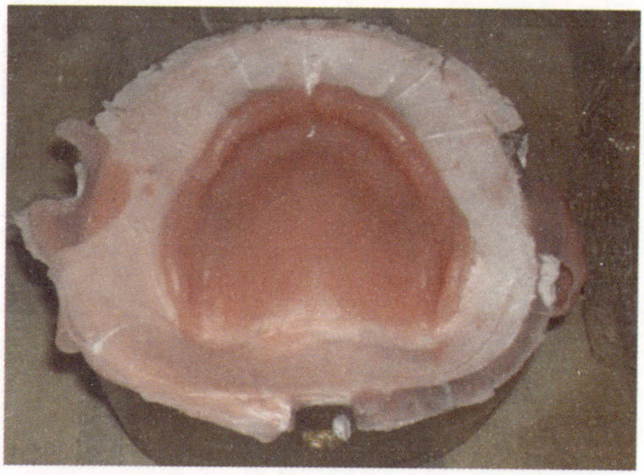

Fig. 21.13 Mould space packed with acrylic resin

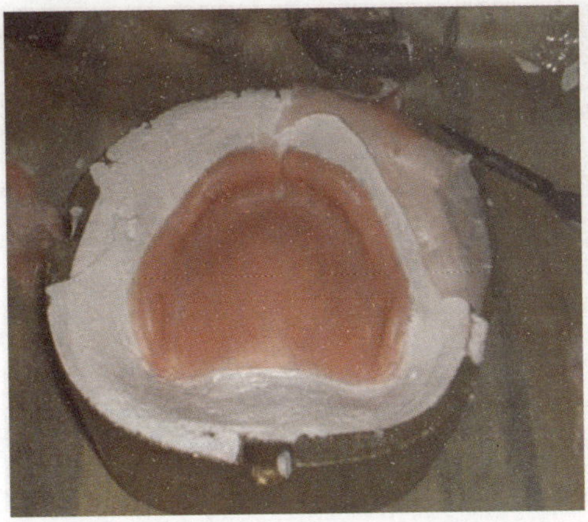

Fig. 21.14 Flash removed with sharp blade

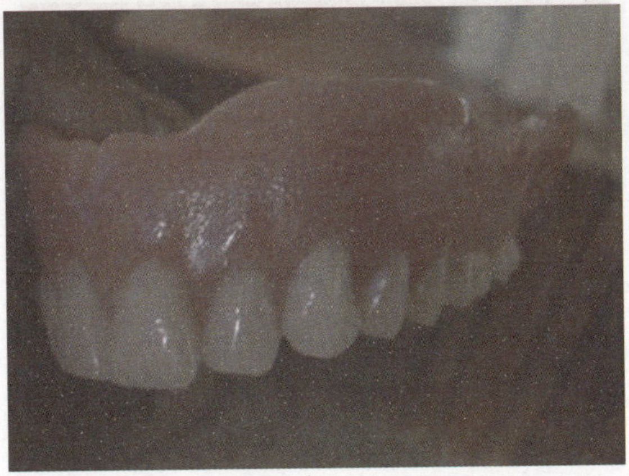

Fig. 21.15 Denture after processing and finishing

Denture repair / reprocessing

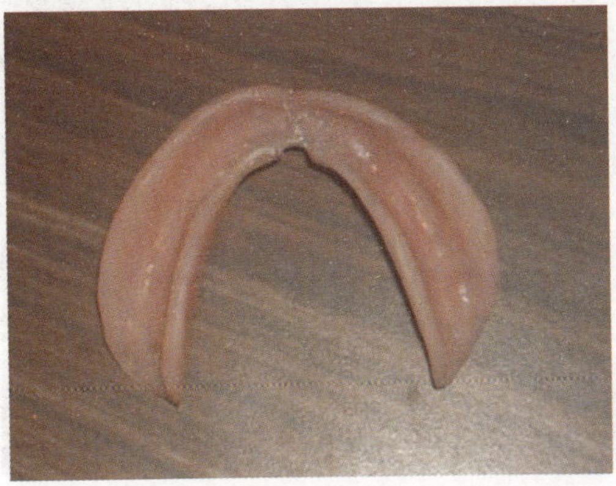

Fig. 21.16 Fractured segments of denture aligned

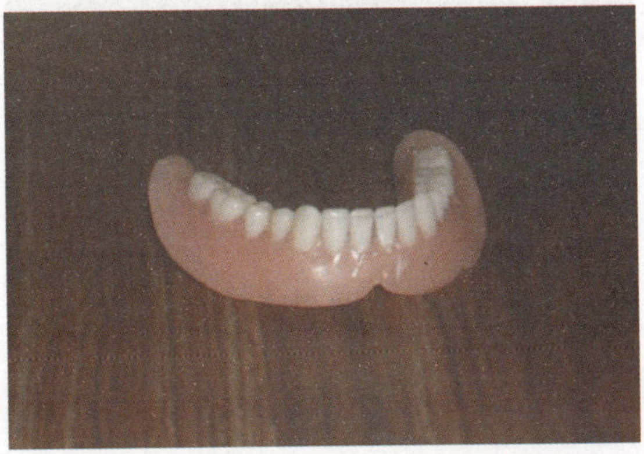

Fig. 21.17 Fractured segments assembled using cyanoacrylate

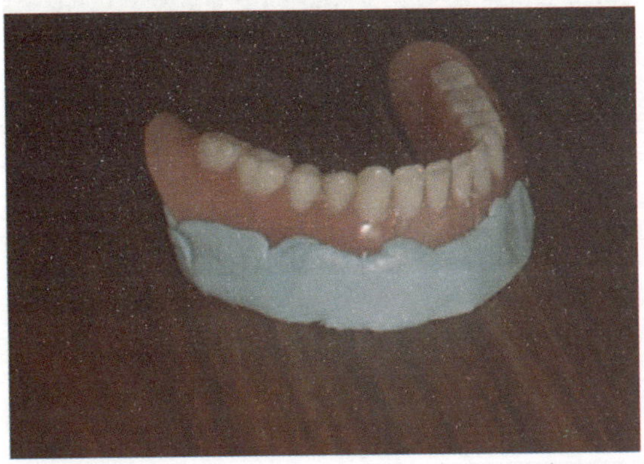

Fig. 21.18 A cast is made out of the denture using silicone putty impression material

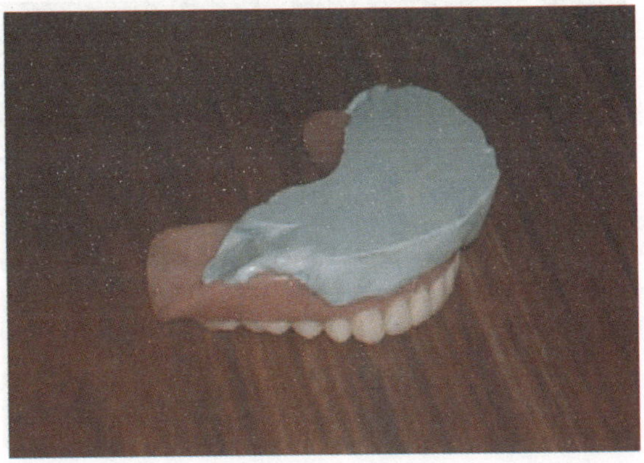

Fig. 21.19 Denture with putty cast

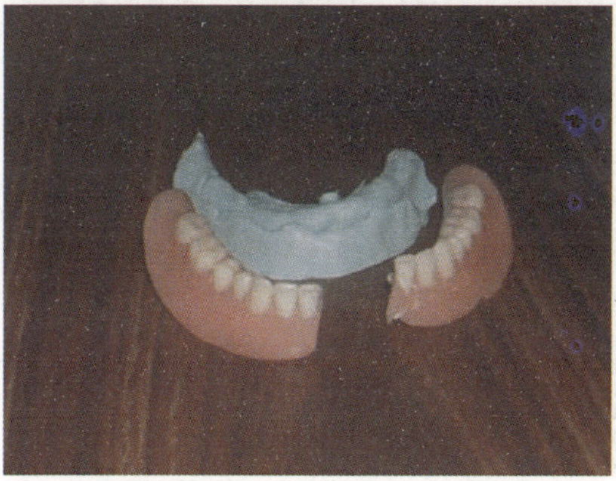

Fig. 21.20 Denture segments separated from the cast

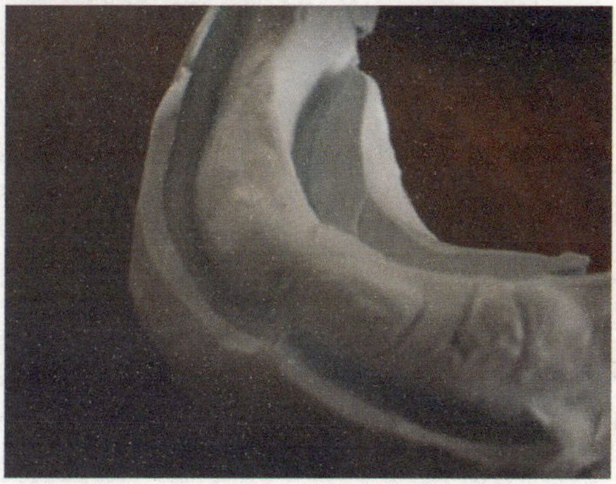

Fig. 21.21 Putty cast

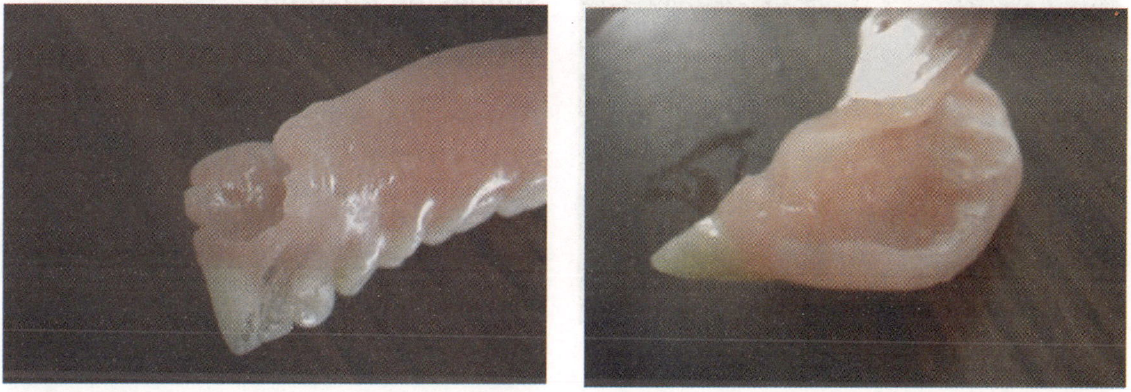

Fig. 21.22 (a) (b) Fractured borders of both the dentures are ground to create space for the repair resin.Retentive grooves also made

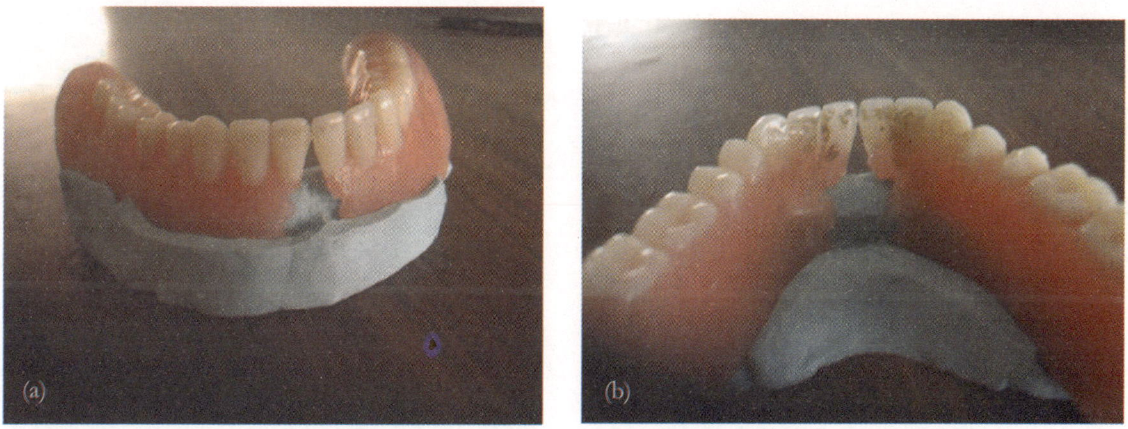

Fig. 21.23 (a) (b) Fractured denture realigned on the cast

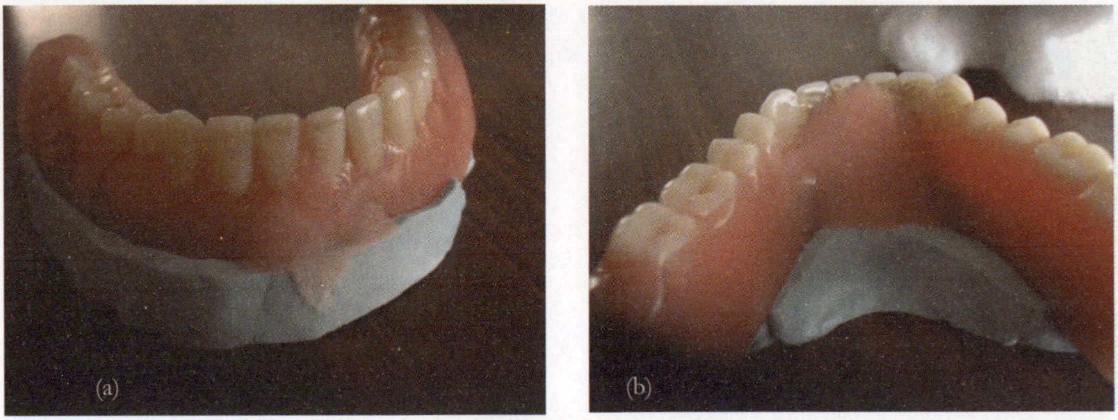

Fig. 21.24 (a) (b) Created gap is filled with autopolmerising acrylic resin

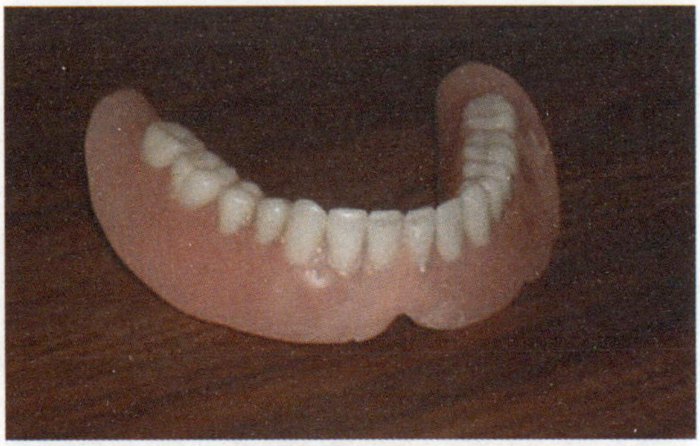

Fig. 21.25 Repaired denture

Suggested Reading

1. Morrow M Robert, Rudd D Kenneth, Eissman F Harold, *Dental Laboratory Procedures: Complete dentures* VolumeI, Mosby, London, pp 284 – 309.
2. Bates F John, Hugget Robin, Stafford G D, *Removable denture construction,* 3rd edition,Wright, London, pp 104-15
3. Anusavice, *Phillips' Science of dental materials,* 11th edition, pp 724-37

22

Complaints

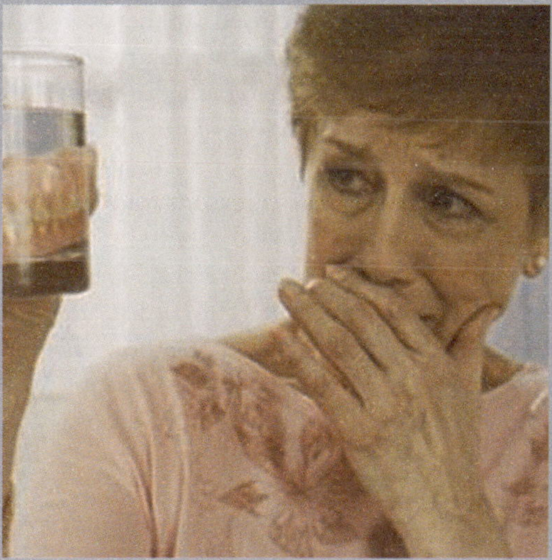

Success of complete denture treatment depends on relieving complaints which are posed at different time intervals

Introduction

Dentures become a success if the complaints are identified and appropriate remedial measures are taken. This chapter deals with the common complaints encountered in complete denture treatment.

Pain

Complete dentures are made of rigid material and they function over soft or firm tissues. While dentures do not change form frequently, tissues alter its shape in course of time. The incompatible texture as well as the time dependant changes can cause discomfort to the wearer almost on a regular basis. Hence dentures are to be attended to with regular frequency to ensure successful functioning.

As and when the dentures are inserted it will stimulate salivary secretion resulting in flooding of the mouth with the saliva and looseness of the denture. In due course of time salivary secretion will get diminished and it will not be a problem to the patient. Pain can appear anytime after the denture is delivered. Commonly it is caused by the over extension of the borders resulting into injury and ulceration. This must be attended to immediately by way of modifying the borders or else it can lead to hyperplastic tissue changes. Poor fit of the dentures and rough fitting surfaces are also reasons for pain. Non compressible areas are to be relieved even during the impression stage. If that is not achieved, inflammation and pain can result. This also needs immediate attention by way of identifying the areas of pressure concentration using pressure indicating paste. If pressure indicating pastes are not available, tooth paste can be used as a substitute.

Incorrect centric occlusion, cuspal interferences, teeth positioned off the ridge, uneven occlusal balance and anterior contact in centric relation are also capable of producing pain because of abnormal stress concentration in areas which cannot tolerate loading. Excessive vertical dimension can cause pain but correction may need a refabrication. Irregular ridges, undercuts and sharp crestal regions will cause injury during function. Careful planning before the commencement of the treatment can eliminate pain due to this reason. Prominent mylohyoid ridge and genial tubercles present in old aged individuals are very difficult situations to be managed. Use of resilient liners and surgical modifications can be thought of. In the area of genial tubercle, the denture border has to be extended to areas where compressible tissue is present.

In advancing age, mental foramen will be present nearer to the crest of the ridge and during mastication there are chances for the nerve to get compressed. Tingling and itching sensation of the lower lip is a manifestation of nerve compression . Addition of resilient liners and surgical repositioning of the nerve are the treatment of choice. If the mandibular denture is over extended in the retromylohyoid region, it can compress or injure the superior constrictor muscle and it will lead to pain during swallowing. Reduction of the flange is the treatment. Residual pathology like fractured roots, cysts or even impacted teeth can cause pain on wearing dentures. Sharp posterior border of the maxillary denture can cause injury in the posterior palatal region if the patient wears the denture during sleep and snores.

Loose dentures

Maxillary dentures generally provide good retention but it will become loose if the posterior palatal seal is not successfully made. Over extended and under extended borders can make dentures loose. Mandibular dentures can become loose very easily because the area of coverage is highly limited. If the posterior teeth are not set in the neutral zone there is every likelihood that dentures become loose. Lingually placed posteriors can restrict the movement of tongue and dentures will become loose when the tongue moves. Occlusal discrepancies and very high occlusal plane can also make the dentures very loose. If there is dryness of mouth due to lack of saliva, dentures may become loose. This problem is present in irradiated patients, heavy smokers and in those who regularly take antihypertensive drugs. If the lips are very tight it will tend to unseat the mandibular denture. It will happen when the mandibular anteriors are placed too far labially. If denture bases are not adapted properly to the tissues, they become unstable and there by causing looseness. An accurate impression and an accurate cast can eliminate this defect. Even a well fitting denture will have a space of 100 microns. A space more than that are subject to pooling of saliva, collection of food debris and microbial growth.

Faulty esthetics

Esthetics limitations of complete dentures must be discussed prior to the treatment and extensive trial sessions are to be conducted to avoid esthetic dissatisfaction. Patients may also have unrealistic expectations on the esthetics of the dentures. Patient should be able to appreciate esthetics of the contour of soft tissues i.e., external appearance and aesthetics of smile. Over supported and under supported facial features and increased or decreased vertical dimension can cause esthetic loss. Wrinkles on the skin cannot always be eliminated by increasing the fullness of the dentures. If the vertical dimension is too low, chances of getting angular chelitis are more.

Aesthetics of smile mainly depend upon the maxillary anterior teeth and their placement. Midline of the face should coincide with the midline of the dental arch. Anterior segment and mouth should maintain golden proportion. Visibility is also a matter of dissatisfaction and any attempt to reduce visibility arbitrarily will alter the eccentric occlusal relations.

Defective speech

Speech will be altered if vertical dimension is increased, palatal contour is deficient, tongue is restricted, arch form is not following the neutral zone, lingual flanges are thick, posterior palatal seal area is poorly developed and if the patient is having poor neuromuscular skill.

Inefficiency

If the patient is not in a position to chew, it may be considered as inefficiency. Discrepancies in vertical dimension and centric relation can cause inefficiency. Worn off teeth, zero degree posteriors, lack of occlusal balance, occlusal plane set at a higher level can also cause inefficient dentures. Some patients may complain that the teeth are very dull. Correcting the reason will make the dentures efficient. However efficiency should be evaluated not immediately after delivery of the denture but after observing for a few months because inexperience on the part of the patient will also be interpreted as inefficiency.

Nausea and gagging

Over extended posterior limit of maxillary dentures commonly cause this. Thick posterior borders and loose denture will also initiate gagging. Some patients may have certain uncommon belief about dentures and gagging in them may be purely psychogenic.

Fibrous Hyperplasia

Denture induced fibrous hyperplasia is a hyperplastic reaction of the oral tissues to the continuous wearing of ill fitting dentures. This is also known as epulis fissuratum, denture hyperplasia, denture stomatitis and inflammatory hyperplasia. When the denture impinge and traumatize the mucosa usually buccal or labial to the ridge, this lesion appears. The constant friction on the vestibule causes hyperplasia of the connective tissue and it develops into pleats of tissues around the offending flange. Usually it is painless. The denture flange must be modified and if required the tissue can be surgically eliminated.

Microbial Infection

Poor oral hygiene decreases the wash out of debris from the oral cavity. This in turn facilitates the growth of fungi and other microbial organisms. Candida albicans aggravates the hyperplastic and edematous reactions of the mucosa. Papillary hyperplasia of the palate can be due to poor oral hygiene. Diabetes and smoking habit can also be attributed to this. Patient must be instructed to clean the vestibules, retromylohyoid region and palate thoroughly. Ridges must be massaged with fingers and soft brush. Topical and systemic administration of antifungal drugs is also indicated.

Uncommon complaints

1. Whistling – This is due to high vault palate. It can be corrected by modifying the palate by adding more resin.
2. Ear ache – Decreased vertical dimension and occlusal prematurities may cause pain in the TMJ and which will be manifested as ear ache.
3. Food and saliva under the denture – There is no specific solution to this problem. Once the patient gets experienced, the complaint will disappear. This may be due to border deficiency. Patients will gain confidence to manage such situations in course of time. Tissues may also adapt more closely.
4. Loss of taste – This will be felt in the initial phases but soon will disappear.
5. Sneezing and coughing – During sneezing and coughing, dentures get unseated and patients must be warned to keep palm in front of the mouth.
6. Cheek biting – Lack of horizontal overlap in the posterior region, decreased vertical dimension and buccal placement in the posterior teeth are the common causes. Modification of posterior teeth vertical height will eliminate the complaint.
7. Drooling of Saliva - If the vertical height is not adequate, saliva may get pooled and can cause drooling.
8. Inability to eat meat - Usually seen when the teeth are worn off or when monoplane occlusion is used. Experienced patients can manage.
9. Clicking of teeth -Increase in vertical dimension and use of ceramic teeth can cause clicking.
10. Allergy - Allergy to acrylic can cause oedema and ulceration. Usually it is due to the pigment present in the denture base resin and the residual monomer. If denture bases are made in clear acrylic and processing done adequately, acrylic allergy can be eliminated.

Dentures can provide successful service if the maintenance is done adequately for that both the patients and dentists have to put an effort. Properly cleaned dentures well attended periodically can provide long duration of service making the patient forget the handicap of edentulism.

Classification of post insertion denture problems:

I. Complaints about comfort of the denture:
   1. Sore spots
   2. Burning sensation
   3. Redness
   4. Pain in TMJ
   5. Tongue and cheek biting
   6. Swallowing and sore throat
   7. Nausea and gagging
   8. Deafness
   9. Fatigue of the muscles of mastication.

II. Complaints about function of the denture:
   1. Instability or poor fit
   2. Interference
      a) When swallowing
      b) Clicking

III. Complaints about esthetics:
   1. Fullness under the nose
   2. Depressed philtrum or naso-labial sulcus
   3. Upper lip sunken in
   4. Too much of teeth exposed
   5. Artificial look

IV) Complaints about phonetics:
   1. Whistle on "S" sounds
   2. Lisp on "S" sounds
   3. Indistinct "TH" and "T" sounds
   4. "T sound like "TH"
   5. "F" and "V" sounds indistinct

Table I: Complaints about comfort of the denture, causes and treatment:

	Complaint	Causes	Treatment
1 Sore spots	A. Sore spots in the vestibule.	a. Overextension b. Unpolished or sharp edge	a. Adjust denture (disclosing wax). b. Polish denture borders.
	B. Sore spots posterior limit of the maxillary denture.	a. Posterior valve seal too deep b. Sharp valve seal c. Overextension	a. Identify area with disclosing wax (PIP) and relief high pressure area. b. Round off sharp areas. c. Adjust peripheral extension.
	C. Single sore spots over ridge.	a. High occlusion in that area b. Bubbles of acrylic	a. Check with articulating paper and adjust the occlusion. b. Inspect the denture under good light to detect surface roughness then remove and polish lightly.
	D. Soreness under labial flange.	a. Excessive overbite b. Habit-mastication in protrusive relation c. Overextended labial flange	a. Reseat maxillary anterior teeth. b. Train the patient to masticate in centric relation. c. Adjust peripheral extension.
	E. Soreness under lingual flange of mandibular denture.	a. CO not on harmony with CR (drives mandibular denture forward) b. Overextended lingual flange	a. If only slight, if can be corrected, record, remounting & selective grinding. b. Apply pressure indicating paste to denture periphery, adjust peripheral extension.
	F. Generalized soreness over the alveolar ridge.	a. Excessive vertical dimension b. Inaccurate denture base	a. If the occlusal plane of the upper is judged to be correct, make a new lower denture to the decreased vertical dimension, otherwise, new upper and lower dentures. b. New dentures, but the old ones can be rebased if the occlusion is adequate.
2. Burning sensation	A. Anterior hard palate & anterior alveolar ridge areas.	• Pressure over the anterior palatine foramen	• Relief over the foramen.
	B. Rugae, lip & side of the tongue.	• Climacteric, anxiety& ariboflavinosis	• Large dose of vitamin B-complex, taking the denture out, and holding a piece of ice in the mouth will provide a temporary relief.
	C. Premolar to molar area	• Pressure on the posterior palatine foramen	• Relief area over the foramen.
	D. Lower anterior ridge	Pressure on the mental foramen	Relief over the foramen.

Complaint	Type	Cause	Treatment
3. Redness	A. Fiery redness of all tissues contacted by denture, including tongue and cheeks.	Denture base allergy (uncommon)	Remake the denture & use metallic denture base.
	B. Redness of the denture bearing tissues.	Ill-fitting denture Avitaminois	Remake or rebase the denture. Employ vitamin therapy regime.
4. Pain in TMJ		a. Insufficient vertical dimension of occlusion. b. CO not in harmony with CR. c. Arthritis. d. Trauma.	a. Increase vertical dimension. b. Correct occlusion by selective grinding. c. Treat with analgesics. d. Treat with analgesics.
5. Tongue and cheek biting		a. Posterior teeth edge to edge (insufficient horizontal overlap). b. Over-closure c. Changes in the occlusal plane leading to cheek and tongue biting. d. Posterior teeth too far buccal leading to cheek biting. e. Posterior teeth too far lingual (reduction of tongue space) leading to tongue biting. f. Loss of muscle tonus (Lax cheek) leads to cheek biting. g. Tongue biting may occur in patient with epilepsy.	a. Re-contour buccal surface of mandibular molars & premolars to increase the horizontal overlap (buccal overjet). b. Restore the vertical dimension. c. New denture with proper occlusal height. d. Re-contour buccal surface of the upper molars, in some case it may be necessary to remove the last molar tooth. e. Re-establish adequate tongue space. f. Build out thin denture base or extent the under-extended borders. g. Treat the cause.
6. Swallowing and sore throat	A. Maxillary denture	i) Over extension of posterior border. ii) Too thick posterior border.	a. i) Adjust posterior border extension. ii) Thin posterior border.
	B. mandibular denture	i- Overextension of the posterior lingual flange area. ii- Too thick lingual posterior flanges.	b. Reduce thickness or adjust posterior lingual flange area.
	C. Insufficient vertical dimension of occlusion		c. Increase vertical dimension.
	D. Excessive vertical dimension of occlusion		d. Reduce vertical dimension.
	E. Posterior teeth set inside the ridge (tongue is crowded).		e. Re-set teeth in correct position.
7. Nausea and gagging	A. Immediately upon denture placement.	a- Maxillary denture: i) Overextension ii) Too thick posterior border	a. Adjust denture or thin posterior border. b. Reduce thickness of disto-lingual flange. c. Prescribe a mild tranquilizer.
		b- Mandibular denture: i) Distolingual ii) Flange too thick	
		c- Psychogenic factors	
	B. Delayed (2 weeks to months) after denture placement.	a- Incomplete border seal allowing saliva under the denture. b- Faulty occlusion causing denture to loosen and allowing saliva under the denture.	a. Improve border seal. b. Correct occlusion.

8. Deafness		Over closure of vertical dimension.	Increase vertical dimension.
9. Fatigue of the muscles of mastication	Vertical dimension.	a- Excessive vertical dimension of occlusion. b- Insufficient vertical dimension of occlusion.	a. Reduce vertical dimension. b. Increase vertical dimension.

Table II: Complaints about function of the denture, causes and treatment

	Complaint	Potential causes	Treatment
	a- When not occluding	a. Overextension of denture borders and posterior limit. b. Under extended denture borders. c. Loss of posterior valve seal: i) Valve seal on hard palate. ii) Posterior limit not in the hamular notches. iii) Insufficient valve seal. d. Dehydration of tissue due to alcoholism. e. Flabby tissue displaced when making impression. f. Under-filled buccal vestibule.	a. Adjust denture border extension. b. Correct with auto-polymerizing acrylic resin but check with compound for diagnostic purposes. c. Improve posterior palatal seal. d. Remove the cause. e. Correct surgically-change. f. Correct the flange thickness.
	b- When occluding in centric	a. Malocclusion: i) High occlusion in premolar area. ii) Premature individual tooth contact. iii) High occlusion in one side of the arch. b. Poor denture foundation (flabby tissues) c. Incorrect tooth position (teeth set too far buccally). d. Centric occlusion not in harmony with centric relation. e. Non-yielding area in hard palate (torus palatinus).	a. Selectively adjust the occlusion. b. Correct surgically-change denture. c. Reset teeth in correct position. d. Selectively adjust the occlusion. e. Provide sufficient relief.

1- Instability or poor fit	A- Looseness of maxillary denture:	c- Dislodgement of maxillary denture during function	a. Overfilled buccal vestibule. b. Over extension in the hamular notch area. c. Inadequate notches for frenum attachment. d. Excessively thick denture base over the disto-buccal alveolar tubercle. e. Placing the maxillary anterior teeth too far labial. f. Placing the maxillary posterior teeth too far buccal. g. Placing the posterior palatal seal too deep. h. Lack of occlusal harmony	a. Allow proper flange thickness. b. Correct border extension. c. Allow sufficient clearance for frenum attachments. d. Reduce the thickness of the distal ends of the buccal flanges. e. Reset the teeth. f. Reset the teeth. g. Identify pressure area with disclosing wax, provide sufficient relief. h. Correct occlusal disharmony by selective grinding.
		d- When incising food	a. Loss of posterior valve seal. b. Anterior teeth placed too far labially. c. Poor denture foundation. d. Improper incising habits	a. Improve posterior palatal seal. b. Reset teeth in correct position. c. Correct surgically0change denture. d. Train patient to masticate in centric.
		e- When yawing or opening wide	a. Denture base too thick in buccal posterior area. b. Denture over-extended in hamular notch area.	a. Reduce thickness of denture base. b. Shorten denture until pterygo-mandibular ligament doesn't exert tension on posterior border when mouth opened wide.
		f- When talking	a. Inadequate posterior palatal seal. b. Overextension in the posterior region.	a. Increase posterior palatal seal with auto-polymerizing acrylic resin. b. Adjust the posterior overextension.
		a- Peripheral overextension.	a- In the masseter groove area. b- In a lateral direction beyond the external oblique ridge. c- In the lingual flanges. d- In the retromolar pad.	Adjust the denture accordingly.
		b- Tight lips.		a. Remake with the lower anterior teeth set more lingually, with a labial concavity on the denture & with maximum extension in the region of the retromolar pad. b. Vestibuoplasty may be considered.
		c- Lower posterior tilted teeth or set lingually leading to cramping the tongue.		Reduce the width of the lower posterior teeth by grinding off the lingual cusp.
		d- Under-extension & lack of peripheral seal.		Correct the under-extension.

	e- Placing the occlusal plane too high.		• Remake the denture with proper occlusal planeheight.
	f- Improper contour of the polished surface.		Re-contour the polished surface.
	g- Lack of saliva.		Palliative treatment such as artificial saliva.
2- Interference	A- When swallowing	a- Maxillary denture too thick or overextended in posterior region. b- Mandibular denture too thick or overextended in posterior lingual region. c- Insufficient vertical dimension of occlusion. d- Excessive vertical dimension of occlusion. e- Incorrect tooth position.	a- Reduce thickness or adjust posterior region. b- Reduce thickness or adjust posterior lingual flange area. c- Increase vertical dimension. d- Reduce vertical dimension. e- Reset teeth.
	B- Clicking	a- Excessive vertical dimension. b- Denture with poor retention & stability. c- Cuspal interference. d- Excessive incisal guidance.	a. Reduce vertical dimension- use acrylic resin teeth. b. Rebasing or remaking the dentures. c. Eliminate cuspal interference. d. Correct occlusion.

Table III: Complaint about esthetics, causes and treatment:

Complaint	Potential causes	Treatment
A- Fullness under the nose	Labial flange of the upper too long or too thick.	Reduce length or thickness of labial flange.
B- Depressed philtrum or naso-labial sulcus	Labial flange too short or too thin.	Increase length or thickness of labial flange.
C- Upper lip sunken in	Maxillary anterior teeth set too far lingually.	Reset anterior teeth labially.
D- Too much of teeth exposed	a- Excessive vertical dimension. b- Incisal plane too low. c- Cuspids and lateral too prominent.	a. Reduce vertical dimension. b. Reset teeth at higher plane. c. Correct tooth prominence.
C- Artificial look	a- Technique set-up (teeth are too regular in alignment. b- All teeth same shade. c- Lack of grinding incisal edges and angles.	a. Set up individualized (by rotating & shortening few teeth). b. Choose different shades. c. Grind incisal edges and angles to give a more individualized appearance.

Table IV: Complaints about function of Phonetics, causes and treatment:

A. Whistle on "S" sounds	Too large air space on the anterior part of the palate.	Reshape the anterior part of the palate by thickening denture base.
B. Lisp on "S" sounds	Too small anterior air space.	Thin palato-lingual area.
C. Indistinct "TH" and "T" sounds	Inadequate inter-occlusal space.	Reduce thickness of palatal of maxillary denture and lingual of mandibular denture base, reduce vertical dimension.
D. "T sounds like "TH"	Upper anterior teeth too far lingually.	Reset teeth buccally.
E. "F" and "V" sounds indistinct	Improper position of the upper anterior teeth either vertically or horizontally.	Reset teeth either vertically or horizontally so that they contact the lower lip at its highest point during these sounds.

www.medkaau.com/album/download.php?image_id=439.....

Suggested Reading

1. Miller Ernst, *Clinical management of denture induced inflammation,* J Prosthet Dent 1977; 38 (4): 362-65.
2. Palmer John, *Structural changes for speech improvement In complete denture fabrication,* J Prosthet Dent 1979; 41(5): 507- 10
3. Jeganathan S, Payne J A, *Common faults in complete dentures : A review*, Quintessence International 1993; 24(7): 483-87
4. Morstad A T, Peterson A D, *Postinsertion denture problems.* J Prosthet Dent 1968; 19(2): 126-131
5. www.medkaau.com

23

Denture adhesives

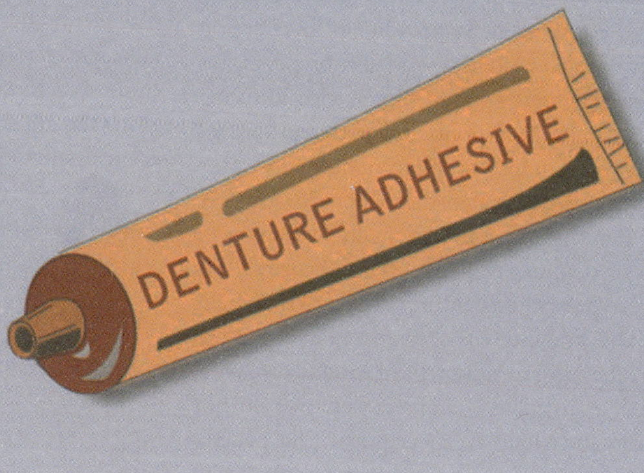

Use of denture adhesives is no more considered as a sign of professional incompetence. In fact denture adhesives improve the functional efficiency of complete dentures. Excessive use of denture adhesives containing zinc causes toxicity usually associated with numbness and tingling of hands and legs

People began using denture adhesives in the late eighteenth century but dental literature makes no mention of these products until the nineteenth century. The first U.S patent for a denture adhesive was issued in 1913. Despite their widespread use, dentists continued to maintain a negative attitude towards denture adhesives. However it is generally accepted that denture adhesives improve denture retention and stability and thereby enhance function. Satisfying the expectations of many patients for optimal denture retention and stability is often beyond the technical skills of even the most accomplished practitioners. Discussing and implementing the judicious use of denture adhesives may satisfy patients' expectations and achieve the intended treatment goals.

Kapur after conducting an extensive study concluded that denture adhesives increased denture retention unequivocally, thereby improving the incisive ability of the denture wearer. Tarbet and colleagues found that adhesives improved chewing ability, confidence, comfort and reduced wobbling of the denture. Boone in an extensive review on this subject found that there was no scientific evidence on the adhesive causing tissue irritation and bone resorption. There was no evidence of oral pathosis also. Chew and colleagues have noticed considerable improvement in retention and stability of both well fitting and ill-fitting dentures but they exerted their greatest effect with ill-fitting dentures. Adisman et al pointed out that adhesives act as a cushion under complete dentures. Grasso and colleagues demonstrated that when an adhesive was used, significant improvement in resistance to movement of dentures in all directions occurred. It is appropriate to prescribe a denture adhesive to augment retention and stability of conventional complete dentures. Adhesives are indicated for routine use when appropriately constructed complete dentures do not satisfy stability and retention expectations of the patient. Denture adhesives may also prove psychologically beneficial when the patient requires supplemental retention and stability, particularly during times of public interaction. Denture adhesives are not indicated to provide retention for ill-fitting prostheses. When properly managed, adhesives enhance the interfacial surface tension occurring between the denture base and supporting soft tissues by (1) improving the adhesive, cohesive, and viscosity characteristics of the interfacial film layer, particularly in saliva-deficient patients, and (2) eliminating voids occurring in the interfacial space in the absence of absolute adaptation of the denture base to the bearing tissues. In addition to improved retention and stability, denture adhesives have been shown to reduce mucosal irritation, reduce food impaction beneath the denture base, improve chewing efficiency, increase bite force, improve functional load distribution across the denture-bearing tissues, and facilitate the psychological well-being of the patient. For patients with xerostomia, the use of a well-hydrated denture adhesive provides a cushioning or lubricating effect, reducing frictional irritation of the supporting soft tissues and preventing further tissue dehydration.

Composition

The composition of most modern denture adhesives includes constituents that promote bioadhesion via carboxyl groups once the adhesive is hydrated. Two commonly employed active ingredients in denture adhesives are polyvinyl methyl ether maleate (PVM-MA) and carboxymethylcellulose (CMC). Once placed on the intaglio surface of the denture, the adhesive material must be substantially hydrated in order to achieve optimal performance. Calcium and zinc salts are added to improve adhesiveness. Other components include the following:

Thickening agent	-	Cellulose
Antibacterial agent	-	Hexachlorophefle
Filler	-	Magnesium oxide
To reduce surface tension	-	Sodium lauryl sulphate.
Flavour	-	Pepper mint oil

Mechanism of action

The material swells 50 - 150 % by volume in the presence of water, filling in spaces between prosthesis and tissues. The forces required to pull two disks apart is directly proportional to the viscosity of the liquid between them. Saliva increases the viscosity of the adhesive. The ingredients containing carboxyl groups such as CMC, PVM-MA produce stickiness through covalent bonds formed on hydration.

Advantages of using denture adhesives

1. Generate increased sense of security and comfort
2. Allow greater occlusal pressure.
3. Reduce wobbling of dentures and food particle collection under dentures.
4. Act as cushion, reducing the transmission of pressure and friction to the rnucosa.

Disadvantage

It can encourage the prolonged used of ill-fitting dentures.

Proper use of adhesives can be defined as follows:

- They must not be used as far as possible on ill-fitting dentures
- They must be used on the fitting surface. Care should be taken not to apply them on the borders. (if applied on the borders peripheral seal is affected)
- A thin layer of adhcsive is adequate
- In compromised patients antimicrobials like Nystain and Clotrimazole can be mixed with the adhesive powder/paste.
- The dentures must be cleaned daily using a denture cleanser.

Myths about denture adhesives

- Use of denture adhesives will reflect poor technical skill of the dentist
- Denture adhesives will increase vertical dimension at occlusion
- Denture adhesives have no role on properly made well fitting dentures
- Denture adhesives can induce bone resorption and oral pathoses

The myths associated with denture adhesives have little scientific background. It is high time we changed our negative attitudes towards denture adhesives. It is our responsibility to be knowledgeable and caring enough to assist each patient in adapting to dental prosthesis. This requires recommendation of denture adhesives and counseling on their proper use. Most denture wearers, at one time or another, have attempted to use adhesive to facilitate comfortable denture function. Unfortunately, the concept that "more is better" does not hold true for denture adhesives.

After providing the denture, the denture wearer should be given along with the instructions a prescription containing the following.

1. A denture brush or tooth brush — to be used along with a detergent or a cleanser.
2. Denture cleanser — most of the denture cleansers obtain the cleansing action through the liberation of effervescent oxygen. Denture to be immersed in a solution of denture cleanser once in a week for 8 hours.
3. Denture adhesive — A powder form or a paste form of denture adhesive may be used compulsorily in the initial phases of denture wearing. This will improve the confidence level of the denture wearer.
4. Pain relieving gum paint/gel — Denture wearer can expect to have pain and bruises over the sulci and ridges and it is desirable to paint the painful areas with these gels.
5. Multivitamin multimineral support — In order to ensure a healthy maintenance of the tissues of the edentulous individual who is nutritionally handicapped, vitamins and minerals can be prescribed. It will also help the individual to pass through the stressful initial period of denture wearing with much ease and comfort. A patient explaination of the prescription will be a highly relieving finale to the treatment process where in the individual has been continuously asked to comply with specific exercises which anyone would feel strange.

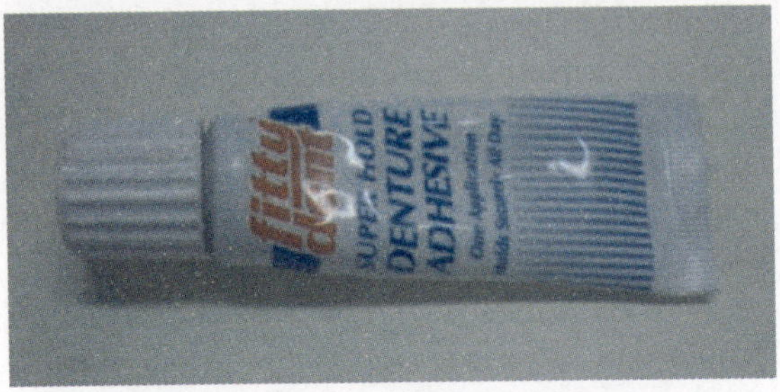

Fig. 23.1 Commercially available denture adhesive

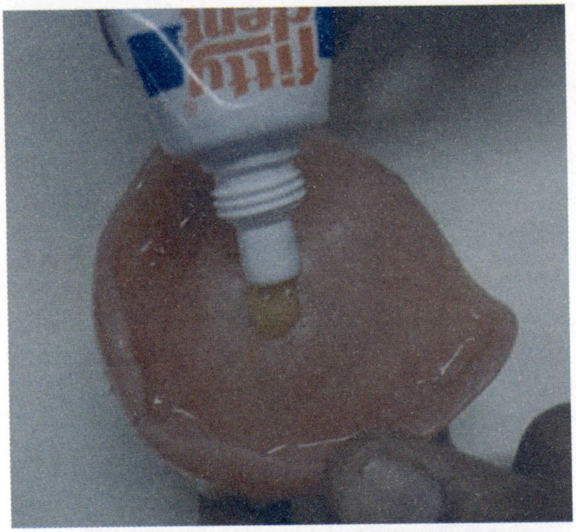

Fig. 23.2 A small amount of the paste should be dispensed onto the clean and dry fitting surface of the denture

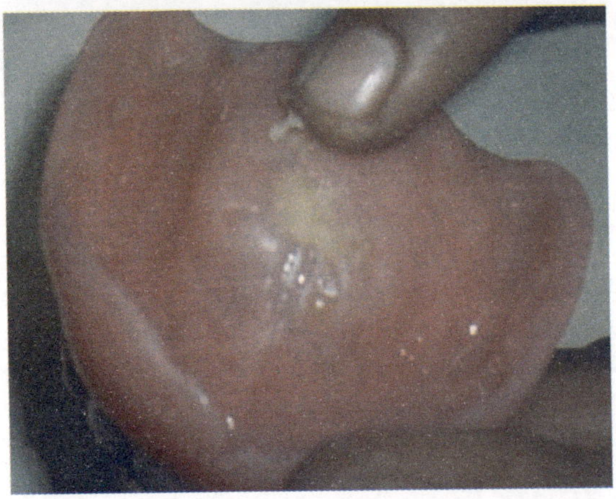

Fig. 23.3 Once dispensed onto the denture, the patient should evenly dispense the paste over the entire intaglio surface of the prosthesis with a clean, dry finger. This will result in a thin, even layer of adhesive

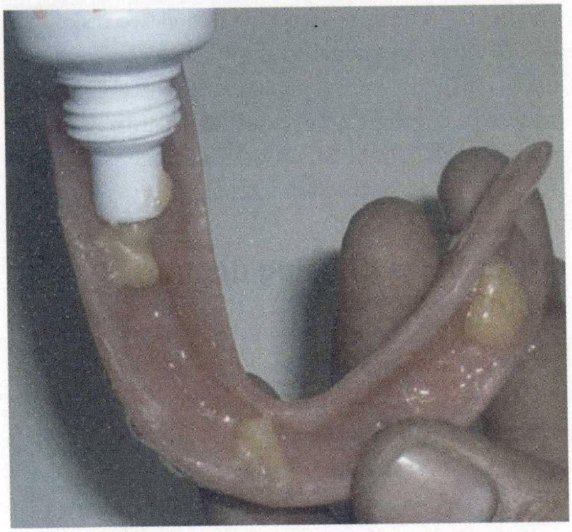

Fig. 23.4 For mandibular denture very small amounts can be dispensed in one or two places along the crest

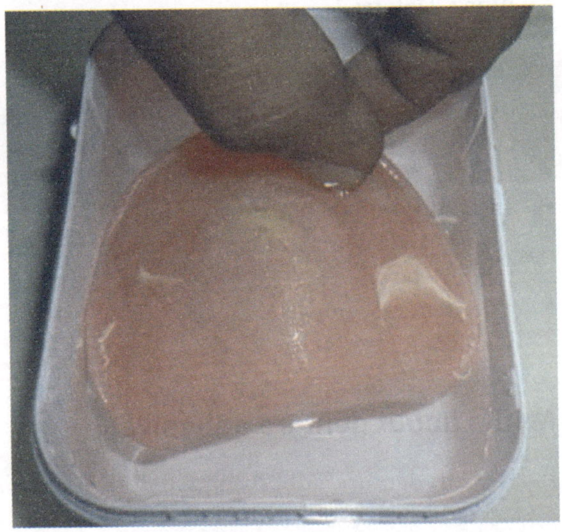

Fig. 23.5 The denture is submerged in a container of cool water to maximally hydrate the adhesive. The denture should remain submerged in water for approximately 20-30 seconds. The denture is then placed in the mouth and firmly seated with finger pressure for approximately 10 seconds.

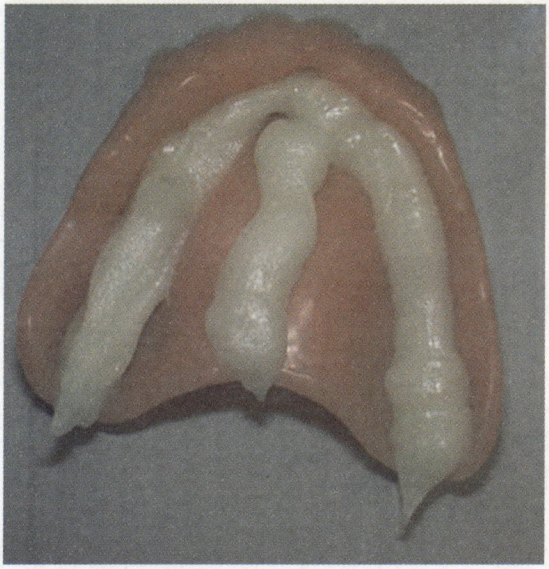

Fig. 23.6 Excessive use of denture adhesive

Aftercare is the silent support to every successful denture.

Correct technique of applying denture adhesive is illustrated from Fig. 23.1-23.6

Suggested reading

1. Gunnar E. Carlsson : *Prosthodontics-Principles and Management Strategies.* Mosby-Wolfe, USA.
2. Shay, K. *Denture adhesives. Choosing the right powders and pastes.* J Am Dent Asso 1991;122:70-76.
3. Slaughter, A.; Katz, R. V. and Grasso, J. E. *Professional attitudes toward denture adhesives: A Delphi technique survey of academic prosthodontists.* J Prosthet Dent 1999;82:80-89.
4. Tarbet, W. J. and Grossman, E. *Observations of denture-supporting tissue during six months of denture adhesive wearing.* J Am Dent Asso 1980;101:789-791.
5. Tarbet, W. J.; Silverman, G. and Schmidt, N. F. *Maximum incisal biting force in denture wearers as influenced by adequacy of denture-bearing tissues and the use of an adhesive.* J Dent Resear 1981;60:115-119.
6. Polyzois, G. L. *An update on denture fixatives.* Dent Update 1983;10:579-580, 582-573.
7. Adisman, I. K. *The use of denture adhesives as an aid to denture treatment.* J Prosthet Dent1989 ;62:711-715.
8. Grasso, J. E.; Rendell, J. and Gay, T. *Effect of denture adhesive on the retention and stability of maxillary dentures.* J Prosthet Dent 1994;72:399-405.
9. DeVengencie, J.; Ng, M. C.; Ford, P. and Iacopino, A. M. *In vitro evaluation of denture adhesives: possible efficacy of complex carbohydrates.* Int J Prosthodontics 1997;10:61-72.
10. Grasso, J. E. *Denture adhesives: changing attitudes.* J Am Dent Asso 1996;127:90-96.

24

Relining

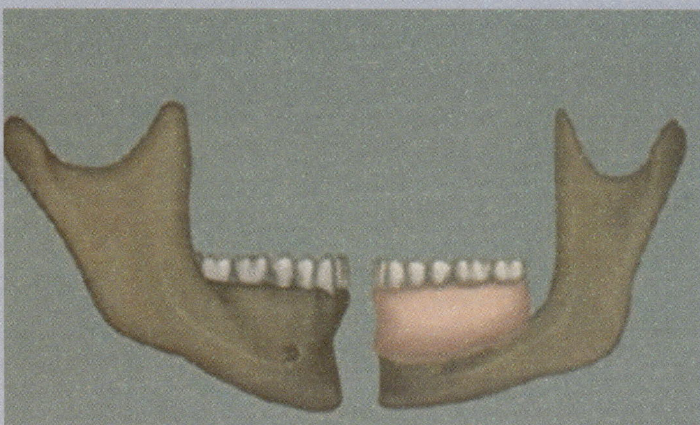

This is a a process that ensures intimate denture tissue interface

Relining in complete dentures

Even the most carefully fabricated complete dentures can produce adverse changes in the supporting tissues. Denture base materials are also subjected to change in due course of time. Eventually the fit of the denture is affected. To avoid remaking and to prevent further damage to the tissue, impression surface of the denture is modified through relining so that better fit is ensured matching to the altered supporting tissues. Relining procedure is the most commonly prescribed interventional procedure that involves the addition of a new layer of material to the existing denture base. According to Glossary of Prosthodontic Terms (GPT) 8, the procedures used to resurface the tissue side of a removable dental prosthesis with new base material, thus producing an accurate adaptation to the denture foundation area are called relining.

Diagnosis

Patients who have worn dentures for a long time usually seek dental care when the dentures are not well fitting, causing soreness, unable to chew well, and when the height of the lower third of face is reduced. These difficulties may have been caused due to two reasons viz occlusal discrepencies that existed at the time the dentures were made or,changes in the denture bearing area. It is essential that the cause be determined before any attempt is made to correct them.

Dentures with built-in errors in occlusion cannot be compensated by relining. Occlusal correction will be the treatment of choice. If the dentures are not stable because of preexisting occlusal errors, they get unseated with minimal force and the supporting tissues may show signs of irritation or inflammation predominantly on one side of the mouth than on the other. In such cases, use of dentures has to be discontinued for 1 or 2 days and a reevaluation of the dentures with pressure indicator paste is carried out. Modifications of the dentures are carried out accordingly. Clinical remount and occlusal adjustments can also be carried out. These procedures will eliminate the cause of the oral discomfort and make the dentures comfortable and serviceable without relining.

A change in the basal seats of the dentures usually is revealed by looseness and movement of the prosthesis on clinical examination, general soreness and inflammation, discernible loss of the occlusal vertical dimension and compromised esthetics. Overextension of denture flanges can cause ulcerations or hyperplastic tissue in the sulci. If the supporting tissue is traumatized,correction of the extension of dentures and surgical modifications to eliminate the hyperplasia may be necessary before relining impressions are made. Resorption of the bone of the maxillae usually permits the upper denture to move up and back in relation to its original position. Patients may complain of pain in the anterior vestibule, below the nose. However, the occlusion also may force the maxillary denture forward. The lower denture usually moves down and forward, but it may move down and back relative to the mandible as resorption occurs.

Indications for relining

1. Immediate dentures are relined after three to six months.
2. When the residual alveolar ridges have resorbed and the adaptation of the denture bases to the ridges is compromised.
3. When the patient cannot afford the cost of having new dentures constructed.
4. When the construction of new dentures with the accompanying series of appointments can cause physical or mental stress, such as for geriatric or chronically ill patients.

General Considerations

A thorough examination of the patient and of the existing dentures must be carried out before commencing therapy. The following points should receive special attention.

1. The occlusal vertical dimension should be satisfactory.
2. Intercuspal position should match with centric relation

3. The appearance must be accept¬able to the patient and dentist. The size, shape, shade, and arrangement of the artificial teeth must be satisfactory.
4. The posterior limit of the maxillary den¬ture should be adequate.
5. The border extensions, appropriate.

Contraindications: The dentures should not be relined when one or more of the following conditions do exist.

1. Excessive amount of resorption has taken place.
2. Presence of abused soft tissues. Relining is not indicated until the tissues recover and return as closely as possible to the normal form.
3. Patient's with temporo-mandibular joint problems. Until accurate diag¬nosis and treatment of the problem has been undertaken, relining is contrain¬dicated.
4. Dentures with poor esthetics or unsatisfactory jaw relationships, creating speech problems.
5. Presence of osseous undercuts, until surgical removal and healing occurs, relining need not be considered.

Relining procedures

Dentures can be relined either using chairside or laboratory technique.

Chairside technique :

Space for relining material is created by removing the denture base material from the tissue surface of the denture , while keeping three specific areas viz one in the anterior and two in posterior – are kept intact to serve as stops. If the denture stability is compromised and the fitting surface is worn off, stops have to be createdby placing putty impression material.

Relining with putty stops :

The denture surface is thoroughly cleaned. Tray adhesive is applied in three select areas- one in the anterior region and two in the posterior region of the intaglio surface. Putty elastomeric patches of 10 mm are placed in these areas and the denture is pressed against the residual ridge. The mandibular denture is stabilized first by asking the patient to close in centric occlusion. Once putty is set, the denture is removed and the excess material flown is removed with a sharp knife. Then denture relining material (acrylic based) is mixed and applied on the intaglio surface avoiding the putty stops . The denture is then placed over the ridge and the patient is asked to bite against the opposing denture. Denture is removed after solidification of the reline material. The putty stops are removed and in that place, reline material is applied and the denture is reseated. This completes the relining of one denture. The opposing denture can be relined similarly.

If the dentures are stable preparation of stops are not made with putty, instead the intaglio surface of the denture is relieved by 2mm except in three areas – one in the anterior and two in the posterior region. These areas will act as stops. After grinding, the intaglio surface is cleaned and the denture relining material (acrylic based) is mixed and applied avoiding the stops. The mandibular denture is stabilized by asking the patient to close in centric occlusion. Once reline material is set, the denture is removed and the excess material flown is trimmed. The opposing denture is relined similarly.

Suggested readings

1. Zarb, Bolender, *Prosthodontic treatment for edentulous patient,* 12th edition St. Louis, Mosby publications, 2004, Pp 471 - 480.
2. Winkler S, *Essentials of complete denture Prosthodontics,* 2nd edition, India, A.I.T.B.S publishers and distributors, 2009, Pp 341 – 360.
3. Morrow, Rudd, Rhoads, *Dental laboratory procedures,* Volume 1, 2nd edition, Missouri, Mosby publications, 1996, Pp 364-383.
4. Rahn AO, Heartwell CM, *Textbook of Complete dentures,* 5th edition, 1993,USA, pp 425-431
5. Kim et al, *Effect of Relining Method on Dimensional Accuracy of Posterior Palatal Seal. An In Vitro Study,* J Prosthodont 2008, 17:211–8
6. Assery M.K, *Chair side denture relining with VLC resin -new materials report,* The Saudi Dental Journal,1991; 3:35-41.

Method 1

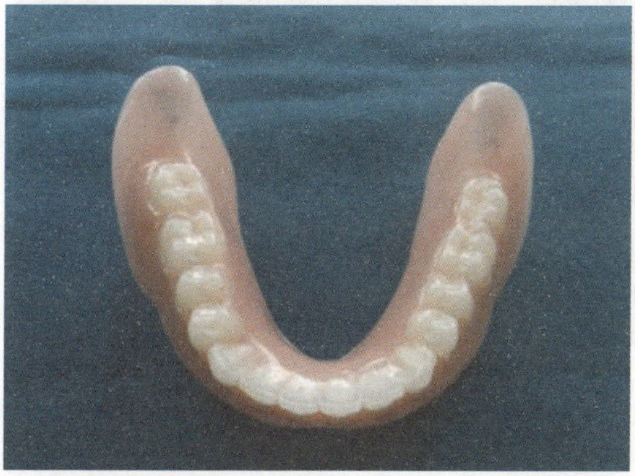

Fig. 24.1 Mandibular denture

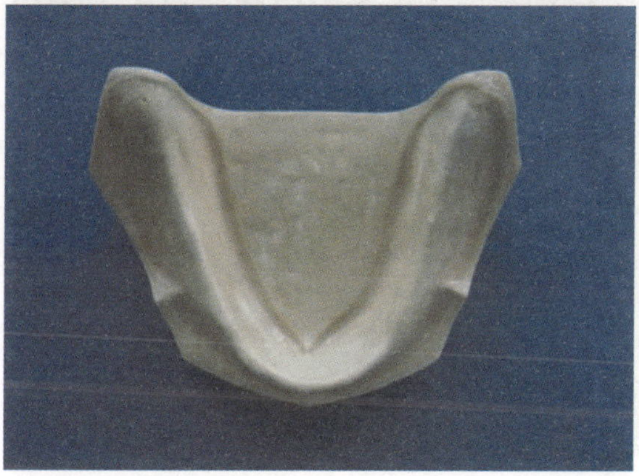

Fig. 24.2 Mandibular cast

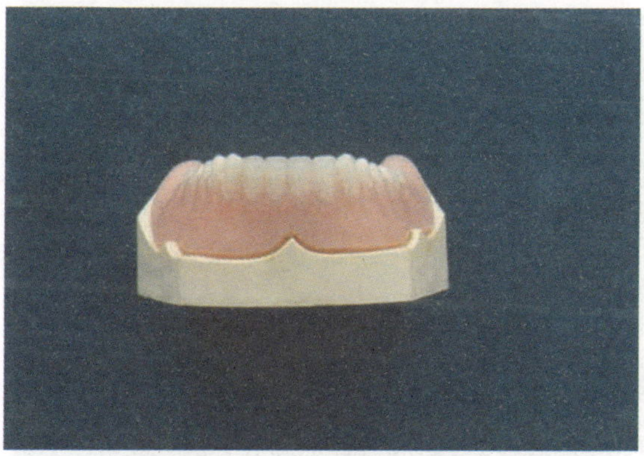

Fig. 24.3 Space observed between the cast and the denture

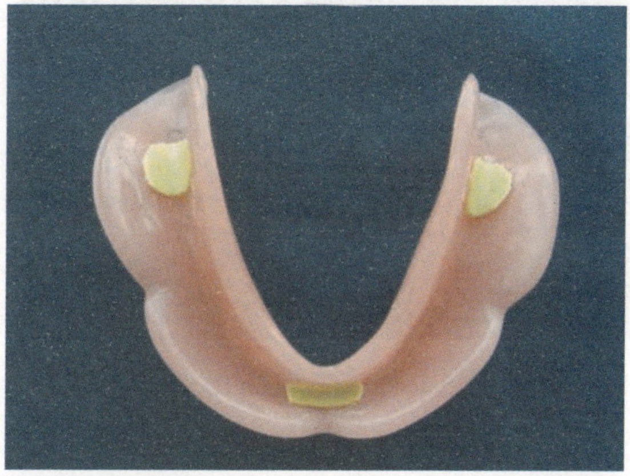

Fig. 24.4 Putty stops

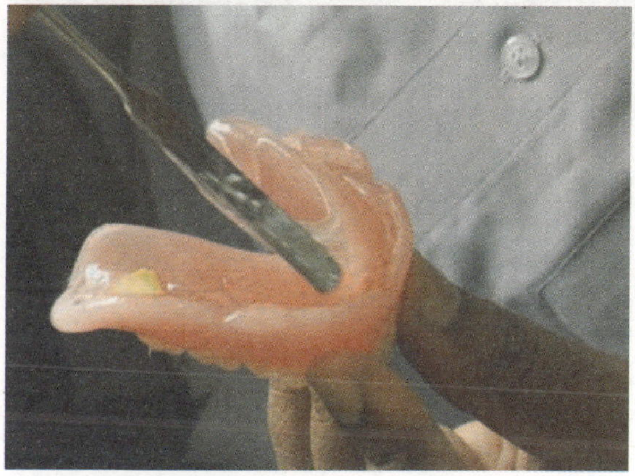

Fig. 24.5 Reline material applied on the intaglio surface of the denture

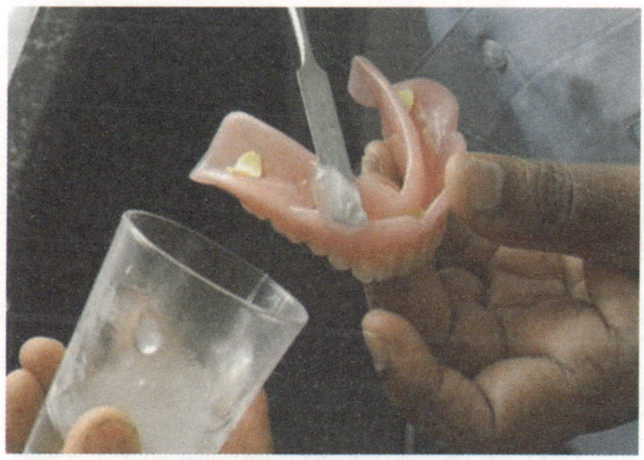

Fig. 24.6 Acrylic based denture relining material applied on the denture border area

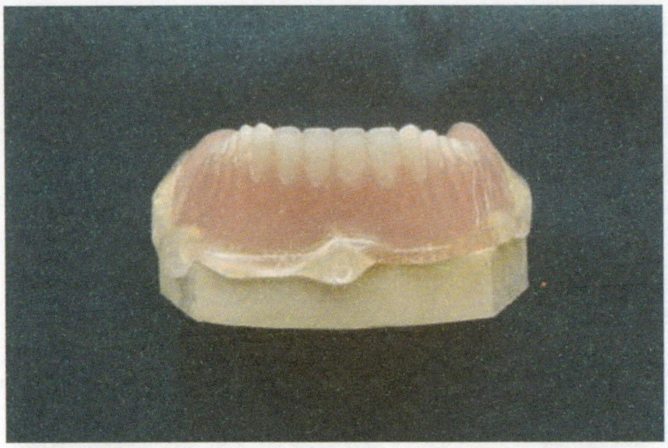

Fig. 24.7 Relined denture seated on the cast

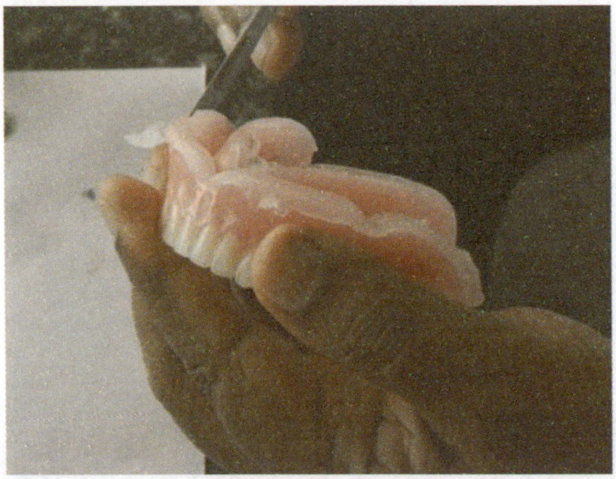

Fig. 24.8 Excess reline material removed with sharp knife

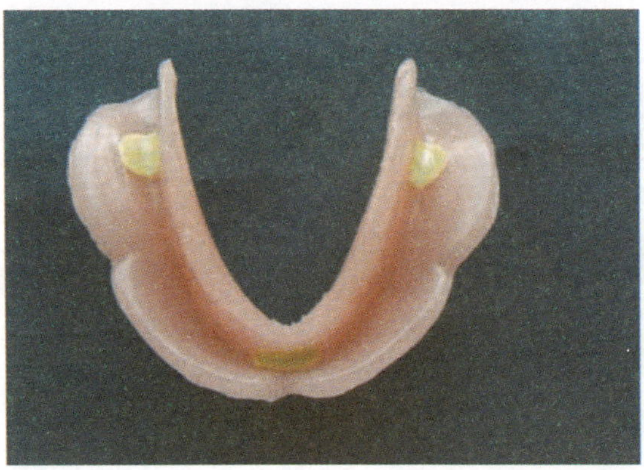

Fig. 24.9 Putty stops exposed

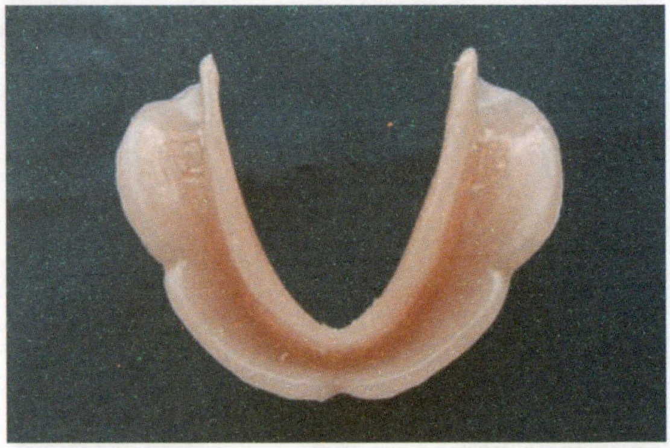

Fig. 24.10 Relined denture after removal of putty stops

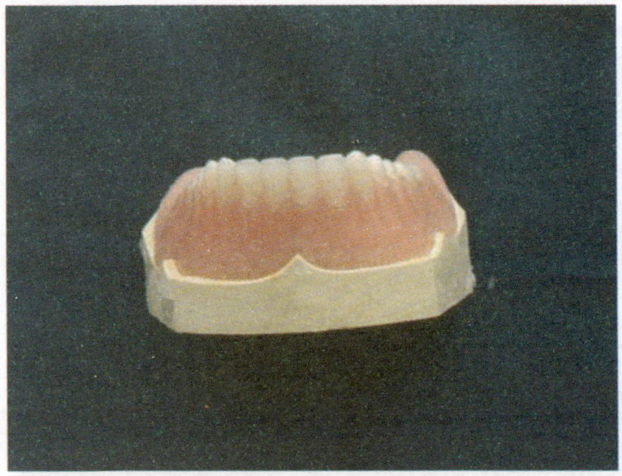

Fig. 24.11 Reline material placed in the region of putty stops

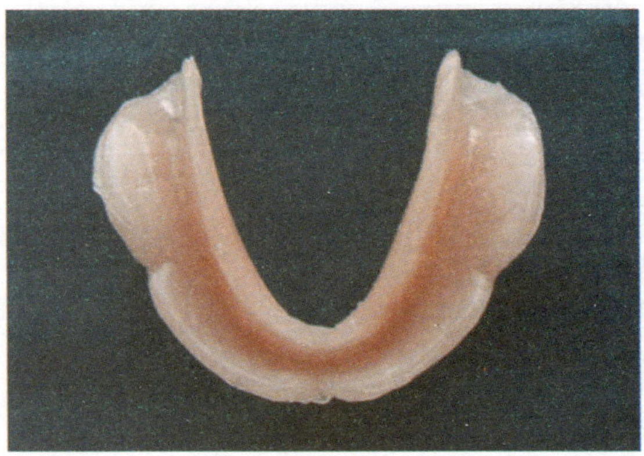

Fig. 24.12 Relined mandibular denture

Method 2

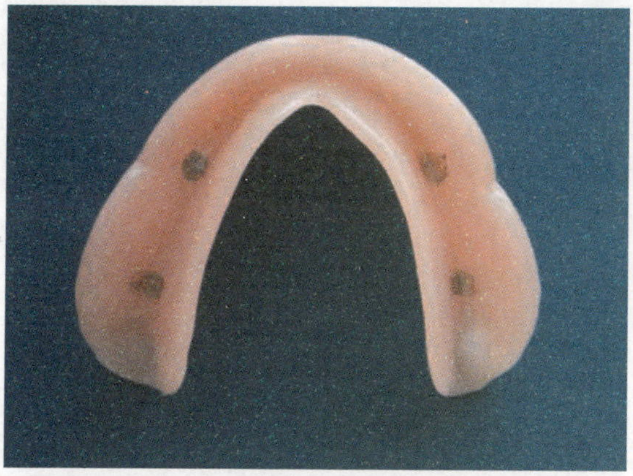

Fig. 24.13 Stop regions marked

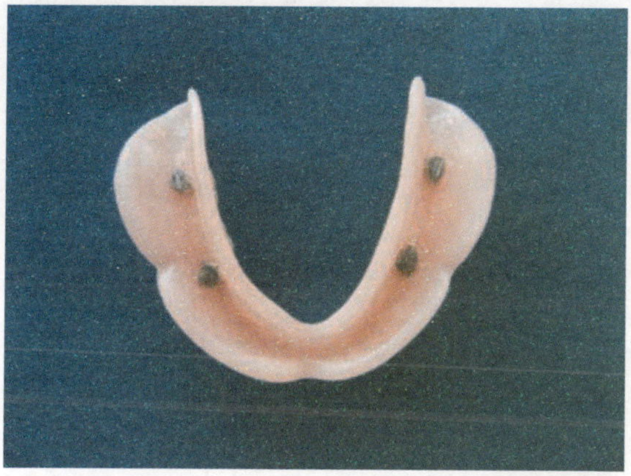

Fig. 24.14 Surface uniformly ground excepting the marked stop areas

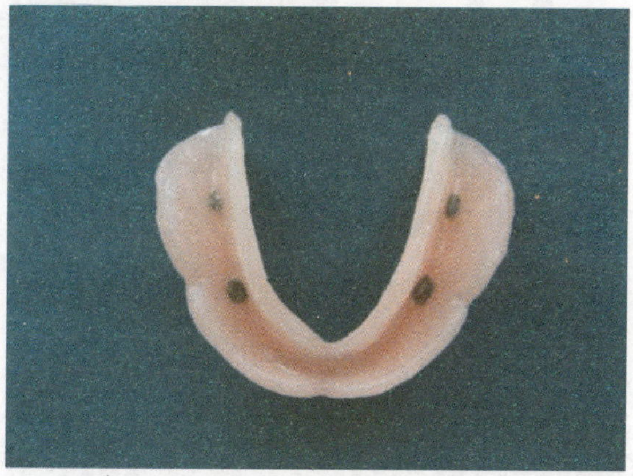

Fig. 24.15 Denture relined and the stops are exposed

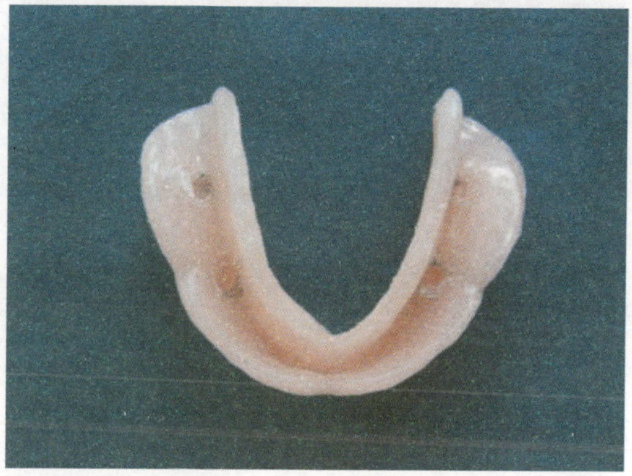

Fig. 24.16 Stops removed with tungsten carbide trimmer

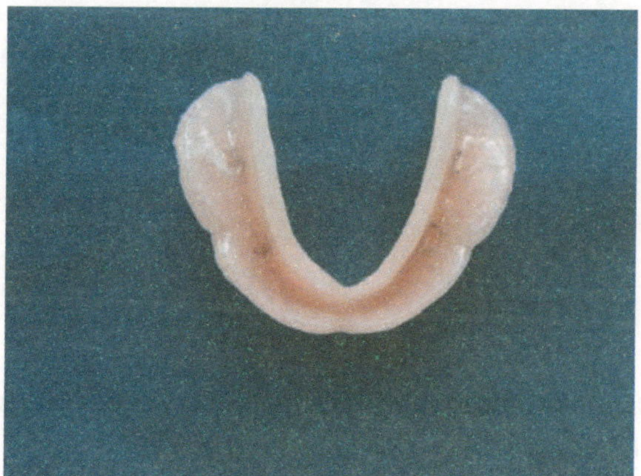

Fig. 24.17 Denture reline complete

25

Immediate dentures

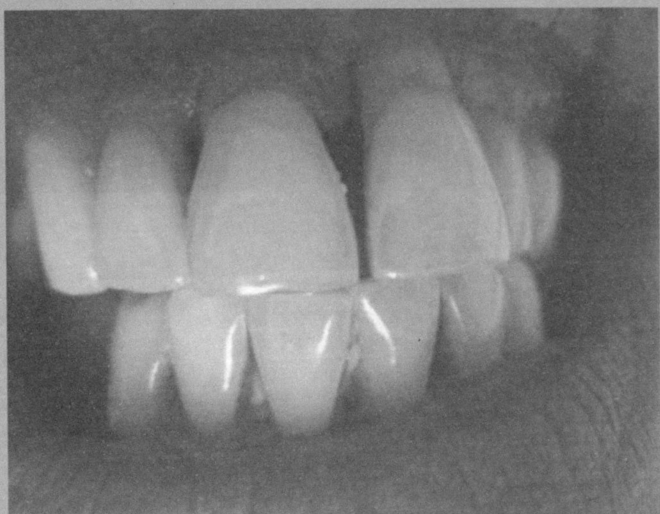

Patients who cannot compromise with the phase of edentulism require immediate dentures

A partially edentulous situation where existing teeth cannot be preserved because of compromised health generally requires dental extraction and complete dentures. (fig.25.1) But many individuals cannot accept the phase of complete edentulism especially the long healing phase. For them immediate complete

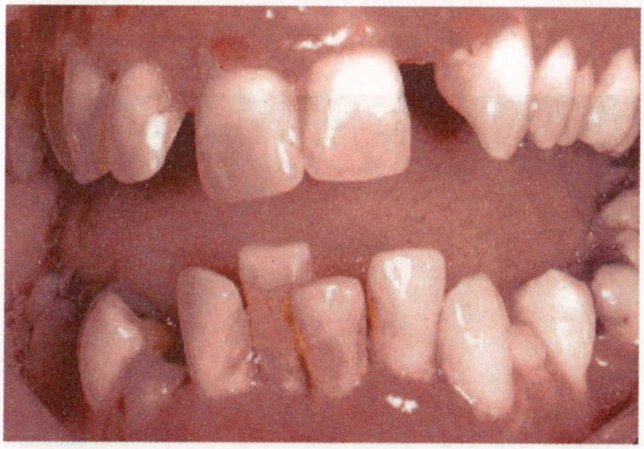

Fig.25.1 Periodontally compromised teeth. a candidate for complete immediate denture

denture is a boon. Immediate dentures are prepared before dental extraction and the dentures are inserted soon after dental extraction. Immediate denture acts as a bandage of the extraction wound, controls bleeding, avoids food particles from entering the tooth sockets, protects blood clot and promotes rapid healing. Immediate denture maintains the facial appearance as well as circumoral support, muscle tone, vertical dimension of occlusion, jaw relationship, and face height. The tongue will not spread out as a result of tooth loss. It is easier to duplicate (if desired) the natural tooth shape and position, plus arch form and width. If desired, the horizontal and vertical positions of the anterior teeth can be replicated accurately.Irrespective of the fact that the ridges are subjected to early function, less resorption takes place and the resultant ridges are better preserved and adapted to supporting a complete denture. Overall, the patient's psychological and social well-being is preserved.

The procedure is time consuming and requires more appointments especially during the adjustment phase. There is no opportunity to observe the anterior teeth at the try in appointment, hence the esthetic result cannot be evaluated until the dentures are inserted.

The immediate denture may be subjected to relining or refabrication in six months to one year following insertion. The dentist should inform the patient of this prior to the start of the treatment. Due to increased treatment time, postoperative adjustments and the need to remake or reline the denture, the treatment becomes expensive.

Method

Review of medical and dental history, clinical oral examination and radiographic evaluation is the first stage. Mounted diagnostic casts help in evaluation

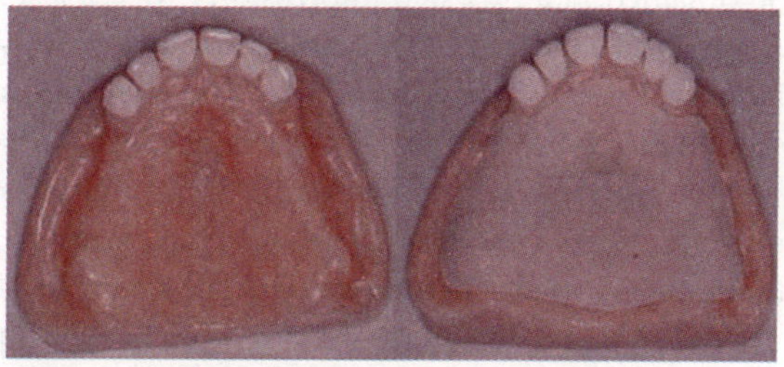

Fig.25.2 Posterior teeth are extracted and allowed to heal. Custom made tray to cover the edentulous areas

of tooth position, occlusal plane discrepancies and presence of undercuts. Posterior teeth are extracted in advance and any needed preprosthetic surgery performed at the initial surgery appointment. (fig.25.2) If first premolars can be preserved along with the anteriors, maintenance of vertical height becomes easy. However they have to be modified to match with centric relation. A healing period of 8 to 12 weeks is allowed prior to starting impression procedures. Initial impressions are made with alginate in a stock tray.

Cast is prepared. The teeth are covered with double thickness of baseplate wax which provides space for the impression material around the teeth. A custom tray is fabricated with autopolymerising acrylic resin. The tray is placed in the patient's mouth and checked for correct extension. Border moulding is done with silicone putty. Final impression is made with light or regular body silicone. Impression can

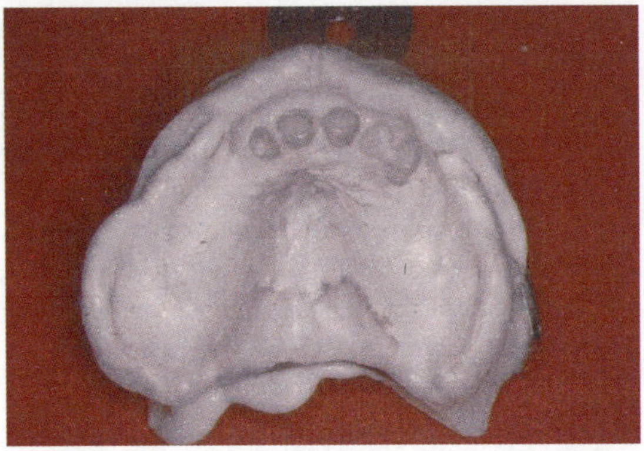

Fig.25.3 Border moulded impression of the edentulous area is picked up by an over impression made in a stock tray.

be obtained in a two step impression process also. A preliminary cast is made and a custom tray is fabricated that covers only the posterior edentulous section of the cast. Tray is border moulded with silicone putty and impression of the edentulous area is made in light or regular body silicone. An over impression is made in alginate in stock tray. (fig.25.3)

After alginate sets the stock tray is removed along with custom tray which is embedded in the impression. The impression is poured with dental stone.

Registration of jaw relations

Transfer base is prepared in autopolymerising acylic resin and wax rims are prepared at the edentulous areas. Maxillary cast is mounted on the articulator using face bow. Occlusal vertical dimension can be established easily if patient has posterior teeth to serve as occlusal stops. Phonetic evaluation of closest speaking space can provide added information on the validity of vertical dimension. If patient has no posterior teeth to serve as stop, vertical dimension is determined as in the case of a completely edentulous individual. The mandibular cast is mounted using centric relation record.

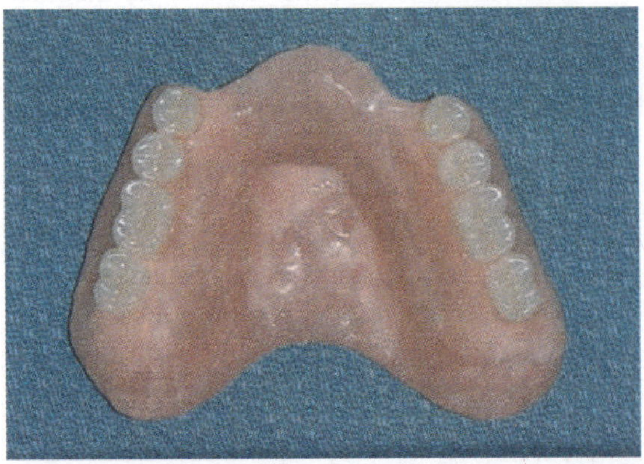

Fig.25.4 Trial denture- posteriors only

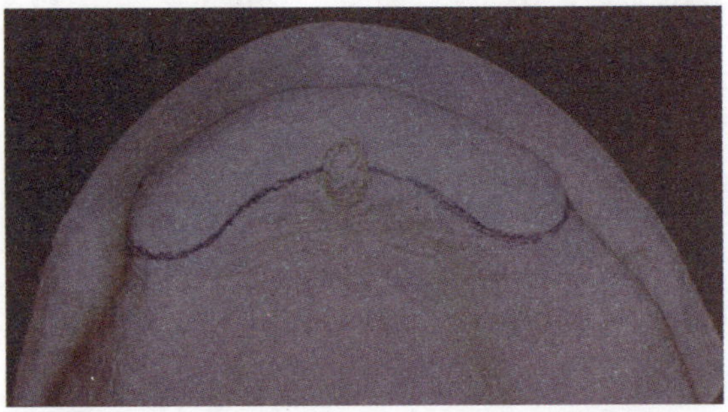

Fig. 25.5 Anterior teeth were removed and the cast is modified

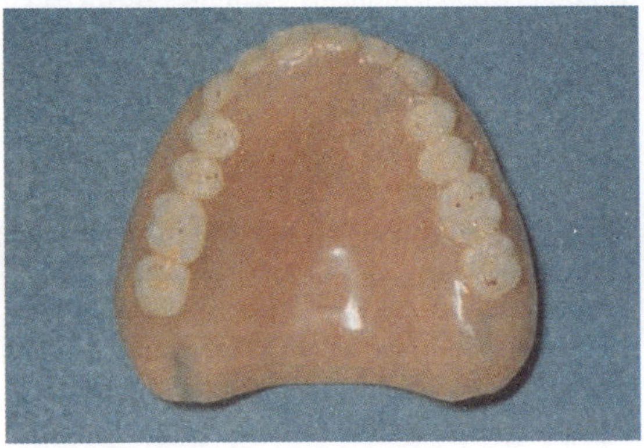

Fig. 25.6 Anteriors are arranged on modified cast and processed

Tooth selection and arrangement

The existing dentition is utilized in selecting the shade and mold of the teeth. Posterior teeth are arranged first and they ensure multiple holding contacts (fig.25.4). Anterior teeth contacts are usually avoided at centric relation to simulate the complete denture situation. Verification of centric relation and vertical dimension is done as in complete dentures.

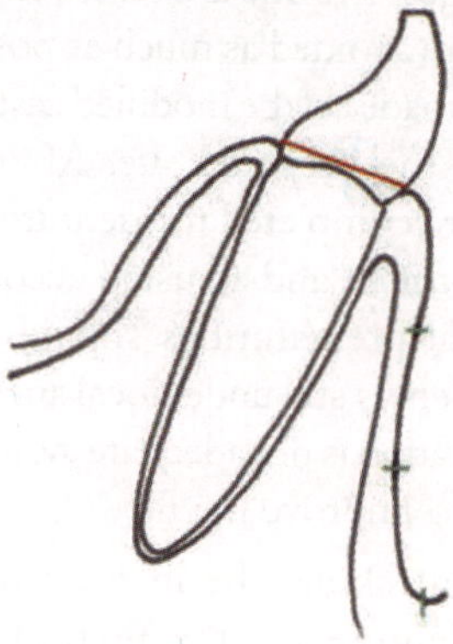

Fig.25.7 Remove tooth at gingival level

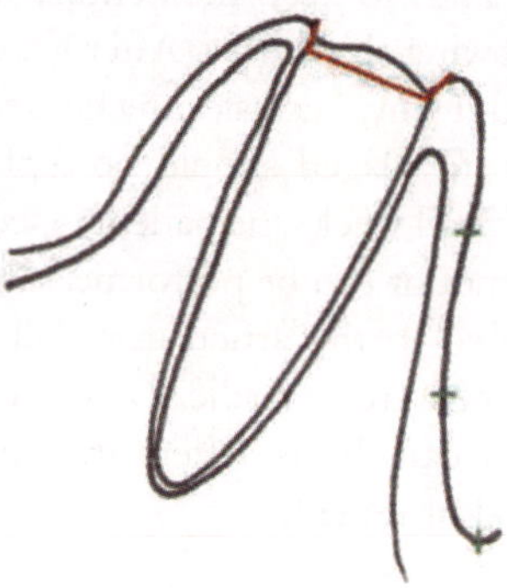

Fig.25.8 Recess Socket 1 mm

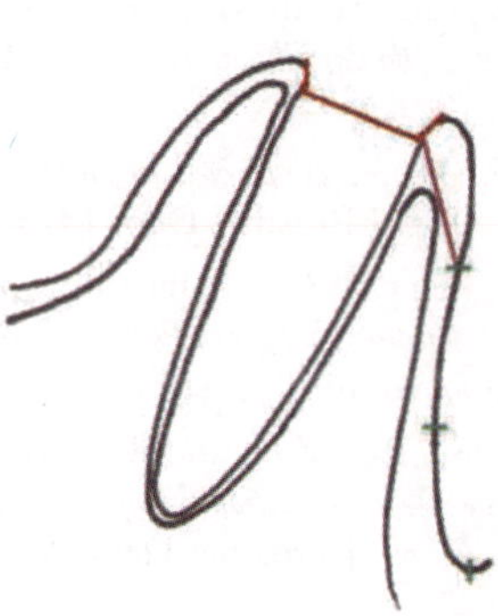

Fig.25.9 Labial edge recess to incisal third mark

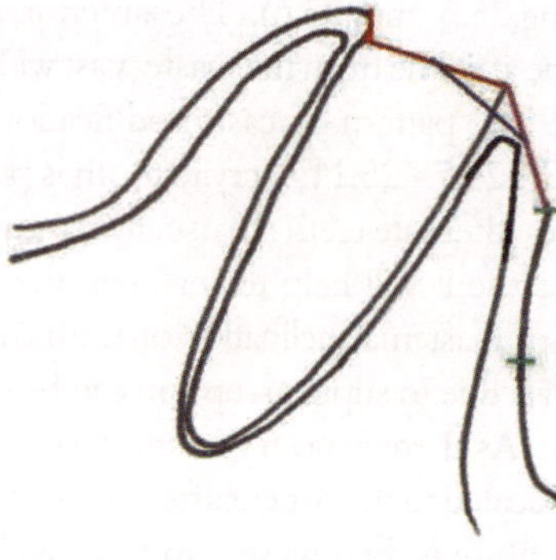

Fig.25.10 Mid-point recess to mid-width labial cut

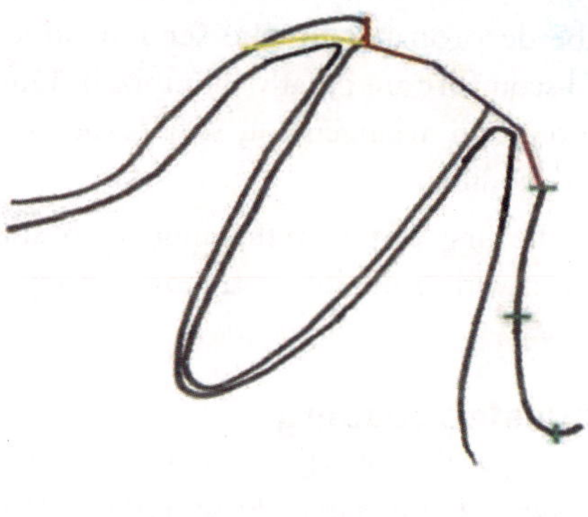

Fig.25.11 Round off labial to middle third, sand smooth

Arrangement of anterior teeth

After posterior try in appointment, anterior teeth are arranged (fig.25.5 and 25.6). The anterior teeth are removed one at a time from the master cast with a rotary instrument. The pattern of cast modification is given in figures. fig. 25.7 - 25.11 Acrylic tooth is positioned in that place. Alternate teeth are usually removed in the process because it will help to maintain the position. Correction of diastema, inclination of teeth and change in incisal level due to supra eruption can be corrected at this stage. As there is no try in stage, changes must be communicated to the patient after the posterior trial. The trial denture is then waxed up to provide proper contour and thickness of denture base, followed by the processing.

Insertion of immediate denture

There are two options, viz a) the teeth are extracted and immediate denture is inserted, Otherwise b) the teeth to be extracted can be root canal treated and on the day of denture insertion all the teeth can be decoronated. In the second option, pain and discomfort are greatly minimized. During the anterior teeth arrangement, soft tissue areas need not be modified.

In the first option remaining teeth should be removed with a minimum trauma. Bony spicules and sharp edges of bone are removed. Use of flaps and sutures are avoided as much as possible. A clear surgical stent made on the modified cast will be useful in evaluating the prepared site. After the surgical procedures are completed the denture is positioned and checked for fit and adjusted accordingly. Then gross occlusal prematurities should be corrected while the patient is still under local anesthesia. If the denture adaptation is not adequate tissue conditioner can be used to improve the fit.

The patient should be instructed to wear the immediate denture for the first 24 hours and a check up is done after that. Occlusion is checked. The denture is carefully removed and the tissues are evaluated for ulceration from denture pressure. After 48 hours the patient is seen again. The patient is instructed to clean the dentures several times a day and to keep the denture during night for the following three days. After a week sutures are removed if any, occlusion rechecked and tissue conditioner if placed should be replaced at this stage. After 3 – 4 weeks the patient is seen again and a clinical remount can be performed and occlusion can be refined in the articulator. Till six months resilient linings are periodically repeated. By that time tissue usually heals. Afterwards the denture is either relined or remade.

Suggested reading

1. Heartwell C., and Salisbury F. W., *Immediate complete dentures: An evaluation.* J Prosthet Dent 15:615-624, 1965.
2. LaVere A. M., and Krol A. J., *Immediate denture service.* J Prosthet Dent 1973;29:10-15.
3. Campagna S. J., *An impression technique for immediate dentures.* J Prosthet Dent 1968;20:196-203.
4. Jerbi F. C., *Trimming the cast in the construction of immediate dentures.* J Prosthet Dent 1966;16:1047-1053.
5. Payne S. H., *A transitional denture.* J Prosthet Dent 1964;14:221-230.
6. Demer W., *Minimizing problems in placement of immediate dentures.* J Prosthet Dent 1972;27:275-284.
7. Chierci G., Parker M. L., and Hemphill C. D., *Influence of immediate dentures on oral motor skill and speech.* J Prosthet Dent 1978;39:21-28.
8. Passamonti G., Kottrajarus P., Gheewala R.K., Clark R.E., and Manness W. L., *Effect of immediate denture on maxillomandibular relations.* J Prosthet Dent 1981;45(2):122-26.
9. Morrow R. M., et al. *Immediate interim tooth-supported complete dentures.* J Prosthet Dent 1973;30:695-700
10. Tallgren A., Lang B. R. and Miller R.J. *Longitudinal Study of Soft-tissue Profile Changes in Patients Receiving Immediate Complete Dentures.* Int J Prosthodont 1991;4:9-16
11. Gardner L.K., Parr G.R., and Rahn A.O., *Modification of Immediate Denture Sectional Impression Technique using Vinyl Polysiloxane.* J Prosthet Dent 1990;64:182-184

26

Single complete dentures

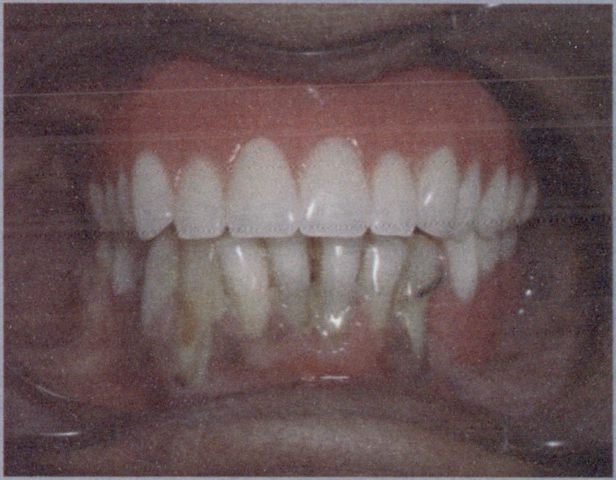

Fabrication of single denture requires special skill in designing the occlusal scheme

Single complete denture is a complete denture that occludes against some or all of the natural teeth, a fixed restoration, or a previously constructed removable partial denture or a complete denture. Single dentures are more often fabricated in the maxillary arch, as these teeth are usually lost before their mandibular antagonists. Mandibular single dentures should rarely be considered, unless a means of stress reduction can be used - a processed resilient denture liner, overdenture or implant retained denture. Otherwise rapid and severe residual ridge resorption can result from the forces on the mandibular ridge. Single dentures tend to be difficult to fabricate for the following reasons:

1. More force from the opposing natural dentition tends to displace the denture and cause fracture due to flexure.
2. Greater forces from the natural dentition, especially, anterior teeth tend to result in severe residual ridge resorption, making denture retention and stability more difficult yet. (Combination Syndrome)
3. Tooth malpositions like extrusion, tipping and rotations cause the denture to be less stable and difficult to get balanced articulation
4. Supra-eruption of the opposing natural teeth produces an in harmonious occlusal plane, and minimizes the vertical space for setting the opposing denture teeth.

Treatment differs from normal complete denture therapy. Occlusal adjustment of natural teeth may be required to level the plane of occlusion by reducing severe curve of Spee (Fig 26.1), leveling steps in the occlusal plane caused by supraeruptions (Fig 26.2) and alter the contour of rotated teeth to permit bilateral contacts on flat surfaces.

A single complete denture may oppose any one of the following conditions viz natural teeth, a partially edentulous arch in which the missing teeth have been or will be replaced by either fixed or removable partial dental prosthesis or an existing complete denture. Treatment planning depends mainly upon the clinical situation which is presented by the patient. They can be any one of the following:

- Maxillary denture opposing natural mandibular teeth (commonest)
- Mandibular denture opposing natural maxillary teeth (very rarely)
- Maxillary denture opposing a combination of natural teeth with either fixed or removable partial dentures
- Single denture fabricated against an existing denture
- Maxillary complete denture opposing implant supported prosthesis

Commonly occurring conditions are explained below.

Complete maxillary denture opposing natural mandibular teeth

This situation is complicated by an uneven support. Mean mucosal denture bearing area of edentulous maxilla is 23 cm^2 and edentulous mandible is 12 cm^2. Where as the mean surface area of total periodontium of maxillary dentition and mandibular dentition is 45 cm^2 each. The patient can generate heavy occlusal forces, due to the existence of opposing natural teeth. The mucosa (denture foundation tissue) is unsuitable to resist high occlusal forces from the opposing natural teeth, which results in advanced bone loss of the residual alveolar ridges. This particular situation can fall into the following categories:

1. Opposing full natural mandibular dentition (Shortened Dental Arch)
2. Opposing natural mandibular posterior teeth (Kennedy Class IV)
3. Opposing natural mandibular anterior teeth (Kennedy Class I)
4. Opposing bounded edentulous space with modification spaces (Kennedy Class III)
5. Opposing implant supported prostheses

Mandibular occlusal plane is generally determined by arbitrary anatomic guides:

- Lower lip line at rest
- Corners of the mouth (mesial slope of mand. canine)

- Equatorial plane of the tongue
- ½ to ⅔ height of retromolar pads

The common problem posed is that of occlusal discrepancies and is far from ideal. Teeth are malopposed, tipped, rotated and/or extruded. First molars and second premolars are often lost making the remaining molars tilt mesially and distal halves supra-erupt. The poor quality of the resulting occlusal plane, cause interference in protrusive and lateral excursive movement. It will be difficult to achieve balanced occlusion. The expected complications will be loss of denture seal and/or trauma to the residual ridge, accelerated bone loss and soft tissue hyperplasia. Natural occlusal form and morphology usually does not match with that of the denture teeth

Occlusal plane is improved by

a. Enameloplasty (recontontouring/ odontoplasty/ selective grinding)
b. Fixed restorations (onlays, crowns, FPDs)
c. Orthodontic intrusion/ uprighting
d. Removable partial denture/ overlay denture
e. Dental extraction (last choice)
f. Minimizing steep cusps and deep anterior overbite.

In conventional complete dentures, 2 mm of overjet and overbite is dictated by esthetics and phonetics which can be altered easily by the dentist. However, in single maxillary denture, the overjet and overbite is dictated by the position of the existing natural mandibular teeth. Hence, occlusal rim is modified to accommodate the mandibular anteriors and which allows protrusive movement.

Mandibular denture opposing natural maxillary teeth

This situation is the least favoured in single dentures. Preservation of the mandibular ridge against maxillary teeth is possible only with tooth root or dental implant supported dentures. Conventional dentures if designed should at least have a resilient liner to absorb the excessive forces exerted by the natural teeth. Physiologic tolerance of forces of teeth as well as mucosa is given below.

Teeth: upto 300 lbs/inch^2

Periodontal ligament (pdl) width:

0.25 mm (0.15-0.38 mm)

0.21 mm (11-16 years)

0.18 mm (32-52 years)

0.15 mm (51-67 years)

Majority of periodontal fibres are oriented obliquely which can tolerate vertical axial loading approximately 17 times better than lateral non-axial loading. Edentulous mucosa has a width of 1-2mm and can tolerate loading up to 30 lbs/inch^2

Mandibular residual ridge area is comparatively low when maxillary residual ridge area is considered and there is a likelihood of stress concentration on the mandibular ridge. That is why the mandibular single denture is not always favourably considered. However there are certain situations where a mandibular complete denture, opposing upper natural teeth are accepted viz Class III jaw relationship - this occurs when the mandible is larger than normal or the maxilla is smaller than normal and cleft palate

Complete maxillary denture to oppose a partially edentulous mandibular arch and fixed prosthesis

It must be determined first whether fixed restorations are possible in the mandibular arch. If fixed partial dentures are possible, the material used for the fabrication is a matter of concern. If the fixed partial dentures have ceramic occlusals, either porcelain or resin teeth can be used for the maxillary denture. If the maxillary denture has to oppose tooth enamel or gold occlusal surfaces, then gold or resin teeth can be used.

Complete maxillary denture to oppose a partially edentulous arch and a removable partial denture

Remaining mandibular teeth should be in an acceptable state of dental health. The partial denture should meet minimal acceptable requirements. The occlusal plane, tooth arrangement for occlusion, esthetics and the material composition of the removable partial denture should be suitable to be opposed by a complete denture. It is better to construct both the removable partial denture and maxillary complete denture at the same time.

Single complete denture opposing an existing denture

The following questions have to be analyzed before giving a single complete denture opposing an existing complete denture.

- How long has the existing denture been in use?
- Was the denture an immediate insertion at the time of tooth removal?
- Does the denture meet the requirements of an acceptable denture?
- Has the denture opposed another complete denture, a partially edentulous arch that supported a removable partial denture, restored natural teeth, a fixed partial denture?
- Is the operator satisfied to institute complete denture procedures utilizing the existing denture?

Preference should be given for the refabrication of both the upper and lower dentures if the existing complete denture is not satisfactory to be used.

Mouth preparation

In order to obtain balanced occlusion, it is desirable to establish a reasonable occlusal plane in the arch containing natural teeth. Modifications are made in the case of malposed teeth, severely tipped teeth, supra erupted teeth, irregular occlusal plane and less space for teeth

Methods for mouth preparation

In case of single maxillary denture opposing mandibular natural teeth which is the most common situation that a patient presents with, mouth preparation can be done with any one of the following methods described in literature.

Swenson's technique

a. Mount the maxillary edentulous cast and the mandibular cast on a semi-adjustable articulator using an arbitrary facebow and centric relation record at the established vertical dimension of occlusion.

b. Make a protrusive record and set the horizontal condylar guidance (condyle angle).

c. Set the upper artificial teeth one by one on the denture base and adjust the lower occluding stone teeth (by scraping) in order to establish a harmonious occlusal plane. Mark the area of the stone teeth that have been altered.

d. When a favorable occlusal plane and articulation of the teeth have been achieved, the occlusal adjustment is then carried out on the natural teeth in the mouth using the marked diagnostic cast and the trial denture set up as guides.

e. After the occlusal adjustment is been made in the mouth, a new impression of the natural teeth is obtained, a new centric relation record is made, and the new lower cast is mounted on the semi-adjustable articulator.

f. The maxillary artificial teeth are rearranged for harmony in centric relation occlusion and in excursive movements. The next clinical step is the try in of the trial wax up maxillary complete denture.

Yurkstas technique

a. A metal 'U' shaped occlusal template which is slightly convex on the lower surface is used.

b. The template is placed on the occlusal surfaces of the remaining teeth and cusps to be adjusted are identified.(Fig 26.3)

c. Stone cast is modified to an acceptable occlusal relationship and the reduced areas are marked with a pencil. (Fig 26.4)

d. Necessary alterations are done on the natural teeth using the cast as a guide

Bruce technique

a. The lower dentulous and upper edentulous casts are mounted in an articulator with jaw relation records.

b. Necessary modifications are made on the stone cast.

c. An acrylic resin template is fabricated on the modified stone cast (Fig 26.5)

d. Template is positioned in the patient's mouth to check interferences and the interferences are removed by modifying the teeth

e. Process is repeated until the template seats properly.

In general, the mandibular occlusal plane is modified first. If the anterior teeth are supra erupted, the incisal plane has to be brought down. (Fig 26.6) The overjet and overbite of the maxillary single denture will be dictated by the lower natural anterior teeth. Most often 2mm of overjet is difficult to obtain and hence the vertical overlap is also restricted. An edge to edge position can be obtained and is usually accepted.

In order to establish a reasonable occlusal plane, either the occlusal surfaces of the posterior teeth has to be built using restorative materials or reduced by enameloplasty. To build the occlusal surfaces a diagnostic wax up is done,(Fig 26.7) duplicate cast obtained (Fig 26.8,26.9) and a vaccuform template is made on this duplicated cast (Fig 26.10). Using this template, the occlusal surfaces can be built using composite restorative material (Fig 26.11, 26.12). For enameloplasty, a wax or vaccuform template can be made use of. The cusps of lower posterior teeth which are above the decided occlusal plane are marked with a pencil. For making wax template one layer of modeling wax is adapted on to the occlusal surface of the teeth extending to occlusal thirds of buccal and lingual surfaces and then the marked areas are exposed using a sharp instrument. (Fig 26.13) The wax/ vaccuform template is then transferred in to the patient's mouth and the cusps that are exposed are trimmed to the level of the wax (26.14-26.15). The altered surfaces of the teeth are finished and polished. An impression is now made and this cast is mounted against which the maxillary teeth are arranged.

Impression procedure

For edentulous arch preliminary impression is made with putty consistency elastomer, impression compound or irreversible hydrocolloid in a stock tray. Border molding is done with putty or green stick compound. Final impression is done with light or regular body elastomer. If hyperplastic tissue is present, the custom made tray is spaced or windowed over the flabby tissue and the impression is completed with light body elastomer.

Jaw relations

Face bow transfer, establishment of vertical dimension and registration of centric relation are similar to those followed in conventional complete dentures. In conventional complete dentures, the anterior plane of the maxillary occlusal rim determines the position of the maxillary anterior teeth. The posterior plane of the occlusal rim is made parallel to the camper's plane. However in maxillary single denture opposing mandibular natural teeth, the occlusal plane is dictated by the lower natural teeth. The mandibular anteriors are accommodated within the maxillary occlusal rim so that vertical overlap is included. (Fig 26.16 A,B) For this purpose, a window is created in the anterior region of the maxillary occlusion rim. In maxillary single denture, the posterior occlusion rim helps in establishing the vertical dimension. (Fig. 26.17)

Methods to achieve a harmonious balanced occlusion

1. Functional chew in technique
2. Articulator equilibration technique

1. Functional chew in technique

This is a method of recording functional occlusal paths. For this technique to be successful, record bases should have good stability, patient should have good neuro-muscular control and mental competence to effectively co-operate.

a After making impressions and casts, make occlusion rims in impression compound at the proper location.

b Transfer the cast and occlusion rim to an articulator.

c Compound maxillary occlusal rim is trimmed buccally and lingually so that occlusion is free in lateral excursions and at the same time the vertical height is maintained.

d Place soft carding wax on the rims and the patient is instructed to perform chewing movements

e Carding wax gets functionally molded whereas the compound rim in the central fossa maintains the vertical dimension.

f The generated occlusal rim is removed from the mouth and stone is vibrated into the wax path of the cusps and this record is secured to the lower member of the articulator.

g This lower stone path is what the upper teeth are set to and is in harmony with the condylar path.

h The upper posterior teeth are set against the lower stone model.

i The maxillary anterior teeth are checked for esthetics.

j After esthetics is approved at the try-in, lower cast chew in record is secured and all the interfering spots are ground. Thus in centric and in eccentric movements maximum bilateral balanced occlusion is established.

2. *Articulator equilibration technique*

This technique is preferred when denture bases are not stable and the neuro-muscular control of the patient is poor.

a Upper cast is mounted on the articulator using face-bow

b The lower cast is related to the upper by centric interocclusal record at an acceptable vertical dimension.

c The bucco- lingual position of the teeth and their relation to the upper arch is studied. Cusp-fossa relationship is maintained as far as possible.

d At the time of wax try-in, eccentric records are made, condylar inclinations are set and the posterior teeth are balanced.

e After denture is processed, it is again related to the mounted lower cast with a new centric interocclusal record. The condylar inclinations previously determined are reset on the articulator.

f Once the centric holding stops are re-established by selective grinding balance is achieved.However, perfectly balanced occlusion in all eccentric positions may not be possible in many cases when working with natural teeth in one arch.

Tooth material

Acrylic is the most preferred material of choice when teeth are selected. Ceramic teeth are selected when the opposing teeth are made of ceramic. The wear of acrylic teeth was compensated previously with amalgam inserts and by incorporating gold occlusal surfaces. However present day cross linked acrylic/composite resin teeth will not wear off that easily. Composite resin occlusal resin inserts are also recommended. A limited wear of teeth in single denture ensures harmonious relationship in due course of time.

Potential adverse treatment outcomes

Most common adverse sequelae are

1. Kelly's combination syndrome
2. Denture fracture
3. Tooth wear

Kelly's Combination syndrome

A series of destructive changes occurring in the jaws of the patients wearing a complete maxillary denture opposed by mandibular natural teeth as well distal extension partial denture(Kennedy Class I) has been described as "combination syndrome".

Description of features

Kelly (1972) put forward five features of combination syndrome.

- Loss of bone in anterior maxilla and subsequent replacement with flabby fibrous tissue.
- Down growth of the tuberosities
- Papillary hyperplasia of the palate
- Lower incisor supraeruption
- Bone loss under the removable prostheses.

Saunders et al (1978) added 6 more additional features

- Loss of vertical dimension
- Occlusal plane discrepancy
- Anterior spatial repositioning of the mandible

- Loss of stability and refabrication of the existing dentures
- Epulis fissuratum
- Periodontal problems of the remaining teeth

Mechanics

Kelly - Bone loss in the anterior maxilla is the first to occur

Saunders – Bone loss under the removable prosthesis was the root cause for the problem

Sequence of events

Continued bone loss under the removable prosthesis causes decreased occlusal load posteriorly. In an attempt to chew food, the patient tends to bring the mandibular arch forward. This results in mandibular natural anterior teeth applying load on the premaxillary region manifesting in resorption of bone in the anterior maxilla. As the fulcrum of rotation is in the cuspid – bicuspid region, the maxillary denture rotates upward in the anterior region and downward in posterior region resulting in change in occlusal plane. This causes negative pressure in the posterior palatal seal area because of which the tuberosity area grows down and papillary hyperplasia of the palate is also observed. This chain of events ultimately causes loss of stability of the denture. Resorption in the anterior maxilla causes labial flange to irritate the labial mucosa and produces epulis fissuratum. Lower anterior supra erupts and poor oral hygiene contributes to periodontal problem.

Systemic and dental considerations

a. Systemic factors - like diabetes and osteoporosis increases the rate of resorption of the bone.

b. Dental factors- In case of class III jaw relationships, there will be increased pressure in the anterior maxilla.When lower anteriors are retained for a long time, the patient is accustomed to bite in the anterior region.

Treatment planning

a. Prevention

- Retain weaker posterior teeth by using combined endodontic and periodontic techniques.
- Endosseous endodontic implants are used in the posterior mandibular region
- An overlay denture on the lower may avoid the combination syndrome

b. Modifications in removable partial denture and complete dentures

Kelly – advocated covering of retromolar pad to have stability of the lower removable partial denture.

Schumitt – advocated construction of lower removable partial denture first and then to construct the upper complete denture

c. Choice of occlusion

- Anterior teeth only for esthetics and phonetics.
- Posterior occlusion free of supra contacts during centric and all eccentric positions.
- During protrusive movement, there should be minimum contact in the anterior region, when posterior teeth are in contact.

d. Overdentures

- Lower anterior teeth are treated endodontically and their height is reduced.
- This can be used for proprioceptive sensation of the lower jaw and prevents resorption of the underlying bone.
- Langer advocated use of "stud attachments" in overdenture.

e. Implant – supported prosthesis

Implants can be placed in the posterior region of the mandible to decrease the residual ridge resorption

f. Surgical consideration

Kelly advocated surgical excision of the maxillary tuberosity fibrous growth to establish proper occlusion.

- Treating the combination syndrome requires recognition of the factors involved.
- Frequent recalls visits and check ups with frequent relining to compensate for the resorption especially in the lower distal extension prosthesis.
- Educating the patient about the possible outcome of the treatment and better understanding of that patient cooperates with the dentist.

g. Denture fracture

Specific conditions that can cause denture fracture are :

a. Heavy anterior occlusal contact
b. Deep labial frenal notches
c. High occlusal forces due to strong mandibular elevator musculature.

If the clinician is unable to control these factors or the fracture potential is high, a cast metal base is best used to resist deformation and fracture.

Maintenance visit

Patient's with mandibular Kennedy Class I /II removable partial denture opposing single maxillary denture have to be recalled every six months and verified for occlusal contact relationships. If a space is developed between the upper and lower posterior occlusal surfaces, relining of lower partial denture is advocated. Also the condition of the supporting tissues has to be evaluated and treated accordingly.

Rationale for implants

Implant retained overdentures for the maxilla will provide improved stability, enhanced function and reduction in the irreversible bone loss

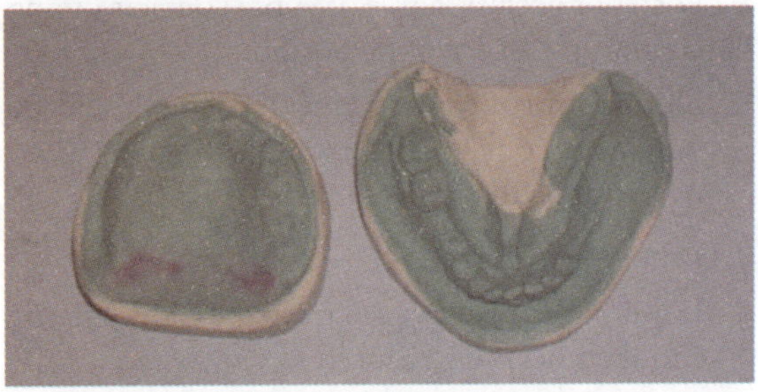

Fig. 26.1 Upper and lower casts

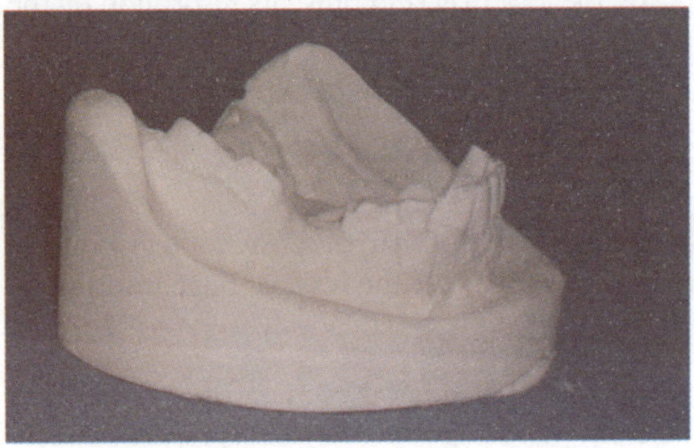

Fig. 26.2 Duplicated mandibular cast

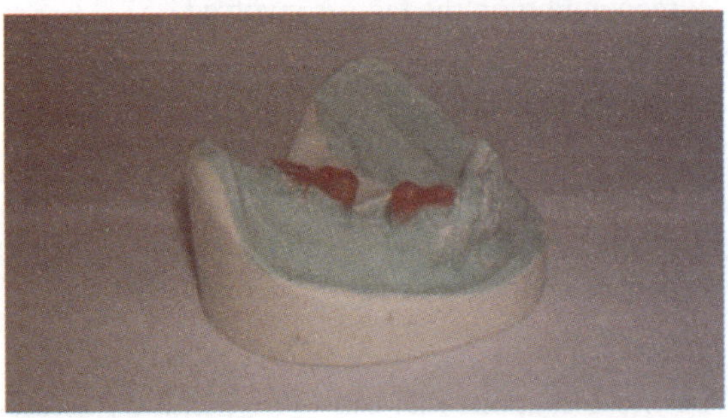

Fig. 26.3 Diagnostic Wax-up for occlusal correction

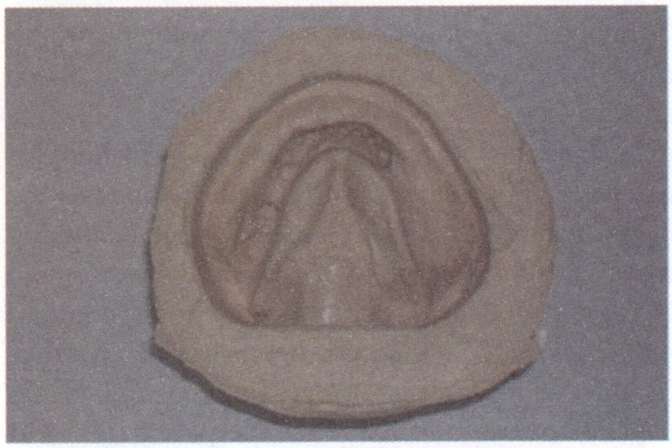

Fig. 26.4 Alginate mold of Waxed-up cast

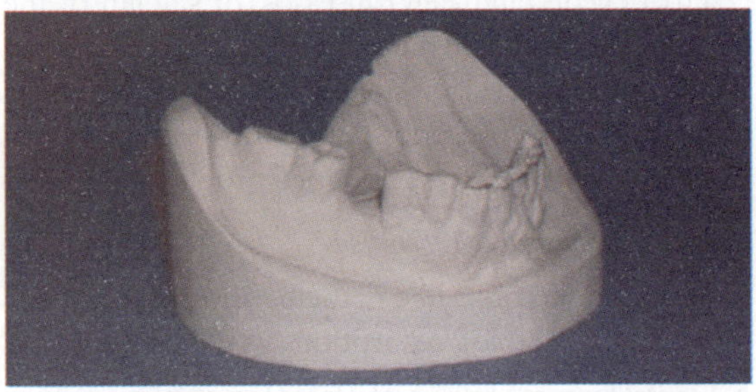

Fig. 26.5 Duplicated cast with marking for reduction of incisal edges

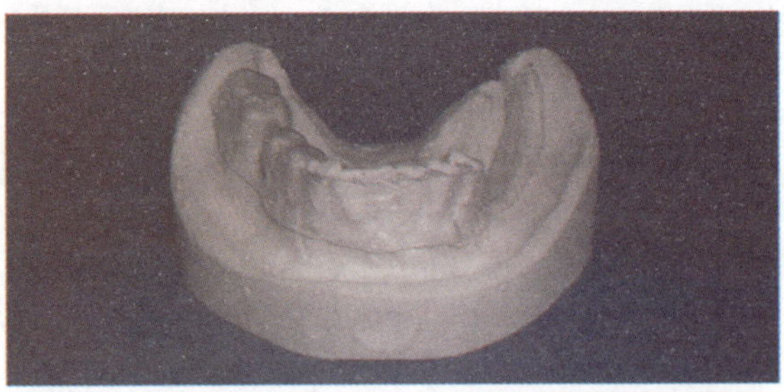

Fig. 26.6 Vaccuform Template

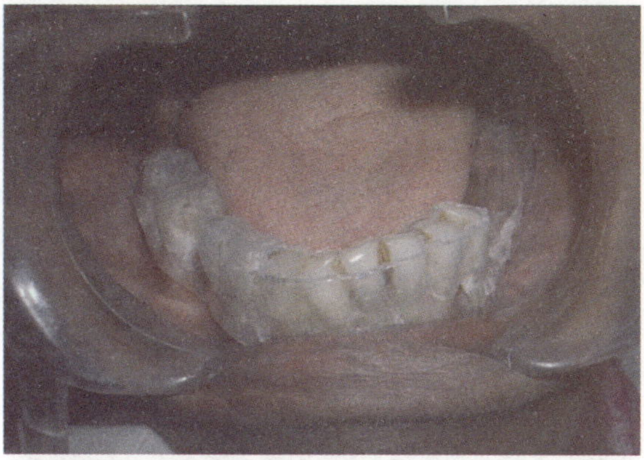

Fig. 26.7 Template inserted in the mouth showing reguired amount of addition in posteriors and reduction in anteriors

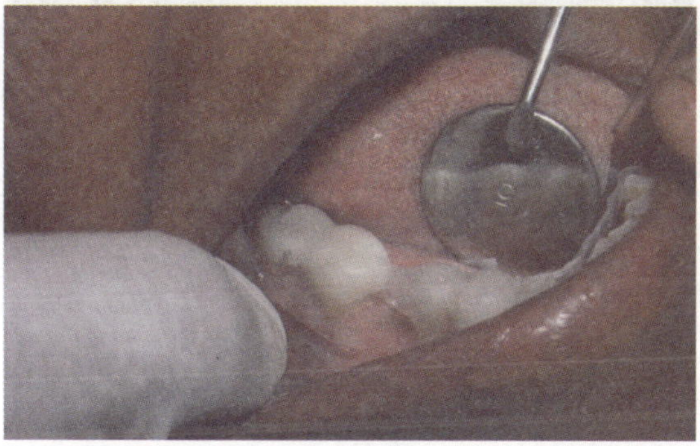

Fig. 26.8 Composite build-up on posteriors

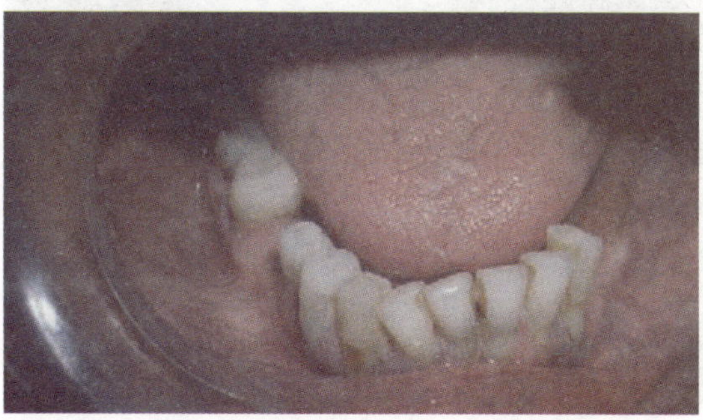

Fig. 26.9 After occlusal correction

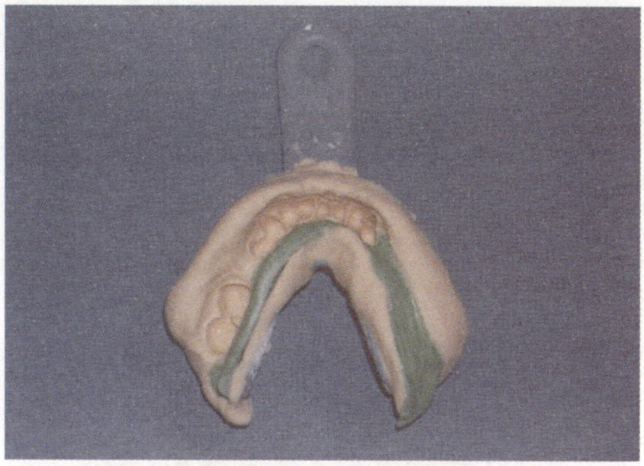

Fig. 26.10 Lower impression

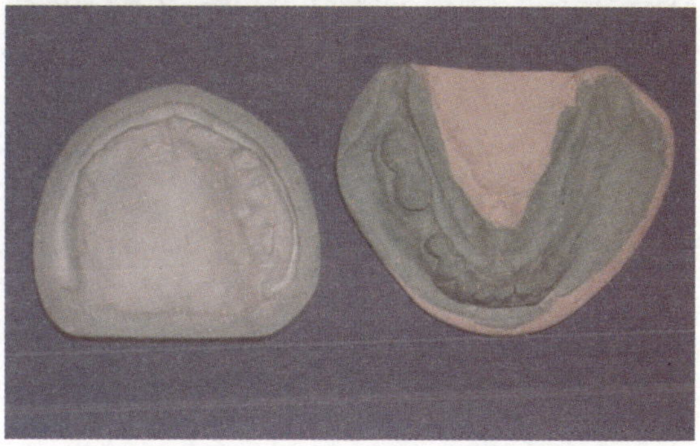

Fig. 26.11 Upper and Lower Master Casts

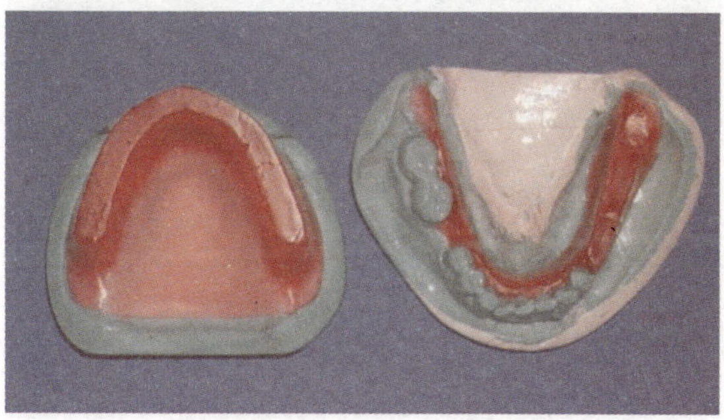

Fig. 26.12 Record bases and Occlusal rims

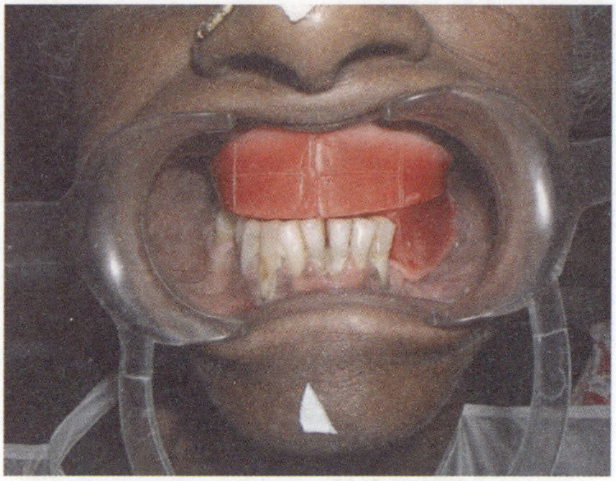

Fig. 26.13 Jaw relation – Intraoral view

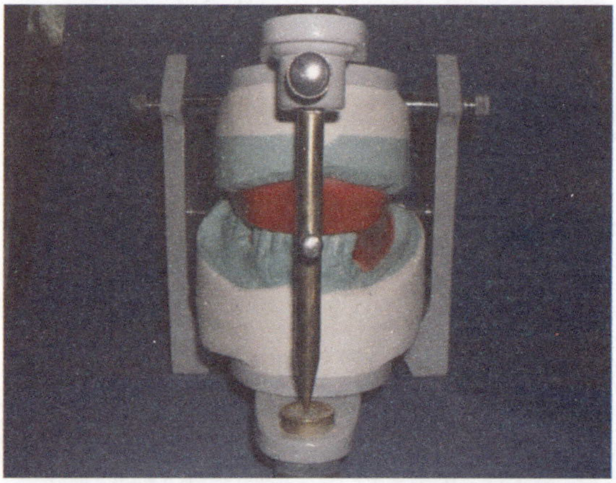

Fig. 26.14 Mounted casts – Frontal view

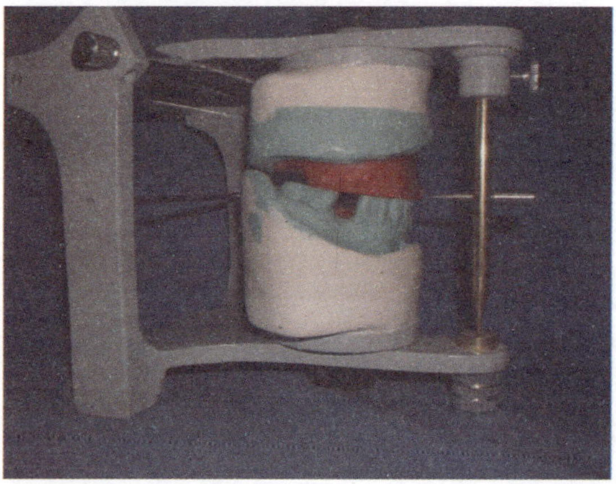

Fig. 26.15 Mounted casts – Right lateral view

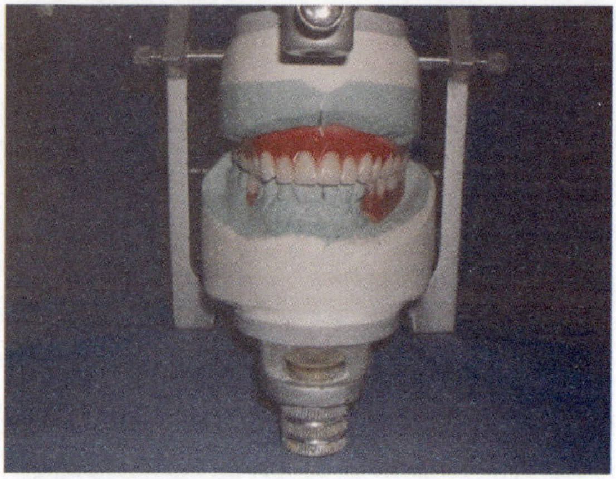

Fig. 26.16 Trial Denture – Frontal view

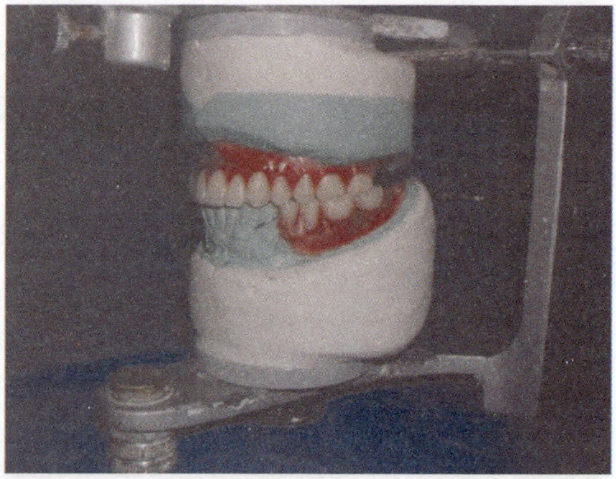

Fig. 26.17 Trial Denture – Left lateral view

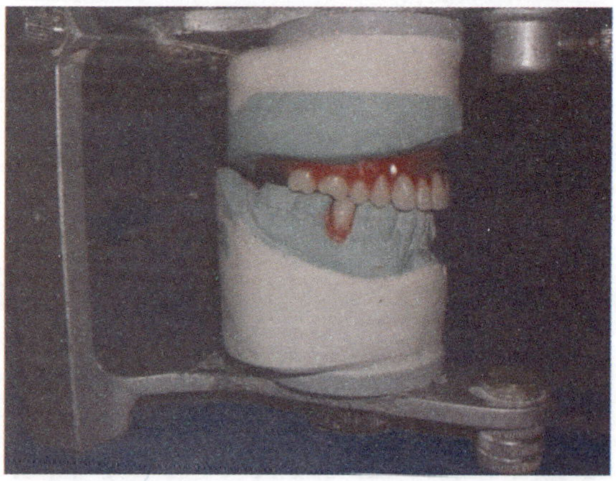

Fig. 26.18 Trial Denture – Right lateral view

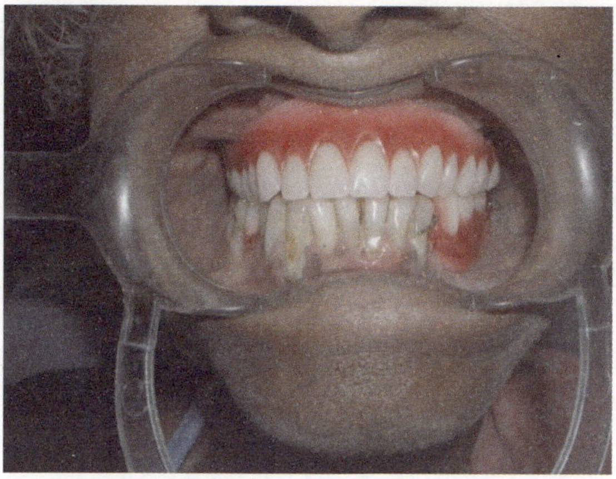

Fig. 26.19 Wax try-in Frontal view

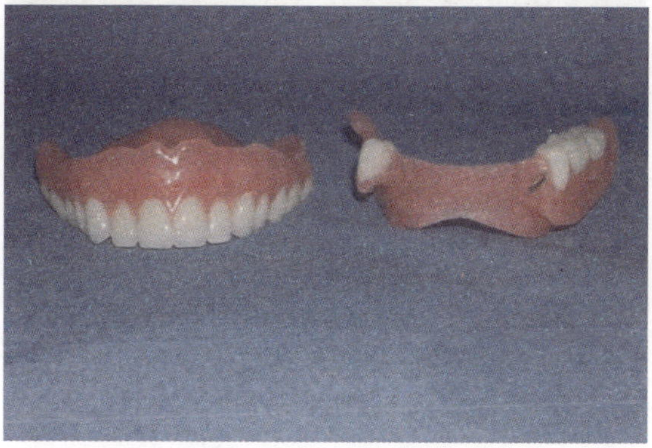

Fig. 26.20 Final Prosthesis

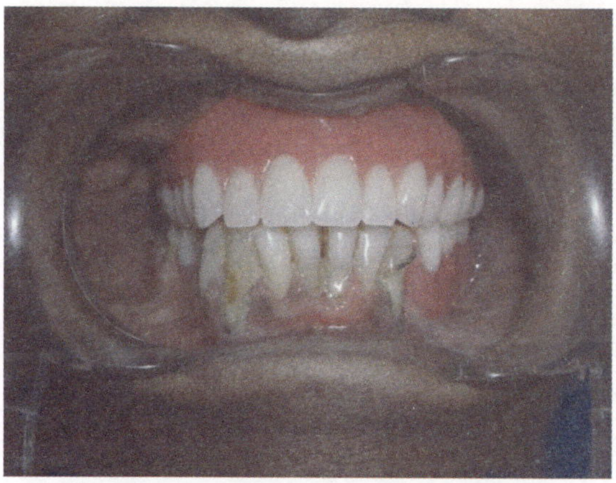

Fig. 26.21 Denture insertion – Frontal view

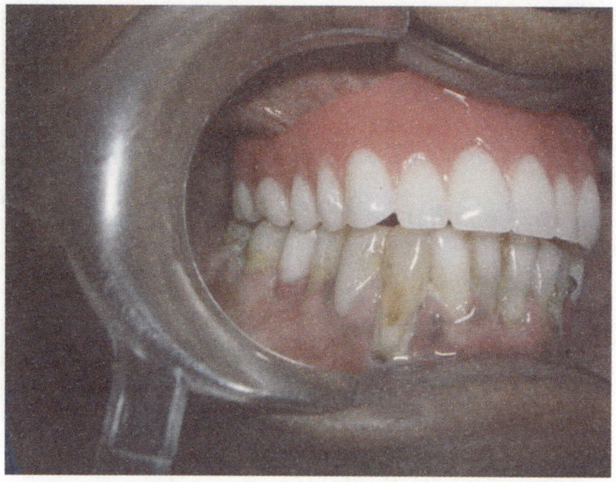

Fig. 26.22 Denture insertion – Right lateral view

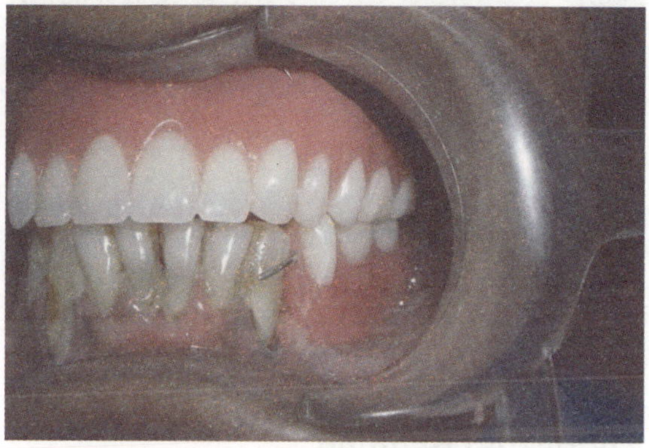

Fig. 26.23 Denture insertion – Left lateral view

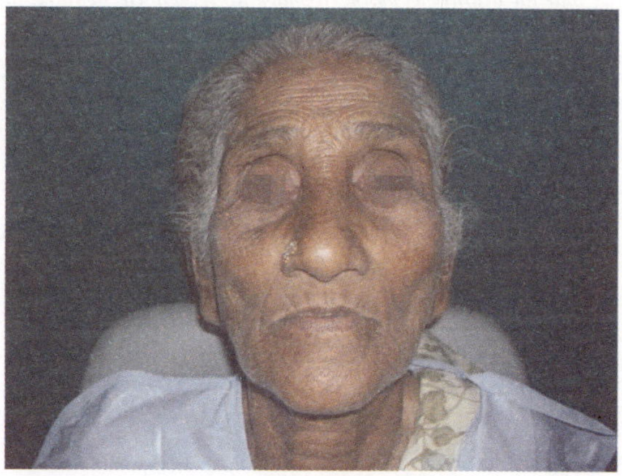

Fig. 26.24 Preoperative frontal view

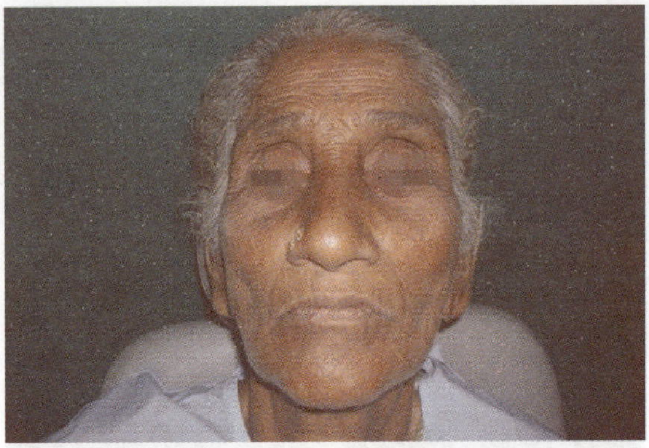

Fig. 26.25 Postoperative frontal view

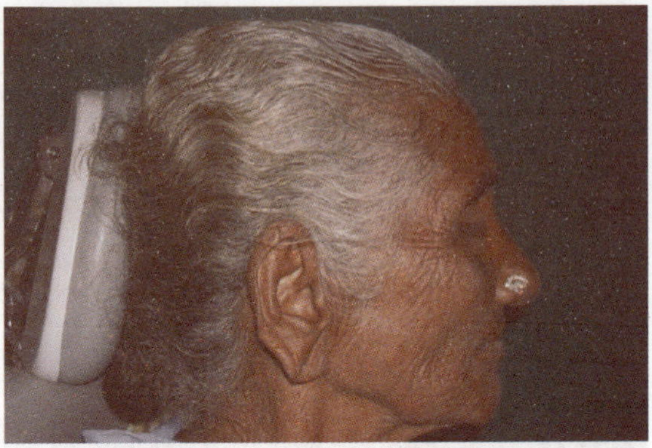

Fig. 26.27 Postoperative lateral view

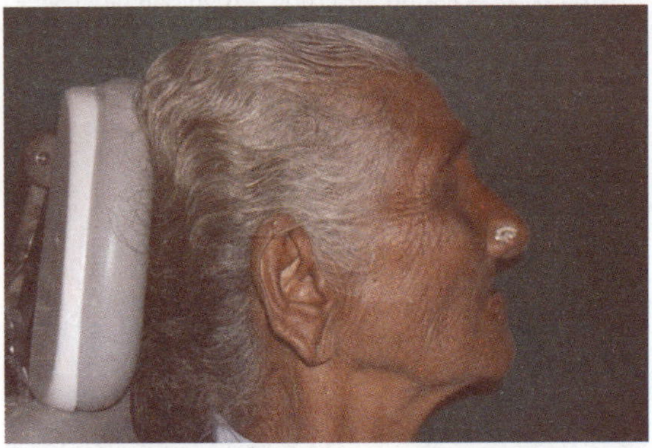

Fig. 26.26 Preoperative lateral view

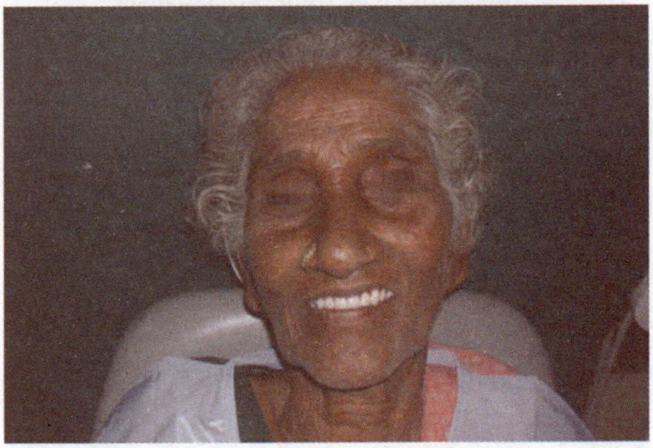

Fig. 26.28 Postoperative front view

Suggested Reading

1. Arthur O Rahn, Charles M. Heartwell, *Textbook of complete Dentures,* Edition 5, London, 1993
2. Ellsworth Kelly, *Change caused by a mandibular removable partial denture opposing a maxillary complete denture.* J. Prosthet. Dent 1972; Vol 27; No.2
3. George A. Zarb, Charles L.Bolender, Judson C. Hickey, Gunnar E. Carlsson: *Boucher's prosthodontic treatment for edentulous patients,* Edition 10, B.I Publications Pvt. Ltd.
4. John J. Sharry, *Complete denture prosthodontics,* Mcgrawhill book Company, Inc. 1962
5. Robert G. Vig, *A Modified Chew – In and Functional Impression Technique.* J. Prosthet Dent 1964; Vol 14; No2
6. Sheldon Winkler, *Essentials of complete Denture Prosthodontics,* Edition 2, Ishiyaku Euro America Inc.
7. Yair Langer et al, *Modalities of Treatment for the combination syndrome.* J Prosthet Dent 1995; 4(2); 76-81
8. Driscoll et al, *Single maxillary complete denture,* Dent Clin N Am 2004; 48: 567–583
9. Saunders et al, *The maxillary complete denture opposing the mandibular bilateral distal-extension partial denture: Treatment considerations.* J Prosthet Dent 1979;41: 124-128.
10. Schmitt S M, *Combination Syndrome: a treatment approach:* J Prosthet dent 1985;54(1):664-71
11. Palmqvist S, Carlsson E, Owall B, *The combination syndrome: A literature review* J Prosthet Dent 2003;90:270-5
12. Smith P W, McCord J F,Grey N J A: *Combination syndrome revisited;* CPD Dentistry 2001; 2(3):96-101
13. Shen K, Gongloff RK. *Prevalence of the "combination syndrome" among denture patients.* J Prosthet Dent 1989;62:642-4.
14. Gupta S, Lechner SK, Duckmanton NA. *Maxillary changes under complete dentures opposing mandibular implant-supported fixed prostheses.* Int J Prosthodont 1999; 12:492-7

27

Over dentures

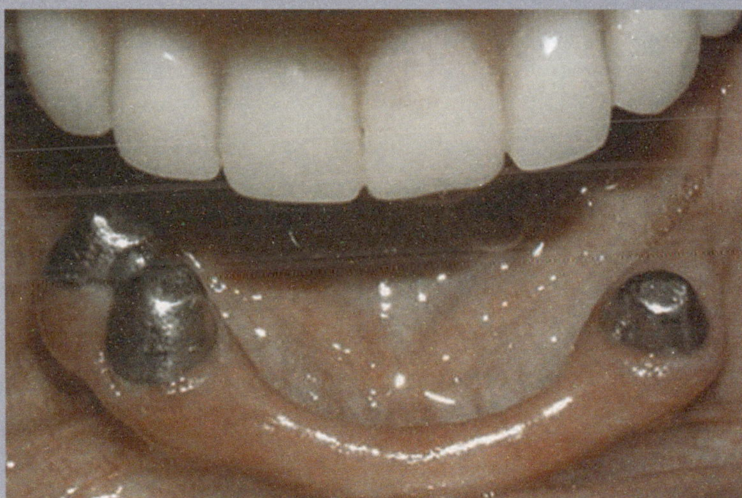

Natural teeth components are used to provide functional advantages to the dentures

Overdentures are removable dentures that are placed over natural tooth roots or implants. They can be either interim restorations or definitive prosthesis. Over dentures gain additional support from the roots or implants compared to conventional complete dentures.

Tooth supported overdentures appear as complete dentures and enclose within its borders both residual ridge and supporting tooth roots. These roots are usually endodontically treated and generally used for support rather than for directly retaining the prosthesis. The retained roots which serve as over denture abutments preserve the residual alveolar ridge surrounding them and provide support and retention to the complete denture prosthesis better than the ridge that would progressively resorb. The amount of resorption is eight times less in overdentures when compared to conventional complete dentures. Retaining teeth for overdenture abutments is most critical in areas with a high probability of residual alveolar resorption and in patients who have a history that would indicate high risk for residual alveolar bone loss. Overdentures may have improved masticatory competence because of the retention of partial proprioception by way of the remaining periodontal ligament of the abutment teeth.

In implant supported overdenture, the treatment plan ranges from two implants to completely implant supported. Patients with mandibular overdentures retained by two implants had higher satisfaction scores than complete denture patients. Anterior mandibular bone under an implant overdenture may resorb as little as 0.5 mm over a five year period, whereas resilient overdenture design may cause 2 to 3 times the resorption in the posterior mandible as compared to the complete denture.

Indications for overdenture

1. Patients with few remaining natural teeth .
2. Patients with poor prognosis for routine complete dentures.
   - High palatal vault
   - Xerostomia
   - Poor mandibular ridges
   - When high rate of resorption is expected
   - When opposing natural teeth are present
   - Smaller dental arches
3. Patients with congenital or acquired intraoral defects.
   - Partial anodontia
   - Cleft palate
   - Microdontia
   - Amelogenesis imperfecta
4. In case of severe attrition, vertical height can be restored with an overdenture .
5. Very young patients facing total extraction.
6. Patients with few remaining natural teeth.
7. Low caries index and good oral hygiene.

Contraindications

1. High caries index and poor oral hygiene
2. When the abutments have a doubtful prognosis
   - when endodontic treatment is not possible
   - when periodontal therapy and reduction of crown root ratio does not improve the periodontal health.
3. Failure to establish a sufficient zone of attached gingiva
4. Unco-operative, terminally ill or senile patients

Classification of overdentures

I. Tooth supported overdentures

a. Noncoping

b. Coping

c. Attachments

II. Implant supported overdentures

I. Tooth supported overdentures

a. Noncoping overdentures

Selected abutments are reduced to a coronal height of 2 to 3 mm and then contoured to a convex or dome shaped surface. Most teeth require endodontic therapy followed by amalgam or composite restoration.

b.Coping overdentures

A coping is a thin covering. The abutment teeth may be covered with copings to give better protection against caries. Cast metal copings with dome shaped surfaces and chamfer finish lines at the gingival margins are made and cemented.

c. Attachments

The attachments essentially increase the crown-root ratio and then torque or apply horizontal or vertical dislodging forces to the root abutments. Here, low caries index, proper home care, periodontal health and inter ridge distance are absolutely necessary.

Coping Types

A coping fitted to a prepared abutment is called a primary coping. The sleeve, or coping, that fits over this primary coping is referred to as a secondary coping.

There are four basic types of primary copings viz long copings (6-8 mm), medium copings (4-6mm), medium-short copings (2-4 mm), short copings (1-2 mm)

a. Long Copings (6-8 millimeters for vital teeth)

The long coping is an excellent restoration, applicable to many overlay techniques. It may be used simply to provide stability and retention under a telescopic overdenture.

b. Medium Copings (4-6 millimeters for vital and non-vital teeth)

Medium sized copings may be used with vital teeth where the pulp has receded or with non vital teeth having adequate bone support. Medium sized copings are not generally designed as individual copings for retention of the overlay prosthesis. They are generally connected with some type of bar attachment or they may also be used with auxiliary plunger or pressure button attachments. They are conical with greater taper on all surfaces, particularly the facial surface when used with bar attachments. If used with a plunger button attachment, the surface engaged by the plunger is flattened.

c. Medium short copings (2-4 mm for nonvital teeth)

Medium short copings are indicated for nonvital teeth, where a more favorable crown root ratio is desired than that possible with medium or long copings. This coping form (and preparation) is indicated when it is difficult to obtain auxiliary retention of the coping on the abutment with a dowel or parallel pins (the proximal walls of the preparation should be very closely parallel for maximum frictional fit of the coping); numerous neighboring abutments are to be splinted, thus permitting better embrasure formation than possible with very short copings. These copings are also used with bar attachments.

d. Short Copings (1-2 millimeters for non-vital teeth)

Short copings are fabricated to conform to the curvature of the alveolar ridge, with a very low profile. They are indicated for maximum favorable crown-root ratio. Such short copings are particularly suited to various types of stud attachments, but may also be used effectively with many forms of bar attachments.

Mandibular overdentures

Though overdentures are used in both the arches, mandibular complete overdenture are greatly indicated because of the following reasons.

a. Mandibular anterior teeth especially the canines are often the patient's last remaining teeth and retaining these teeth gives the patient and dentist an alternative to edentulousness.
b. Mandibular residual alveolar ridge bone can be extremely prone to resorption, especially for postmenopausal women or patients whose teeth are lost at an early age.
c. Retention for mandibular complete dentures poses a problem for majority of patients.
d. Enhanced proprioception provided by the abutments assist mandibular movements.
e. Less area is available for supporting the mandibular denture compared to the maxilla because of presence of tongue in the lower jaw.

Bilateral abutments

Bilateral abutments are always recommended because they provide equity in support. Proprioception of a unilaterally supported complete overdenture makes it difficult to obtain true centric-relation position. While masticating, patients prefer to make working-side contacts on the tooth supported side which leads to problems in stability and retention. An analogy can be made to driving a car with a flat tire; one area is fully supported while another is without solid support. It is preferable to have both sides of the arch equally supported or unsupported. A combination of two abutments on one side and one on the other side of the arch can be used, as long as the single abutment is not one with compromised support. Usually the teeth retained are bilateral canines or first premolars. Occasionally incisors are also retained.

Factors to be considered in designing mandibular tooth supported over dentures

While designing a mandibular complete tooth supported overdenture, the following factors should be considered:

a. Bilateral abutments have the best potential for providing equity in prosthesis support.
b. Teeth should be evaluated to find out whether they can be successfully treated endodontically.
c. Abutment teeth should have adequate periodontal support. Teeth with mobility make compromised or poor overdenture abutments, especially if bone loss is noticed radiographically. A minimum of 4-6 mm of bone should be present around the abutment tooth.
d. Teeth should have good soft tissue architecture, including minimal periodontal sulcus depth and adequate attached gingiva surrounding the tooth. This is important because of the mechanical demands of the denture base, which rests and gains support from the periodontal soft tissues. Without attached gingiva, periodontal breakdown can be expected, even when the denture base is relieved.
e. The arch should be evaluated to find a path of insertion that requires creation of minimal relief of the denture base. Mandibular anterior teeth exhibit an axial alignment that creates an anterior undercut as compared to the straight vertical path of insertion. Varying the path to a more anterior or posterior alignment can often help matters if the posterior anatomy permits. If the anterior undercuts are unmanageable, it may lead to over relieved, food trapping, dentures. Hence lower first premolar is preferred than canine.
f. Adequate inter arch space is imperative. This is perhaps the single most important factor in patient selection for mandibular complete overdenture. If a patient has a marked Angle's Class III relationship, maintaining mandibular anterior tooth roots may make it impossible for esthetic placement of mandibular anterior artificial teeth. If the mandibular anterior ridge is hypertrophied or tall, maintaining abutment roots may further compromise the vertical dimension of occlusion and lead to an unaesthetic or non functional denture.
g. A good rule for deciding whether saving mandibular teeth as overdenture abutments will lead to problems in vertical space, is to evaluate the ridge in relation to the crest of the lower lip. If the space between the crest of the lower lip and the crest of the mandibular anterior ridge is less than 5 mm and if the inter arch space at rest position is less than 10 mm, over denture treatment should be considered to have a guarded prognosis. In short, if an area of the ridge has too much bone, maintaining teeth as overdenture abutments will further hinder denture fabrication.

Maxillary overdenture

The goal of overdentures in the maxillary arch is to avoid resorption of bone in areas with a high probability Maxillary overdentures are used more frequently to address specific oral situations because maxillary bone loss patterns are different from mandibular patterns. Commonly maxillary complete overdentures are used against mandibular full complement of natural teeth or natural teeth plus a mandibular removable partial denture.

Usually, maxillary anterior teeth such as canines or central incisors are selected for abutments. It is particularly expedient to use the maxillary overdenture because of the following reasons.

Frequently anterior teeth remain in the mandibular arch. The combination of a maxillary complete and mandibular distal extension RPD can lead to a destructive pattern of oral changes referred to as combination syndrome or anterior hyperfunction syndrome. Bone loss from the maxillary anterior residual alveolar ridge leads to maxillary denture instability and subsequent down growth of the maxillary tuberosities, eventually leading to disruption of the plane of occlusion of the dentures and loss of function. By the use of overdenture with anterior abutments, a positive stop in maxillary anterior bone can be created and thereby this vicious cycle can be stopped before it begins.

Even if a tooth supported RPD or a full complement of natural teeth remains in the mandibular arch, maxillary alveolar bone is most likely to be lost anteriorly. In addition, maxillary anterior bone loss is most destructive to denture esthetics and retention. Often, sufficient retention is gained by the bone maintained by saving the overdenture abutments, but if overdenture retention is a problem, the abutment teeth offer the possibility of adding attachments.

Maintenance of natural tooth roots under a complete denture opposing natural teeth may offer the patient additional support in incising. Usually patients with maxillary overdentures and mandibular natural teeth can display an ability to bite and incise foods similar to dentulous individuals. This may be partially due to residual proprioception maintained in the periodontal ligaments of the abutments, although this concept lacks evidence.

Similar to selecting patients for treatment with mandibular complete overdentures, selecting patients for maxillary complete overdentures requires careful evaluation of periodontal factors, both in hard and soft tissue, endodontic feasibility, and interarch space and position factors, both horizontally and vertically.

Patients with marked Angle's Class II configurations or extremely high lip lines as compared to the anterior maxillary bone level will probably have compromised esthetics because of overdenture abutments. The vertical dimension should be assessed to ensure adequate vertical space for anterior artificial teeth, even if a vertical overlap is planned. At least 5mm of space is needed between mandibular incisal edges and maxillary alveolar bone or overdenture abutment root faces. More is needed if a monoplane setup without anterior vertical overlap is planned.

As far as possible, unilateral abutment teeth should be avoided although the palate can offer good support. Occasionally unilateral maxillary overdenture abutments can be considered if all the mandibular teeth present are on the same side of the arch or if there is a need for utilization of attachments. As the use of oral implants becomes more popular, a good and relatively inexpensive indication of them may be to augment existing natural overdenture abutment teeth for balanced support and retention for complete overdentures.

Preparation of overdenture abutments

Once a complete overdenture is planned and teeth are selected as over denture abutments, care must be taken to prepare them to maximize serviceability and to minimize potential problems for the surrounding soft tissue. Factors that must be considered in the design of an overdenture abutment are location, angulation, height relative to other abutments, marginal design, and the potential path of draw relative to soft and hard tissue undercuts. If the tooth is to house an attachment, its size, shape and angulation must be assessed relative to the attachment chosen.

Periodontal considerations

An overdenture abutment can have less optimal periodontal support than a tooth that has to serve as a fixed partial denture abutment. If such a tooth has already received endodontic therapy, there is minimal risk in retaining it as long as it has a reasonable prognosis under axial loading and its loss will not necessitate remaking of the prosthesis. Even periodontally questionable teeth can be used to serve as over denture abutment because such teeth frequently improve periodontally, after removal of the clinical crowns since nonaxial forces disappear and access for oral hygiene improves. However the presence of persistent inflammation and mobility even after scaling and root planing, furcation involvement in molars and pocket depth greater than 5mm should indicate a poor prognosis. The presence of keratinized, attached gingiva is important because it will protect the surrounding tissues when the overdenture ceases to bear on the abutment tooth and begins to bear on the surrounding soft tissue. The periodontal health of overdenture abutments must be maintained not only through good oral hygiene and professional periodontal maintenance but also through careful designing and adjustment of abutment teeth and the denture base. Dome-shaped abutments allow some movement of the prosthesis without periodontal damage. Care must be taken in denture adjustments to avoid over relief near the abutments which can create space for food or plaque accumulation at this critical interface.

Endodontic treatment for over denture abutments

Overdenture abutments generally require endodontic therapy because the entire clinical crown has to be removed. Endodontic therapy for overdenture abutments should proceed in standard fashion, although some clinicians choose to remove some portion of the clinical crown rather than prepare a conventional access opening. Care must be taken to avoid removing the entire clinical crown because the abutment will eventually need to be dome shaped and 2 to 4 mm tall. Crown height is also necessary for application of the rubber dam.When a cariously damaged tooth is used as an overdenture abutment, carious lesions at or below the gingival line can make isolation difficult. Crown-lengthening surgery can be helpful in these cases. At the time of the endodontic procedure, a decision should already have been made concerning restoration of the overdenture abutment. Most abutments will be restored with a simple amalgam filling. These teeth can be filled with gutta-percha to the length of the canal and the access cavity with amalgam. When cast copings retained with posts are planned, an appropriate post space preparation should be done as part of the endodontic procedure. When a tooth with history of endodontic treatment is selected as an abutment and if it is asymptomatic and shows no radiographic signs of endodontic failure such as periapical radiolucencies, the filling does not need to be redone despite suboptimal results. The reason is that unlike endodontically treated teeth that will receive crowns, overdenture abutments teeth offer easy access for retreatment should it become necessary.

Restoration of the abutment

Except for cases in which insufficient tooth structure remains in the root-face area of an overdenture abutment, simple amalgam plug canal filling is usually used for restoration. It is inexpensive and easy to place and can be done at the time of the endodontic procedure, with rubber dam isolation still in place, or done at any time thereafter. The first step in preparation is to use a coarse diamond stone to amputate the clinical crown of the tooth, with about 4mm of coronal height left above the gingival line. Care should be taken to avoid the crown fragment flying off as the amputation is completed. The simplest way to do this is to cut across the tooth mesiodistally just short of completion and snap the crown off with the fingers when proximal enamel has been reached. In cases in which the gingival line is much lower on the buccal than other areas, such as in mandibular canine teeth, this contour should be followed such that the root face (horizontal cross section) will be perpendicular to the occlusal force. The blunt root stump should then be contoured to the gingiva and domed by rounding the tooth structure to the gingival line. At this point, the gutta-percha endodontic fill is usually visible at the center of the root face. A fissure bur is ideal for preparing a Class I-type cavity to receive the amalgam plug fill. The bur should be sunk into the canal to the depth of the bur head and all gutta-percha removed. Retention form is added by fanning the bur only in the buccal-lingual direction to avoid perforation in proximal root concavity areas, especially in canine and bicuspid teeth.The size of the lumen of the preparation should be determined by the size of the canal once all gutta-percha is removed. It needs enlargement only if the smallest amalgam condenser is too large to be used to condense the filling material. The depth of the preparation should be sufficient to place a filling of adequate height, even if the abutments need to be reprepared later because of problems in vertical dimension. After condensation, the restoration should be finished flat to the root-face surface and polished. Usually at a subsequent visit, the margins that were finished to the gingival line might have become supragingival. This is due to resolution of gingival tissue inflammation once the clinical crown is removed. The desired dome shape should be re-established. Plug fillings can also be made in materials other than amalgam, including composites and glass ionomer materials.

Cast copings to restore overdenture abutments

When overdentures were originally popularized, many clinicians recommended covering the root faces of all overdenture abutments with cast copings; however, they introduce added cost and complexity to a restoration. Copings do not add much to the success of either abutment teeth or dentures. They add vertical height to the abutments and also a metal-to-tooth structure interface, usually at a gingival-level margin which can cause or exacerbate periodontal problems. Their presence also limits flexibility in adjustment at the interface between the denture and supporting abutment because only the denture itself can be adjusted once copings are permanently cemented. The major indications for cast copings are insufficient or partially destroyed tooth structure and the necessity for adding precision or semiprecision attachments to abutment teeth. When cast copings are to be made, post preparations are usually done at the time of endodontic therapy. Path of draw of these preparations should be different from the path of draw of the overdenture, especially if attachments are planned. Preparation of the root face for a coping is usually simple, but it must end on tooth structure in every area. In a cariously damaged tooth, tissue management can present a problem. Electrosurgery or diamond stone gingivectomy and subsequent healing is sometimes needed before impression making. Fabrication of the patterns for cast copings may be done with either a direct or indirect technique. If a direct pattern is made, the technique is similar to that for cast post-and-core restorations.

Like all castings, copings should be meticuloulsy fitted. Although castings are finished just at the gingival line which is physiologically acceptable as long as adequate interarch space is available. The faces or occlusal aspects of copings should be similar to the dome-shaped contours of bare root faces.

Overdenture attachments

For positive tooth-to-denture retention mechanical attachments can be used. However support system should be given due consideration as in any other prosthesis. If the over denture is retained with two attachments, the stress of occlusion and the unfavorable leverage would cause the abutments to fail. Ideally, the abutments should have sound periodontal support. Sufficient interarch space should also be available to accommodate the attachment within the denture.

Stud Attachments

These are simple in design, consisting of a male stud type that is soldered to a base. The base is a coping covering the prepared tooth stump and has a post extending into an endodontically treated root canal. Retention is achieved when the male stud engages the female housing that is either embedded in the acrylic of an overdenture or soldered to a substructure in the overdenture. Studs can be either nonresilient or resilient. Studs are nonresilient when the female housing is rigidly attached to the male. They are resilient if designed with a spring load to provide for a controlled movement.

Gerber attachment

There are two types viz rigid attachment that does not allow for movement of the base and resilient attachment that allows vertical movement.

The rigid type consists of a male post threaded onto a screw attached to a soldering base and a female housing containing a retention spring and ring. The retention is gained by the spring clip in the female housing engaging a groove in the male section.

The resilient Gerber attachment has a soldering base and a male retention post. The overall housing contains a mounting ring, bushing, and a retention ring with a spring assembly that enables the attachment to move in a vertical direction. This enables the appliance to utilize more of the residual ridge for support. However, this attachment is more bulky than most, so adequate interocclusal space must exist for its utilization.

Dalbo attachments

There are three types viz rigid, resilient, and stress broken. All are composed of a male unit that is attached to the tooth and a female housing embedded in the denture base.

The rigid Dalbo attachment has a cylindric male unit with rounded head. The resilient attachment, the smallest and most commonly used of the types, allow vertical and rotational movement of the female around a sphere-shaped male unit made possible because of a relief space between the units.

The stress broken type is similar in design to the resilient type, with the exception that the female housing is longer and incorporates a coil spring.

Ceka attachment

This consists of a male portion affixed to the tooth and has a rounded shape wider at the top and split vertically into four sections. These four sections are flexible and capable of being compressed. Over this fits a female housing or ring.

Zest anchor

This attachment derives its retention from within the root Post preparation is made within the root and a female sleeve is cemented to place. The male portion is a nylon post and a ball head that is attached to the overdenture as a chairside procedure. This post is placed into the sleeve and the overdenture is placed over this with cold-cure resin placed in a recess to accept the male. Its retention to the tooth is gained by the ball head snapping into the undercut in the female sleeve.

The advantages of this attachment are as follows.

a. It overcomes any space problem because the attachment is within the root structure.
b. The leverage on the abutment tooth is negligible, since the point of attachment is actually well below alveolar bone level.
c. The attachment procedure is simple, can be performed quickly at chairside.

The disadvantages of this attachment are as follows:

a. Since no casting or coping usually is made, the root structure and canal itself are susceptible to caries.
b. The nylon studs can be bent, preventing seating of the appliance, especially if several are being used, or they might even fracture.
c. Food debris can find its way into the female housing especially if the patient attempts eating without the denture in place.

Rothermann attachment

This attachment is of two types - one allowing more movement than the other in a vertical and rotational fashion. It consists of a short stud with a groove deeper at one end than at the other, and a retaining C-shaped ring, the ends of the ring, or clip, fitting into the deepest part of the retaining groove. This attachment requires very little space for its utilization and is therefore excellent for cases with little interocclusal space and because of its low height, need not be parallel if more than one is being used. The male stud can easily be attached to a coping with free hand soldering and the female clip is attached to the denture base with cold-cure acrylic either as a laboratory step or at the chair.

Introfix attachment

This is a tall stud attachment composed of a solder base, an adjustable split male post, and a female housing. Its design is simple, providing a frictional retention between male and female. The male has a longitudinal split, so it can be adjusted to gain more or less retention, and it is replaceable, since it is screwed onto the solder base.

Schubiger attachment

This attachment is a permanent form of fixation using a screw system that connects anchor teeth to bar joints and bar units. It consists of a solder base with a screw that can retain and is interchangeable with a Gerber post attachment. This unit is indicated for a bar attachment on teeth with divergent roots. A definite advantage of this attachment is in its convertibility with weak abutment teeth. If one or more of the abutment teeth are lost, the bar attachment can be unscrewed, leaving the solder base and threaded stud that is common to the Gerber stud unit. Therefore, the remaining abutment teeth can easily be converted into retainers for the overdentures by using one of the Gerber attachments.

Quinlivan attachment

This attachment consists of a prefabricated resin ball that is incorporated with the wax-up of post and coping. The completed casting is then cemented into the endodontically treated tooth. A resin female housing is attached to the overdenture with cold-cure resin. Retention is gained by an O rubber ring inside the female that is securedby a small lip at the orifice of the female cap. The advantages of this attachment are as follows.

a. It is easily and economically fabricated.
b. The O ring can easily be replaced if retention lessens because of fatigue of the rubber ring.
c. The housing is free to rotate in all directions, resulting in minimum torque to the tooth
d. Retention is quite satisfactory.
e. The attachment is only 3 mm in height and thus can fit most space limitations.

The disadvantage is wear and possible fracture of the resin housing if much grinding was originally done to fit a limited space.

Magnets

Another type of attachment that can be used in an overdenture design involves the use of magnets. The magnetic retention unit is comprised of a detachable keeper element made of stainless steel that is fixed to the abutment tooth. This can be done by cementing in a preformed keeper after preparation of the tooth, screwing in a preformed keeper, or casting a root cap and dowel keeper and cementing that to place. The denture retention element has paired, cylindrical, cobalt-samarium magnets, axially magnetized and arranged with their opposite poles adjacent. The flat magnet faces are covered on one end by the attached stainless steel keeper and on the other end by thin stainless steel plates. The plates protect the exposed magnet faces against wear and corrosion in the mouth. The denture retention element is cured into the overdenture and gives the over-denture a retentive force of approximately 250 g. This system appears to be a straightforward, inexpensive technique capable of achieving good retentive results. There is no significant external magnetic field associated with the retention units when the denture is seated and no residual magnetic field when the denture is removed.

Bar Attachments

The purposes of the bar attachments are splinting of the abutment teeth. Bar attachments are of two types: bar units and bar joints. Bar units have rigid fixation where there is no movement between the bar and overlying sleeve and therefore can be classified as tooth-borne. Bar joints permit rotational movement between sleeve and bar, utilizing more of residual ridge for support.

Hader bar

This attachment can serve either as a bar joint or a bar unit and can be used as a stud attachment as well as a bar attachment. The system consists of preformed plastic bars and clips. The plastic bar is attached to the coping wax-up and is cast with the coping. The plastic clips can be embedded in the denture base to gain retention. If more retention is desired, the plastic clip can be tranformed into a metal clip. This is often necessary because the plastic clip loses retention rapidly. The bar and clip attachment is bulky and care must be exercised in its placement to allow for space to set teeth.

Dolder bar

This attachment is supplied as both a bar unit and bar joint. The bar unit consists of a performed bar that is soldered to copings on the abutment teeth. Since the bar is preformed it can only approach a close adaptation to the ridge contour because it must remain in a straight line. The shape of the bar has parallel sides with a rounded top. To this fits a sleeve that is embedded in the acrylic over-denture. Retention is due to a frictional fit.

Bar clip

The joint attachment consists of a small U-shaped clip designed to fit over a round wire. There are two sizes available, 11 and 14 gauge, to be used with either a preformed or cast wire of the same gauge. The clip simply is placed on the wire that has been soldered to the post copings. It is then picked up into the denture with cold-cure resin. Means of attachment of the clip to the resin is not provided, so a retentive wire must be soldered to the clip to gain retention in the acrylic. If the clip becomes worn or broken, the involved clip can be ground out of the denture base and a new one inserted.

Ackerman clip and CM clip

Both of these bar joint attachments are similar in design. They consist of a round bar soldered to the post copings and a clip that fits over the bar similar to the Baker clip. Their difference is in the fact that they come equipped with retention wings on the clip for easy engagement into the acrylic of the overdenture. They also supply a spacer so that the clip does not rest directly on the bar, providing for vertical and rotational movement. Because of their small size and ease of fixation, these clips are excellent for over-denture retention when a bar joint system is indicated for use.

Laboratory procedures

The techniques employed in the fabrication of overdentures are almost identical to that of conventional denture fabrication. The only modification is that abutments must be prepared and restored well before the final impression appointment to include the soft tissue changes. During the teeth arrangement, it may become necessary to alter the height or buccal contour of the abutment in the cast to facilitate esthetic tooth placement and necessary adjustments can be made in the mouth later. If copings are used, this may not be possible. Usually on the lingual surface, additional denture base thickness is given to avoid potential breakage.

Stability and retention

Overdenture abutments are frequently two canines or premolars contralaterally placed and which may create a fulcrum for rotation of the denture base into the depressible soft tissue anteriorly and posteriorly. This can cause instability far worse than those of conventional dentures. An obvious solution is to contour the abutments down and out of contact with the denture base, but this might defeat the supporting function of the abutments. However abutments contoured out of contact cause far fewer problems than those contoured too high. If adjusted too short, the abutment teeth will usually supra erupt into contact with the denture base. Frequently in a long-term recall examination of an overdenture patient, abutments will be noted to be significantly above the gingival line. Usually these changes improve rather than harm the retention and stability of the denture, unless maintenance of vertical dimension or occlusal contacts is compromised. Dentures, especially maxillary dentures, are like suction cups. They need to be slightly overseated into depressible tissue to "suck back" and gain retention. If overdenture abutments prohibit this overseating, retention will be affected. It is acceptable to contour abutments or the denture base to relieve contact entirely.

Maintenance and follow up

Once completed, overdentures must be maintained to ensure serviceability. The overdenture concept, with its potential for maintaining alveolar bone adjacent to abutment teeth, can predispose patients to uneven patterns of bone resorption necessitating periodic relines and occlusal maintenance.

Because of the difference in the resiliency of the natural tooth which is 0.1mm and that of alveolar ridge is 0.4mm to 2mm, the relationship of the denture base to teeth and ridge constantly keeps changing under an overdenture. The overdenture needs to be relined in order to correct this.

Equally important is the health of abutment teeth. Overdenture abutments are frequently compromised teeth at the outset, extra care is needed to maintain them for extended periods. Without clinical crowns, these teeth are much easier to clean, but hygiene is still important. Periodontal scaling, root planing, and even surgery may be needed, exactly as though the teeth had remained serviceable in any other capacity. Maintenance of attached gingiva, even via periodontal surgery, seems to be a key element in the long-term retention of abutments. Dental caries susceptibility is increased, both on amalgam plug-restored over denture abutment teeth and at coping margins, because dentin in exposed and susceptibility to smooth-surface caries increase with age. A simple and very effective way to prevent caries is to use topical fluoride gel, usually 1% and 2% NaF acidulated fluorophosphate gel, in the denture abutment depression daily after tooth brushing. Patients with higher caries risk should receive dietary counseling because, unlike other denture patients, continued intake of sugar-sweetened foods may be deleterious.

If an abutment tooth is insufficiently reduced, mobility and discomfort may be evident. This is probably due to the unfavorable crown-root ratio and is easily corrected. On the other hand, abutment teeth may be overreduced. This often results in a proliferation of soft tissue. This condition is best corrected with copings.

Overdenture are inherently weak as the denture base is relatively thin in the areas of the abutment teeth. Breakage is almost controllable by using all resin teeth and a high impact resin for the denture base. Metal bases can be used if the patient is a constant bruxer or a heavy chewer.

Recall examinations for overdenture patients should include evaluation of abutment extrusion, abutment caries, periodontal disease, oral hygiene and fluoride use, prosthesis instability, prosthesis internal wear in abutment areas, oral cancer recall status.

II. Implant supported overdentures

An international group of scientists, researchers, and clinicians developed and published the McGill consensus on the standard of care for edentulous mandibles (McGill 2002). The consensus included a statement that mandibular 2-unit overdentures should be considered as a first choice standard of care for edentulous patients.

After extraction of mandibular teeth there is an average of 4mm vertical bone loss during the first year following treatment. This bone loss continues over the next 25 years with the mandible experiencing a four fold greater vertical bone loss during the first year following treatment. The bone under an overdenture may lose as little as 0.6 mm vertical bone over a five year period and long term resorption may remain at 0.1mm per year. An implant overdenture provides stability of the prosthesis and the patient is able to consistently reproduce a determined centric occlusion. The chewing efficiency is improved by 20% compared with a complete denture. The retention of prosthesis is also enhanced by the mechanical attachment of the implant support system. Implant supported prosthesis do not require labial extensions or extended soft tissue coverage for support, hence gagging and exaggerated facial contours are not encountered. There are two basic ways to treat patients with dental implants in edentulous mandibles: fixed or removable prostheses. If the ridge is broad and U shaped, inter occlusal clearance is greater than 15 mm and Cl II ,III jaw relationship exists, thin gingival biotype, then implant retained removable prosthesis is indicated.

Implant-retained overdentures need to be designed to be consistent with removable prosthodontic principles (buccal shelf and retromolar pad coverage with adequate vestibular extensions) along with implant attachments. This type of prosthesis can be made with nonsplinted retainers/ attachments that allow rotation or with a framework that splints two or more implants with a casting and allows rotation around the bar. Implant-retained overdentures made on four or more implants will be significantly more rigid and exhibit less movement than overdentures made on two nonsplinted implants with resilient attachments. Multiple, splinted implants with bars and attachments are generally indicated in patients who desire rigid prostheses but who present with significant bone loss (great intermaxillary distance). Flanges are generally required in order to provide optimal lip support and appropriate incisal display. This type of restoration may also be indicated in patients with natural or implant-retained, nonremovable prosthesis in the opposing jaw (maxillae). Patients with four implants and rigidly attached overdentures will probably generate large occlusal forces that may fracture an all acrylic resin denture base. An additional design feature for this latter type of patient would include a secondary bar within the denture base or a metal mini-base. Nonparallel implants may also be indications for splinting because resilient attachments have limitations in the amount of angle correction.

Implants of 3.8/4.1-mm diameter and 12-mm depth are used in the anterior to support an overdenture. The width of the ridge crest is at least 6.1 mm measured at or approximately 1 to 2 mm below the crest in the positions where implants are to be inserted.

Most often, one implant is placed about 3 to 5 mm anterior to the mental foramen on each side, usually in the area formerly occupied by the first premolar, and one implant is positioned on each side of the midline, for a total of four implants.

A minimum of 3 to 5 mm of bone is optimal between the distal of an implant and the mental foramen in the mandible. Overdenture abutments are available in heights of 1.5, 2.5, 3.5, and 4.5 mm,

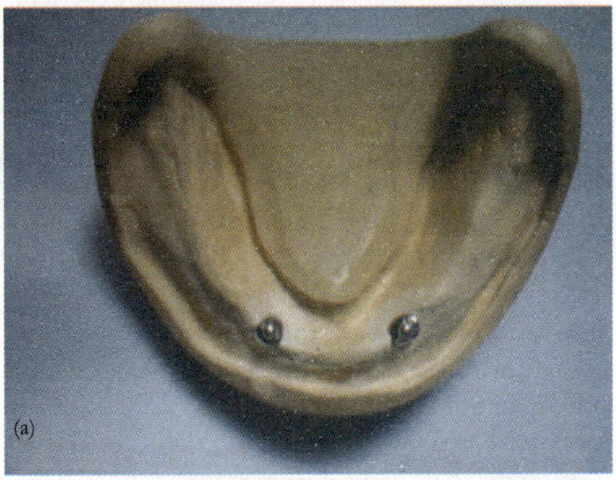

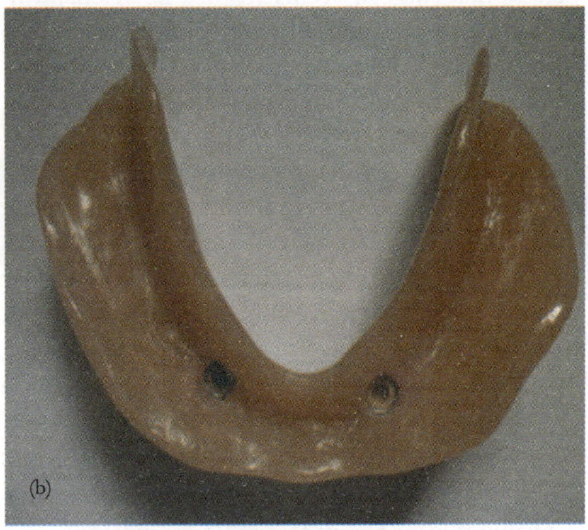

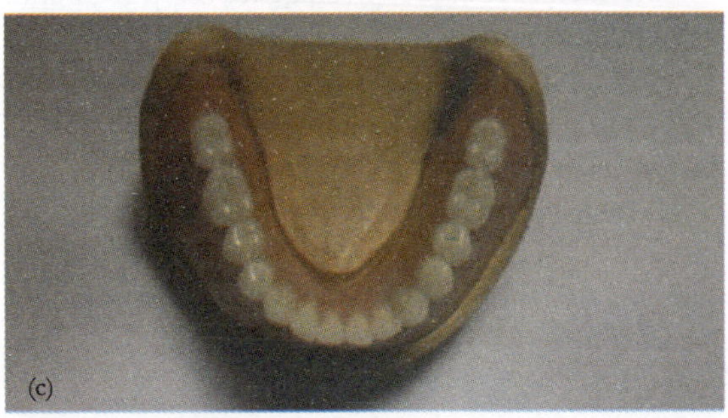

Fig. 27.1 (a) Implant retained over denture
(b) O-rings in lower denture
(c) Denture retained by the implants

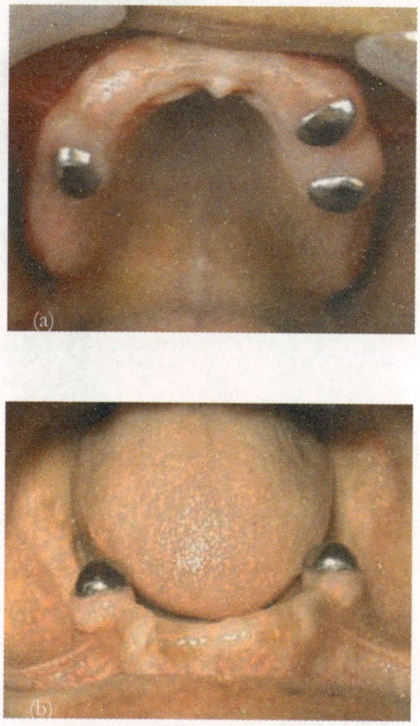

Fig. 27.2 (a), (b) Cast copings cemented to the remaining modified natural teeth which were endodontically treated. These teeth will support the denture

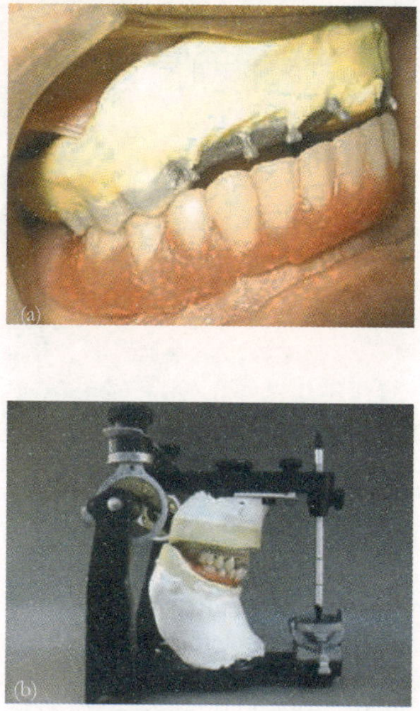

Fig. 27.4 (a), (b) Verification of vertical dimension

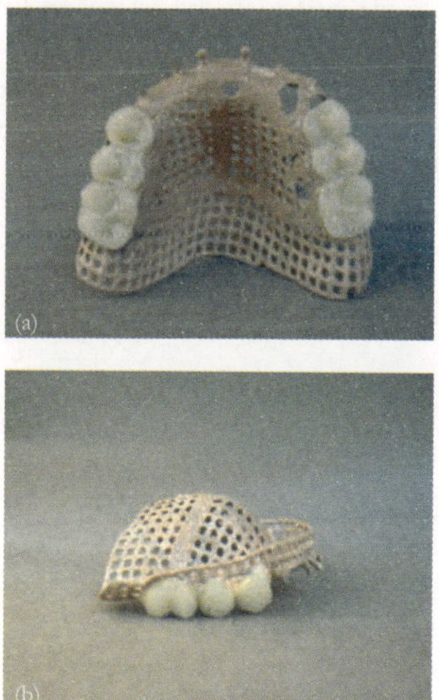

Fig. 27.3 (a), (b) Cast frame work was fabricated with ceramic teeth built directly on the metallic base

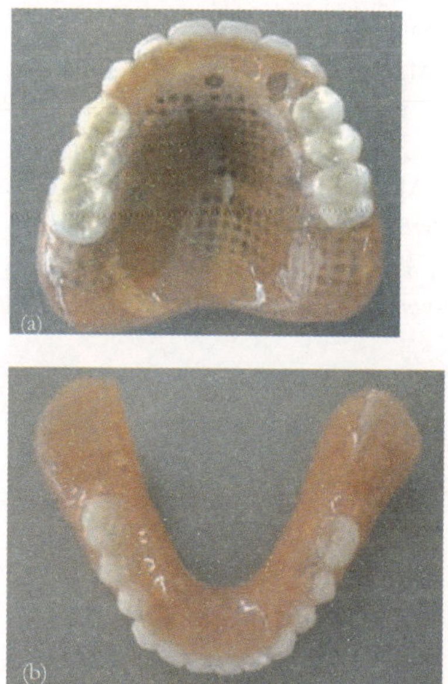

Fig. 27.5 (a), (b) Processed dentures

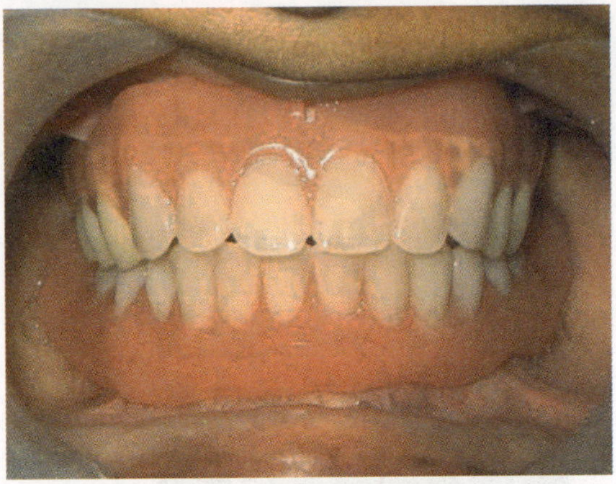

Fig. 27.6 Over dentures inserted

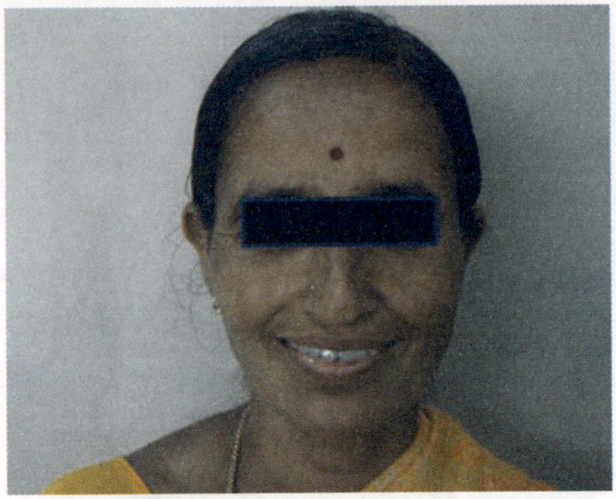

Fig. 27.7 Postoperative view

as are the overdenture abutment analogs, and are supplied with appropriate retaining screws .

Over dentures are well accepted by patients and when indicated, they should be considered as viable treatment options.

Suggested reading

1. Miller P. A. *Complete dentures supported by natural teeth.* J Prosthet Dent 1959; 8:924-928.
2. Morrow R. M.et al. *Tooth-supported complete dentures: An approach to preventive prosthodontics.* J Prosthet Dent 1969; 21:513-522.
3. Morrow R. M., et al. *Immediate interim tooth-supported complete dentures.* J Prosthet Dent 1973;30:695-700.
4. Dodge C. A. *Prevention of complete denture problems by the use of overdentures.* J Prosthet Dent 1973; 30:403-411.
5. Thayer H. H. *Overdentures and the periodontium.* Dent Cli North Am 1980;24:369-377.
6. Crum R. J. and Rooney G. E. *Alveolar bone loss in overdentures - 5 year study.* J Prosthet Dent 1978; 40:610-613.
7. Derkson G. D. and MacEntee, M. M, *Effect of 0.4% stannous fluoride gel on the gingival health of overdenture abutments.* J Prosthet Dent 1982; 48:23-26.
8. Toolson L. B. and Smith D. E. *A five-year longitudinal study of patients treated with overdentures.* J Prosthet Dent 1983;49:749-756.
9. Ullo C. A. and Renner R. P. *Design considerations for a removable partial overdenture.* Compend Contin Educ Dent 1984;5:15-19.
10. Casey D, M. and Lauciello F. R. *A review of the submerged root concept.* J Prosthet Dent 1980;43:128-132.

28

Expected outcome in complete denture prosthodontics - an outline

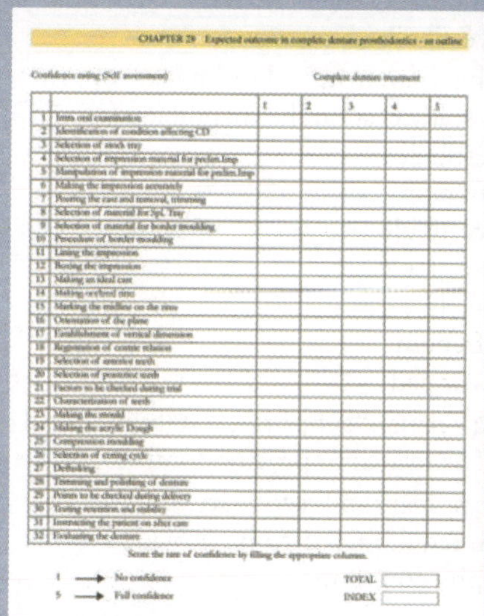

CHAPTER 29 Expected outcome in complete denture prosthodontics - an outline

Confidence rating (Self assessment) Complete denture treatment

		1	2	3	4	5
1	Intra oral examination					
2	Identification of condition affecting CD					
3	Selection of stock tray					
4	Selection of impression material for prelim.Imp					
5	Manipulation of impression material for prelim.Imp					
6	Making the impression accurately					
7	Pouring the cast and removal, trimming					
8	Selection of material for Spl. Tray					
9	Selection of material for border moulding					
10	Procedure of border moulding					
11	Lining the impression					
12	Boxing the impression					
13	Making an ideal cast					
14	Making occlusal rims					
15	Marking the midline on the rims					
16	Orientation of the plane					
17	Establishment of vertical dimension					
18	Registration of centric relation					
19	Selection of anterior teeth					
20	Selection of posterior teeth					
21	Factors to be checked during trial					
22	Characterization of teeth					
23	Making the mould					
24	Making the acrylic Dough					
25	Compression moulding					
26	Selection of curing cycle					
27	Deflasking					
28	Trimming and polishing of denture					
29	Points to be checked during delivery					
30	Testing retention and stability					
31	Instructing the patient on after care					
32	Evaluating the denture					

Score the rate of confidence by filling the appropriate columns.

1 → No confidence

5 → Full confidence

TOTAL

INDEX

This is a self assessment tool to grade the knowledge and skills related to complete dentures

The Edentulous Patient

I. Preliminary impressions and custom impression trays

1. Trace the anticipated extent of the maxillary and mandibular denture borders with a black pencil. Trace the borders of the maxillary and mandibular custom impression tray borders with a blue pencil. And, finally, outline all blockout and relief areas with a red pencil.
2. Describe the technique for custom tray fabrication.
3. Describe the purpose of preliminary impressions and the associated critical landmarks.
4. Identify these anatomic landmarks on the edentulous study cast of the maxilla:
   a. maxillary tuberosity
   b. hamular notch
   c. fovea palatini
   d. rugae
   e. median palatal raphe
   f. maxillary labial frenum
   g. labial vestibule
   h. incisive papilla
   i. buccal frenum
   j. buccal vestibule
5. Identify these anatomic landmarks on the edentulous study cast on the mandible:
   a. labial vestibule
   b. buccal frenum
   c. buccal vestibule
   d. lingual vestibule
   e. buccal shelf
   f. lingual frenum
   g. retromolar pad
6. Define the terms, "support", "stability" and "retention" as related to prosthodontics.
7. Identify the primary and secondary stress bearing areas which require relief to be provided in the custom impression tray.

II. Anatomy for complete dentures

1. Define the muscles of mastication and related muscles:
   a. temporalis
   b. masseter
   c. medial pterygoid
   d. lateral pterygoid
   e. suprahyoids including mylohyoid
   f. buccinator
2. Describe TMJ anatomy, rotational vs. translatory mandibular movements and the muscular involvement in mandibular movement.
3. Describe the role of each of the following intra-oral anatomical structures as it relates to fabrication of a complete denture prostheses:
   a. Areas Related to Support for Maxillary Dentures
      i. residual ridge
      ii. incisive Papilla
      iii. posterior palatine area
      iv. zygomatic process
      v. maxillary tuberosity
      vi. torus palatinus
   b. Limiting Structures of the Maxilla
      i. labial frenum
      ii. orbicularis oris muscle
      iii. buccal frenum
      iv. buccal vestibule
      v. hamular notch
      vi. fovea palatini
      vii. vibrating line
   c. Muscles of soft palate, pharynx, and tongue.
   d. Supporting structures for Mandibular Dentures
      i. crest of residual ridge
      ii. buccal flange area (and buccal shelf)
      iii. bone of Basal seat
      iv. mylohyoid ridge
      v. mental foramen area
      vi. torus mandibularis
   e. Limiting Structure of the Mandible
      i. labial borders
      ii. buccal borders and vestibule
      iii. buccal flange and external oblique ridge
      iv. masseter muscle region
      v. distal extension area
      vi. retromolar region and pad
      vii. lingual border anatomy
      viii. floor of mouth
      ix. mylohyoid muscle and mylohyoid ridge

x. sublingual gland region
xi. alveolingual sulcus
xii. lingual frenum and lingual notch
xiii. lingual flange

III. Final impressions and master casts_

1. Describe the purpose and rationale for making final impressions.
2. Describe how the custom impression tray is utilized in making a final impression.
3. Describe the rationale for border molding of the custom impression tray.
4. Describe how to box the final impression and make the master casts.

IV. Fabrication of record bases

1. Define the term "record base".
2. Describe the function of the record base in complete denture prosthesis.
3. Describe the correct procedure for the fabrication of record bases.

V. Maxillomandibular relations - Facebow transfer and centric relation

1. Define the following terms:
   a. centric Relation
   b. centric Occlusion/Maximum Intercuspation
   c. physiologic rest position
   d. interocclusal distance (freeway space)
   e. vertical dimension at rest
   f. vertical dimension at occlusion
2. Describe differences in the application of the above terms to the dentulous and edentulous patients.
3. Describe the following methods for determining the vertical relations:
   a. facial measurement
   b. physiologic rest position
   c. phonetics
   d. swallowing
   e. muscular proprioception
4. Describe the possible side effects of excessive vertical dimension of occlusion.
5. Describe the possible side effects of insufficient vertical dimension of occlusion.
6. Discuss the significance of the muscles of the head and neck, and their relationship to posture and indirectly to the physiologic rest position of the mandible.
7. List the requirements that always must be fulfilled when a centric jaw relation record is made.
8. List the prerequisites that must be fulfilled prior to making a centric jaw relation record.
9. List the important reasons for registering centric relation.
10. Discuss the methods of recording centric relation.
11. Discuss the methods of recording eccentric jaw relation.
12. Discuss the transfer of these recordings to the articulator.
13. Define the term "facebow".
14. Describe the purpose of using the facebow.
15. Describe the purpose of the anterior point of reference on a facebow.
16. List the conditions where it is essential to use the facebow.

VI. Selection and arrangement of anterior artificial teeth for edentulous patients

1. Describe the following:
   a. selection of tooth shade
   b. selection of size and mold
   c. material selection
2. List the types of occlusal forms available and discuss the methods for arrangement relating to the following:
   a. esthetics
   b. masticatory efficiency
   c. preservation of the remaining oral tissues
   d. east of utilization
3. List the pre-extraction guides for tooth selection.
4. Describe methods to determine the size of anterior teeth.
5. Describe methods for determining the shape of anterior teeth.
6. Describe how stock teeth can be made to look more natural for an individual patient.

7. Explain the dentogenic concept in selecting artificial teeth.
8. Describe the qualities of color.
9. Explain how changes in age affect color of teeth.
10. Explain the purpose of the carved wax occlusion rim.
11. Explain the relation of the artificial teeth to the residual ridge.
12. Explain the relation of the anterior teeth to the incisive papilla.
13. List the guides to replacement of the anterior teeth.
14. List the average dimensions of the maxillary and mandibular wax occlusal rims and record bases.
15. List the muscles that are supported by the anterior teeth.
16. Describe the order of setting the anterior teeth.
17. Describe the effects of inadequate lip support by the anterior teeth.
18. Describe the inclinations of the maxillary and mandibular anterior teeth.

VII. Occlusion Part I: (tooth selection and management and arrangement)

1. Define the term "occlusion".
2. Explain the difference between occlusion and balanced gliding (articulation.)
3. Define the term "tooth arrangement."
4. Explain Hanau's Quint.
5. Describe the aids used to position the posterior teeth antero-posteriorly.
6. Describe the aids used to position the posterior teeth buccolingually.
7. Describe the aids used to position the posterior teeth vertically.
8. Explain how the antero-posteriorly length of the posterior teeth is determined.
9. Describe how the buccolingual width of posterior teeth is determined.
10. Explain how the gingivo-occlusal height of the posterior teeth is determined.
11. Explain how the number of posterior teeth used in tooth arrangement is determined.
12. Explain how the shade of the posterior teeth is determined.
13. Explain on what basis the form of the posterior teeth used in tooth arrangement is selected.

VIII. Occlusion part II

1. Define the term condylar path.
2. List the six factors that govern the establishment of a gliding balanced occlusion.
3. Define the term condylar guidance inclination.
4. Discuss the factors that determine the shape of the condyle path.
5. Describe the configuration of the condyle path.
6. Discuss the methods of registering the condyle path.
7. Explain why condylar guidance is not under the control of the dentist.
8. Identity the three controlling factors or guides on an articulator.
9. Define the term "incisal guidance."
10. Describe what factors determine the steepness of the incisal guide angle.
11. Explain why the incisal guide angle should be kept as flat as possible in complete denture construction.
12. Define the term plane of occlusion. (Plane of orientation or occlusal plane.)
13. Describe how the plane of occlusion is determined.
14. Explain the difference between the plane of occlusion and plane of reference.
15. Explain how the inclination of the plane of occlusion is measured.
16. Explain how the plane of occlusion is located vertically.
17. Describe how the pitch of the occlusal plane both buccolingually antero-posteriorly can be altered to better control the forces of occlusion in complete denture construction.
18. Define the term "compensating curve".
19. Describe the difference between the compensating curve and the curve of Spee.
20. Explain why the antero-posterior curve of the compensating curve is developed when arranging the artificial teeth in a balanced occlusion.

21. Define the term "Curve of Spee".
22. Define the term "Curve of Wilson".
23. Define Christianson's Phenomenon.
24. Explain why the lateral curve of the compensating curve is developed when arranging the artificial teeth in a balanced occlusion.
25. Define the term "reverse curve".
26. Define the term "cusp height".
27. Define the term "cusp angle".
28. Explain how cusp height is determined when arranging artificial posterior teeth.

IX. Occlusion Part III: determinants of occlusion

1. Define the term "Bennett Movement".
2. List the five principal factors or "Laws of Articulation" that govern balancing the occlusion during protrusive movement.
3. Discuss how each of the five principal factors are related to a balanced gliding occlusion during protrusive movement and which ones may be modified or altered in order to produce a balanced gliding occlusion of the artificial teeth.
4. Describe the influence that a high and low incisal guidance inclination has on the cuspal inclination of the teeth.
5. Write the formula for determining the degree of cuspal inclination of any individual tooth to produce a balanced occlusion in either protrusion, or on the working or balancing side.
6. Explain what the Hanau Quint is.
7. Discuss the purpose and meaning of the Hanau Quint.

X. Complete denture occlusion

1. Define the term "anatomic teeth".
2. Discuss briefly the history and development of anatomic teeth.
3. List advantages and disadvantages of anatomic teeth.
4. List the indications and contraindications for using anatomic posterior tooth forms.
5. Define the term "non-anatomic teeth."
6. Discuss briefly the history and development of non-anatomic tooth forms.
7. List advantages and disadvantages of non-anatomic teeth.
8. List indications for the use of non-anatomic teeth.
9. Identify the most important contraindication for the use of non-anatomic teeth.
10. Name the two categories to which all concepts of occlusion for complete dentures can be divided.
11. Discuss the definition of balanced occlusion as defined in the Glossary of Prosthodontic Terms.
12. List purposes of developing a balanced occlusion in complete denture construction.
13. Discuss the concepts of balanced occlusion which use anatomic tooth forms.
14. Discuss the concepts of non-balanced occlusion that use anatomic tooth forms.
15. Discuss the concepts of balanced occlusion which use non-anatomic teeth.
16. Discuss the concepts of non-balanced occlusion which use non-anatomic teeth.
17. Describe the principles upon which the "neutrocentric" concept of occlusion is based.
18. Describe advantages and disadvantages of the "Lingualized" posterior scheme.
19. Identify indications for "Lingualized" posterior occlusal scheme.
20. Identify the functional elements of "Lingualized" scheme.
21. Describe different philosophies of occlusion and their application to the "Lingualized" scheme.
22. List three advantages and disadvantages of porcelain teeth.
23. Discuss the indications and contraindications and for the use of porcelain teeth.
24. List advantages and disadvantages of plastic teeth.

XI. Wax/ esthetic try-in for complete dentures

1. Understand how to test clinically for esthetics, lip support, vertical relation and phonetics.
2. Understand how to evaluate the occlusion of the trial denture.
3. Understand how to make a protrusive record, finalize

the occlusion and perform the final wax-up of the dentures.

XII. Waxing and carving the denture base

1. Describe the proper wax form of the maxillary and mandibular denture bases including labial and buccal borders, palatal form, lingual flanges, and interproximal area.
2. Describe the proper technique for waxing and carving denture bases.
3. Relate denture detail and contours to natural mucosal contours.

XIII. Denture processing

1. Describe the compression molding process on process variables which adversely affect the mechanical and physical properties of the denture.
2. Describe the correct sequence of steps in processing compete dentures with heat curing acrylic resin.
3. Describe the correct sequence of steps in recovery of the prostheses from the gypsum molds.
4. Describe the major causes of error in the above steps.
   a. porosity in acrylic
   b. change in vertical dimension
   c. change in occlusion
   d. lost or missing teeth
   e. broken denture bases

XIV. Denture base chemistry

1. Describe the major requirements of a denture resin.
2. Describe the characteristic of auto, heat, and light-cured acrylic.
3. Describe the "forms' of each "resin system" (auto, heat and light curing), and the chemical composition and function of each component.
4. Compare the three types of polymerization processes (auto, heat and light curing) with respect to:
   a. physical properties
   b. mechanical properties
   c. dimensional accuracy
5. Describe other types of polymers (other than acrylic) used to construct dentures.
   a. polycarbonates
   b. epoxies
   c. polyvinyl
6. Describe the hazards associated with the use of methylmethacrylate monomer.
7. The student will be able to discuss structure property relationships related to polymerization heterogeneities:
   a. crosslinking
   b. residual monomer
   c. radiopacifiers
   d. plasticizers
8. Describe the effect of water on the properties of denture acrylics.

XV. Immediate dentures

1. Define the term "immediate dentures".
2. List indications and contra-indications for immediate dentures.
3. Describe advantages of immediate dentures.
4. Describe disadvantages of immediate dentures.
5. Explain the importance of patient education in the treatment planning, treatment, and follow-up care.
6. List the sequence of appointments for treatment for the immediate denture patient.

XVI. Overdentures

1. Explain how oral examination procedures are used or modified for overdenture patients.
2. List the indications and contraindications for overdenture treatment.
3. Describe advantages and disadvantages of overdenture treatment.
4. Explain the relation of periodontics, endodontics, and restorative dentistry to formulation of a treatment plan.
5. Explain the rationale for chronology of a treatment plan leading to overdenture treatment.
6. Explain the importance of patient counseling on expectation of overdenture treatment.
7. Describe the impression techniques for immediate overdentures and when to apply them.
8. Explain the influence of retaining premolars on impress techniques for immediate overdentures.
9. Describe variations in waxing and flasking procedures for immediate overdentures.

10. Describe the procedures of inserting overdentures and instructing the patient.
11. Explain the rationale of relating overdenture abutments and when and how to alter the denture in the indicated area.
12. Explain the relationship of follow up maintenance to the prognosis of overdentures.
13. Explain the significance of designating overdentures as transitional until a patient has achieved a degree of success with overdenture treatment.
14. Define the term precision attachment.
15. List indications and contra-indications for precision attachment overdentures.
16. List advantages and disadvantages for precision attachment overdentures.
17. List the sequence of treatment for precision attachment overdentures.

XVII. The problem denture patient

1. Describe methods to classify and identify the problem denture patient before initiating treatment.
2. List patterns and tendencies of problem denture patient.
3. Describe influencing factors that affect and determine their attitudes and behavior.
4. Describe some psychological tools to aid in the management of these people.

XVIII. Deflasking and occlusal correction of discrepancies due to processing complete dentures

1. Describe how, by using articulating paper, occlusal grinding and other appropriate methods, to:
   a. Restore the correct vertical dimension.
   b. Establish a widely dispersed series of even centric occlusion contacts.
   c. Provide for smooth and balanced lateral movements.
   d. Mill in minor discrepancies.
   e. Polish the occluding surfaces.
2. Discuss the finishing and polishing procedures utilized in complete denture construction.
3. Demonstrate the finishing and polishing of complete dentures.

XIX. The denture insertion appointment

1. Describe the following:
   a. evaluation and correction of the tissue surface
   b. evaluation and correction of the borders
   c. evaluation and correction of occlusal errors.
   d. instructions given to patients regarding expectations, care and use of the prosthesis
   e. a "clinical remount" is and its rationale

XX. Denture repairs, relines and rebases

1. Describe current practices for repair of dentures.
2. Describe the materials used for denture repairs.
3. Describe the clinical and laboratory procedures for relines and rebases.

XXI. Evaluation of existing dentures

1. Describe how to evaluate the adequacy of existing dentures.
2. Describe when additional diagnostic information is needed.
3. Describe and document when a case is too complex for treatment or has a poor prognosis.
4. Describe the importance of proper informed consent.
5. Describe how to educate the patient concerning unrealistic expectations.

XXII. Immediate dentures

1. Define the term "immediate dentures".
2. List indications and contra-indications for immediate dentures.
3. Describe advantages of immediate dentures.
4. Describe disadvantages of immediate dentures.
5. Explain the importance of patient education in the treatment planning, treatment, and follow-up care.
6. List the sequence of appointments for treatment for the immediate denture patient.

XXIII. Overdentures

1. Explain how oral examination procedures are used or modified for overdenture patients.
2. List the indications and contraindications for overdenture treatment.
3. Describe advantages and disadvantages of overdenture treatment.

4. Explain the relation of periodontics, endodontics, and restorative dentistry to formulation of a treatment plan.
5. Explain the rationale for chronology of a treatment plan leading to overdenture treatment.
6. Explain the importance of patient counseling on expectation of overdenture treatment.
7. Describe the impression techniques for immediate overdentures and when to apply them.
8. Explain the influence of retaining premolars on impress techniques for immediate overdentures.
9. Describe variations in waxing and flasking procedures for immediate overdentures.
10. Describe the procedures of inserting overdentures and instructing the patient.
11. Explain the rationale of relating overdenture abutments and when and how to alter the denture in the indicated area.
12. Explain the relationship of follow up maintenance to the prognosis of overdentures.
13. Explain the significance of designating overdentures as transitional until a patient has achieved a degree of success with overdenture treatment.
14. Define the term precision attachment.
15. List indications and contra-indications for precision attachment overdentures.
16. List advantages and disadvantages for precision attachment overdentures.
17. List the sequence of treatment for precision attachment overdentures.

XXIV. The problem denture patient

1. Describe methods to classify and identify the problem denture patient before initiating treatment.
2. List patterns and tendencies of problem denture patient.
3. Describe influencing factors that affect and determine their attitudes and behavior.
4. Describe some psychological tools to aid in the management of these people.

XXV. Deflasking and occlusal correction of discrepancies due to processing complete dentures

1. Describe how, by using articulating paper, occlusal grinding and other appropriate methods, to:
   a. Restore the correct vertical dimension.
   b. Establish a widely dispersed series of even centric occlusion contacts.
   c. Provide for smooth and balanced lateral movements.
   d. Mill in minor discrepancies.
   e. Polish the occluding surfaces.
2. Discuss the finishing and polishing procedures utilized in complete denture construction.
3. Demonstrate the finishing and polishing of complete dentures.

XXVI. The denture insertion appointment

1. Describe the following:
   a. evaluation and correction of the tissue surface
   b. evaluation and correction of the borders
   c. evaluation and correction of occlusal errors
   d. instructions given to patients regarding expectations, care and use of the prosthesis
   e. a "clinical remount" is and its rationale

XXVII. Denture repairs, relines and rebases

1. Describe current practices for repair of dentures.
2. Describe the materials used for denture repairs.
3. Describe the clinical and laboratory procedures for relines and rebases.

XXVIII. Evaluation of existing dentures

1. Describe how to evaluate the adequacy of existing dentures.
2. Describe when additional diagnostic information is needed.
3. Describe and document when a case is too complex for treatment or has a poor prognosis.
4. Describe the importance of proper informed consent.
5. Describe how to educate the patient concerning unrealistic expectations.

Confidence rating (Self assessment)

Complete denture treatment

		1	2	3	4	5
1	Intra oral examination					
2	Identification of condition affecting CD					
3	Selection of stock tray					
4	Selection of impression material for prelim.Imp					
5	Manipulation of impression material for prelim.Imp					
6	Making the impression accurately					
7	Pouring the cast and removal, trimming					
8	Selection of material for Spl. Tray					
9	Selection of material for border moulding					
10	Procedure of border moulding					
11	Lining the impression					
12	Boxing the impression					
13	Making an ideal cast					
14	Making occlusal rims					
15	Marking the midline on the rims					
16	Orientation of the plane					
17	Establishment of vertical dimension					
18	Registration of centric relation					
19	Selection of anterior teeth					
20	Selection of posterior teeth					
21	Factors to be checked during trial					
22	Characterization of teeth					
23	Making the mould					
24	Making the acrylic Dough					
25	Compression moulding					
26	Selection of curing cycle					
27	Deflasking					
28	Trimming and polishing of denture					
29	Points to be checked during delivery					
30	Testing retention and stability					
31	Instructing the patient on after care					
32	Evaluating the denture					

Score the rate of confidence by filling the appropriate columns.

1 ⟶ No confidence

5 ⟶ Full confidence

TOTAL [ ]

INDEX [ ]

29

Denture care

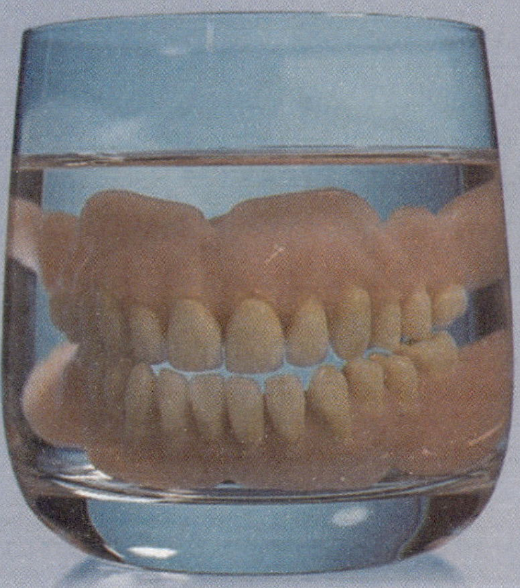

If denture care is neglected, years of successful denture wearing get restricted

Dentures can break, so always fill the sink with water, then clean your dentures over the sink, just in case they slip out of your hands by accident.

Rinse your dentures thoroughly to remove loose food particles. Use cool or warm water. But never use hot water – it can warp your dentures.

Apply a denture cleaning paste to a moistened denture brush or a soft-bristled toothbrush. Do not use ordinary toothpaste, bleach or vinegar unless directed to do so by your dentist.

Brush all surfaces thoroughly. Avoid using brushes with stiff bristles, as they can damage the denture material

Rinse dentures well under the tap to remove all traces of cleaning paste

While you sleep at night, soak your dentures in a denture cleanser recommended by your dentist.

Brush your gums, tongue and palate with a soft-bristled regular toothbrush to remove plaque and stimulate circulation. Then reinsert your dentures.

To give your mouth an extra, fresh clean feeling, rinse with a mouthwash four times a day

A few facts everyone should know about dentures

Dentures don't last forever.

Even if your dentures fit perfectly, you should still see a dental professional regularly.

No one has to know you're wearing dentures.

Denture wearers can eat more normally.

Denture wearers can speak more clearly.

Adhesives can play a role in your denture's fit and comfort.

Never try to make your own denture repairs.

With planning, denture corrections can often be made in one day.

Don't avoid replacing your denture just because you don't want to go thro ugh another long adjustment period.

Over-the-counter and prescription medications can affect dentures.

The denture wearer's lament

Oh, I wish I'd looked after my teeth
And spotted the perils beneath
All the toffees I chewed
And the sweet sticky food
Oh, I wish I'd looked after my teeth

I wish I'd been much more willin'
When I had more tooth there than fillin'
To pass up gobstoppers
From respect to my choppers
Annd to buy something else with me shillin'

When I think of the lollies I licked
And the liquorice all sorts I picked
Sherbat dabs big and little
All the hard peanut brittle
My conscience gets horribly picked

My mother she told me no end
"If you got a tooth, you got a friend"
I was young then and careless
My tooth brush was hairless
I never had much time to spend

Oh I showed them the tooth paste all right
I flashed out late at night
But up-and-down brushin'
And pokin' and fussin'
Didn't seem worth the time-1 could bite

If I had known I was paving the way
To cavities caps and decay
The murder of fillin's
Injections and drillin's
I would have thrown all my sherbet away

So I lay in the old dentist's chair
And I gaze up his nose in despair
And his drill it do whine
In these molars of mine
"Two amalgams" he'll say "for in there"

How I laughed at my mother's false teeth
As they foamed in the water beneath
But now come the reckonin'
It's me they are beckonin'
Oh, I wish I'd looked after my teeth

(Denturists' Association of British Columbia)

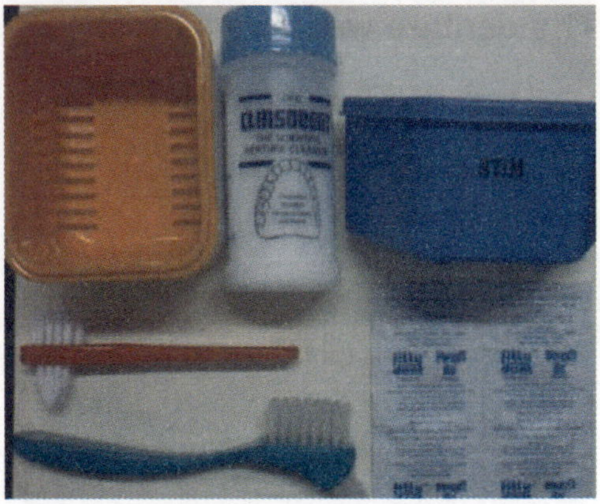

Fig.29.1 Commercially available denture cleansing material

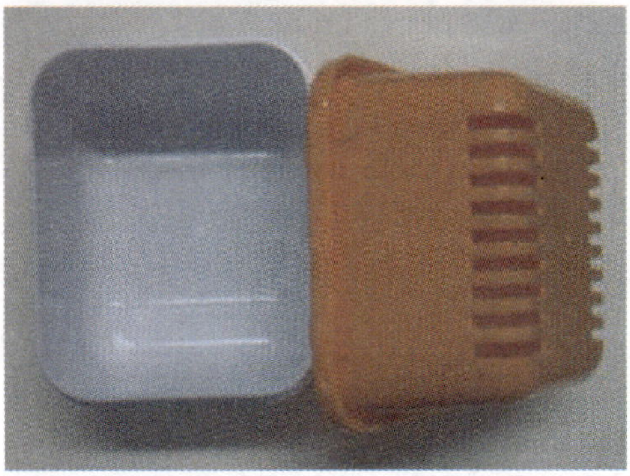

Fig.29.2 Denture cup

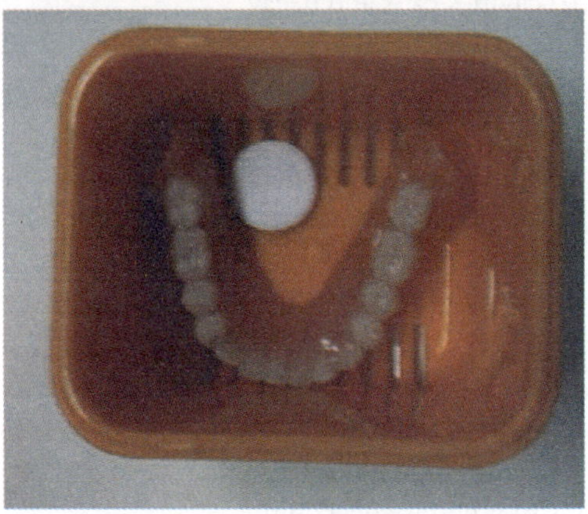

Fig.29.3 Denture cleansing tablet is dropped in the denture cup containing water along with the denture and left overight

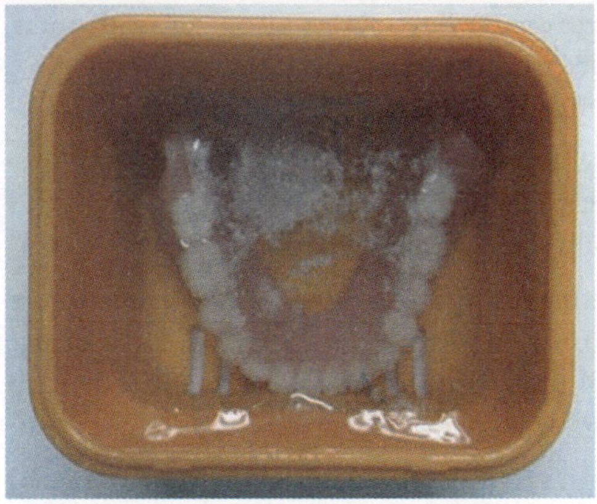

Fig.29.4 The effervescence produced by the tablet will remove food debris

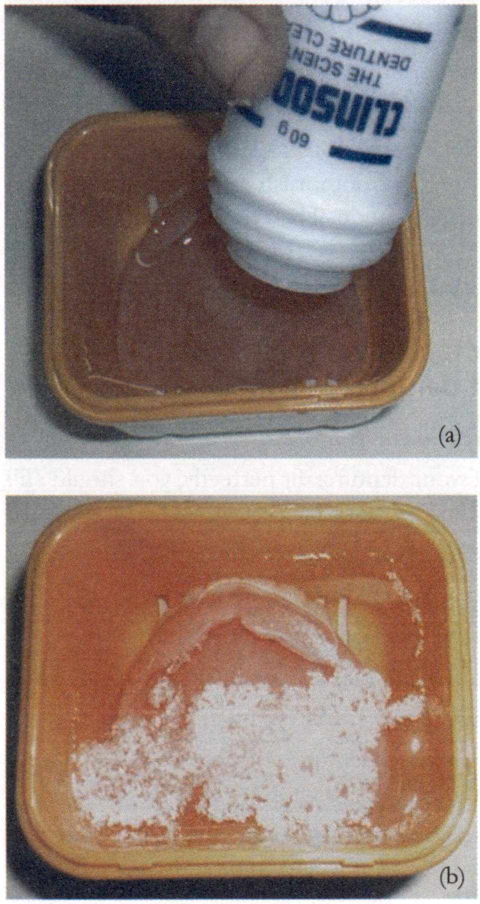

Fig.29.5 Use of denture cleansing powder

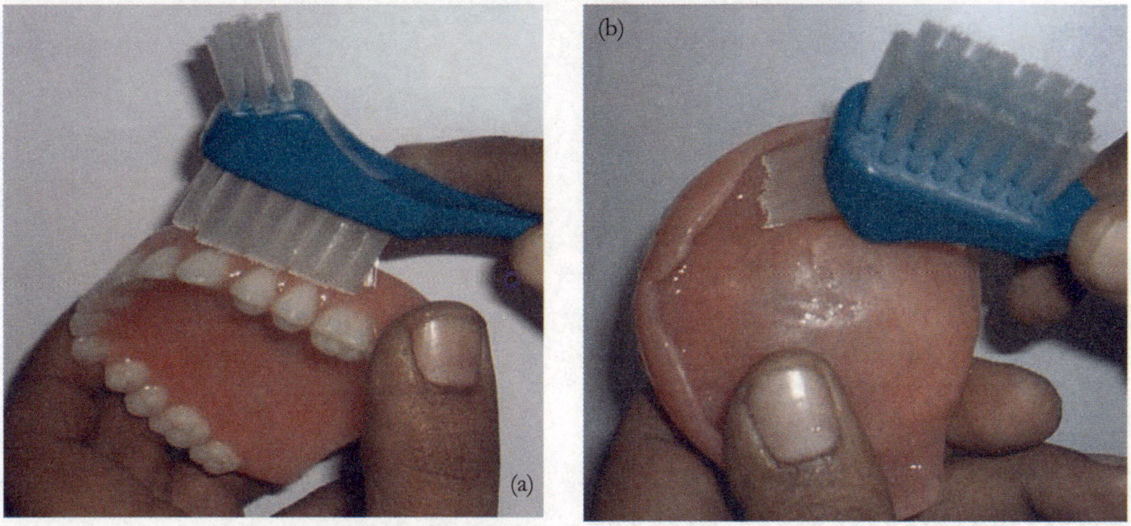

Fig.29.6 (a), (b) Denture brush can also be used to clean the denture

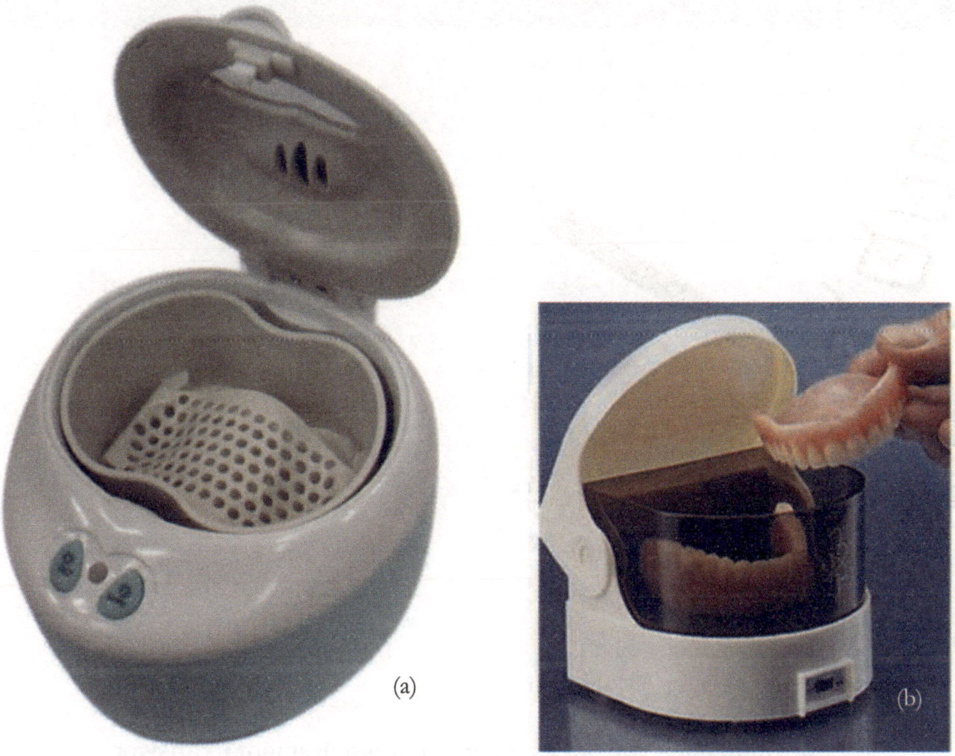

Fig.29.7 (a), (b) Ultrasonic denture cleansers

30

Guidelines for complete denture fabrication

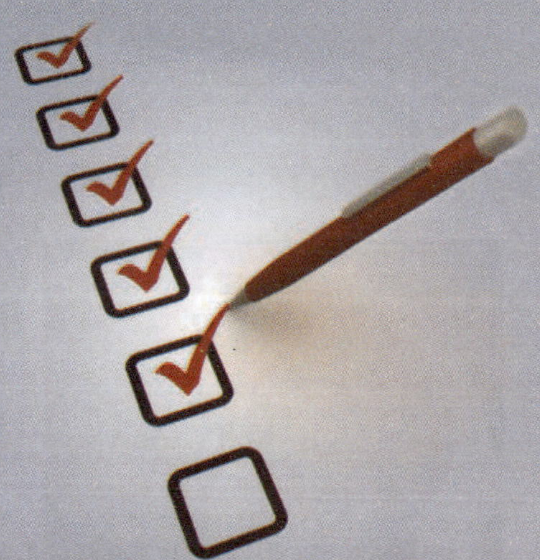

Guidelines will act as a minimum requirement to answer predictability of the treatment

Complete dentures are made to restore normal speech, provide occlusal and facial support and adequate masticatory function. They should have a pleasing appearance, be comfortable to wear, and not prejudice the health of the supporting tissues. There can, however, be no guarantee that they will satisfy all these criteria for patients who have poor denture control skills, inadequate foundations, or intolerance to prostheses. Preparation of the mouth prior to treatment and the design of complete dentures is the responsibility of the dentist.

Clinical procedures

Diagnosis and treatment plan

In order to formulate the treatment plan a medical and dental history should be recorded and a clinical examination carried out, in conjunction with radiographs and casts. Previous dentures should be examined and complaints if any obtained from the patient should be analyzed. Any pathological conditions should be investigated and appropriate treatment provided in order to render the oral tissues healthy before final impressions are made. Any elective surgery should be carried out at an appropriate stage.

Primary impressions

The requirements of the primary impressions are that they should accurately record clinically relevant landmarks of the edentulous mouth without excessive tissue distortion. They should be taken in rigid stock trays modified as necessary to fit the form of the denture bearing area.

Maxillary impressions should record the following:

i) The residual ridge, tuberosities and hamular notches.

ii) Functional labial and buccal sulci, including the freni

iii) The hard palate and its junction with the soft palate.

Mandibular impressions should record the following:

i) The residual ridge and retromolar pads.

ii) Functional labial and buccal sulci, including the freni and the external oblique ridges.

iii) The lingual sulcus, lingual fraenum, mylohyoid ridge and retromylohyoid area. The impression should be recorded with the mylohyoid muscle in a functional raised position.

Where the impression is over-extended in relation to the functional depth of the sulcus, a clear indication should be made on the impression or resultant cast to help the technician in the construction of special trays. Appropriate spaced or close fitting rigid trays should be requested in the laboratory prescription, depending on the type of impression material and technique to be used and the anatomy of the denture bearing area. The site for any stops as well as the amount of spacing should be stipulated by the clinician.

Secondary (final) impressions

These should record the entire functional denture bearing area to ensure maximum support, retention and stability for the denture during use. Each special tray should be examined in the mouth and adjusted as necessary to satisfy the above requirements. To ensure adequate lip and cheek support the maxillary impression should show an intact rounded record of the labial and buccal sulci, allowing relief for the fraena. It should extend posteriorly to the hamular notches and just beyond the junction of hard and soft palates. The mandibular impression should show an intact rounded record of the labial, buccal and lingual sulci, allowing relief for the fraena. It should extend posteriorly to cover the retromolar pads.

Impressions should be boxed or the borders marked appropriately before the casts are poured in order to preserve an accurate record of the functional depth and width of the sulci.

Recording jaw relation (maxillomandibular relation)

The bases which carry the occlusal rims should be rigid and stable. The upper rim is modified to give correct lip support. The incisive papilla provides a useful biometric guide to the prominence of the rim, its centre lying 8-10mm palatal to the labial surfaces of the maxillary central incisors (in the natural dentition). Patients' wishes, or previous satisfactory dentures, may dictate otherwise. The height of the upper rim should be adjusted to indicate the level for the upper anterior denture teeth and the antero-posterior (occlusal) plane made parallel to the interpupillary and alar-tragal lines (unless facial irregularities warrant an alternative).

A central line should be marked on the upper rim. This will usually be coincident with the midline of the face. The tubercle of the upper lip is a useful guide in determining the midline. The occlusal vertical dimension should provide for most patients a minimum interocclusal clearance (freeway space) of 4 mm.

It is established by adjustment of the lower occlusal rim and verified using various techniques of clinical measurement, preferably by affixing adhesive tapes of triangular shape; one on the nose tip and one on the chin. Failure to provide sufficient freeway space may lead to discomfort, pain, and bone resorption while excessive freeway space may lead to discomfort from the temporomandibular joints, cheek biting, angular cheilitis, and poor appearance. Progressive incremental additions of acrylic resin to the occlusal surfaces of existing or diagnostic dentures may be necessary before a satisfactory occlusal vertical dimension can be established.

The horizontal jaw relationship to be recorded at the established occlusal vertical dimension is retruded contact position (RCP). This is a reproducible position at which the denture teeth are placed in intercuspal position (ICP). Once this position can be reproduced, the bucco-lingual width of the occlusal rims should be adjusted to identify the "denture space" (neutral zone). This is important in order to provide tongue space, facial soft tissue support, and denture stability. In some instances functional recording of the mandibular denture space may be appropriate using a suitable impression material on a stable base.

The occlusal rims must be located securely together in RCP in the mouth using an accepted technique. The use of a facebow may be desirable with a semi-adjustable articulator. When semi adjustable articulator is used, it must be programmed to simulate the patients's condylar path, lateral side shift and the incisor teeth relation. For this purpose the casts are mounted on the articulator based on the occlusal rim registration mentioned above and making inter occlusal records both in centric and eccentric positions of the jaw.

The prescription accompanying the registration should give details of mould, shade, material, and manufacturer's brand of chosen teeth. A diagram may help the technician with the arrangement.

The cusp form, material, and size of posterior teeth should be selected. The number of teeth to be used and their anatomical type should be recorded. When setting up the teeth it is usual to limit the lower occlusal table to the horizontal part of the ridge and to avoid placing teeth over an inclined plane.An impression of a previous denture may be helpful to the technician where a particular form of anterior tooth arrangement is to be repeated.

The trial insertion

The occlusal plane, occlusal vertical dimension, and RCP should be verified as correct. Tooth position and arrangement should provide adequate lip and cheek support and tongue space, allow clear speech, and give a pleasing appearance to the patient. Where alterations are required to the horizontal or vertical jaw relationship, a new recording will be required and a re-try necessary. The position of the posterior palatal border of the maxillary base should be examined to ensure it is correctly extended just beyond the junction of hard and soft palate. The fovea palati act as a useful landmark, lying 2-3 mm behind the posterior margin of the hard palate. It is the clinician's responsibility to mark the posterior extent of the denture on the master cast in the appropriate position unless a functional post dam was incorporated into the final impression. The patient should be given the opportunity to see the trial dentures in place at this stage. It is wise for them to agree verbally (and ideally in writing) that the appearance is satisfactory. It is preferred to sign an informed consent at this stage.

Insertion of the dentures

The denture bases should be inspected and any remaining surface blemishes or defects removed. Each denture should be inserted and assessed for retention, extension, appearance, and stability. Factors assessed at the trial stage such as lip support, speech, and horizontal and vertical jaw relationships should be reconfirmed as correct. Articulating paper may be used to examine occlusion and articulation in the mouth, although this should be carried out with caution to avoid errors. A pressure indicating paste or other suitable recording material may be used on the fitting surfaces of the dentures to indicate excessive tissue displacement.

It is recommended that the processed dentures are remounted on the articulator following deflasking (for example using the split-cast method), and the occlusion adjusted. A clinical remount using a check record is a useful method for refining the occlusion, the dentures being remounted on the original articulator and adjustments carried out to provide correct articulation. This could be valuable at the review appointment after the dentures have been worn for a period and the supporting tissues have adapted to them.

Instructions (both verbal and written) on the use and care of dentures should be given to the patient, and a review appointment made approximately one week later.

Inspection and review

At the review appointment, any adjustments should be made to the dentures in the light of the patient's experiences or complaints. The denture bearing areas should be examined for trauma even in the absence of patient complaints. The occlusion and articulation should be examined at this stage. The importance of attending for regular review should be explained to the patient.

Due regard should be given to the disinfection and sterilisation of all materials/ prostheses which pass from clinician to laboratory and vice versa, according to health and safety requirements.

Technical procedures

The clinician is responsible for the provision of complete dentures. At each stage the dentist should provide a clear prescription for the laboratory. If the technical quality of the dentures is inadequate it is the clinician's responsibility to have the problem remedied

Primary casts and special trays

Surface moisture should be removed from the impressions after rinsing and before casting. Plaster of Paris or dental stone is mixed with water. The impressions are cast using vibration to eliminate air bubbles and separated from the cast after 40 minutes. The cast should record the depth and width of the sulci and be surrounded by a "land" width of at least 3 mm. The base should be 1 cm thick at the deepest part of the cast. The "land" area should always be recorded unless the extent of the special tray has been indicated on the impression by the clinician.

Special trays are made according to the clinical prescription, which will stipulate the amount of spacing and stops (if any). Handles must be designed to avoid distortion of the tongue or lips. The periphery of the tray should normally extend 2mm short of the deepest part of the recorded sulcus, or to the indication on the cast made by the clinician. In the maxilla it should extend posteriorly to the hamular notches and fovea palati; in the mandible to the distal aspect of the retromolar pads.

Working casts and registration blocks

Surface moisture should be removed from the final impressions after rinsing and before casting. Dental stone in the correct measure is vacuum mixed with water and the impression is cast. The thickness of the base and the width of the "land" is the same as for primary casts. The base of the registration block should normally be made of a rigid material. Close adaptation of the base to the working cast is essential for stability in the mouth and accurate registration of jaw relations. Registration rims are usually made of wax. The upper block should measure approximately 22mm in height from the deepest part of the labial sulcus. The equivalent dimension of the lower block should measure approximately 18mm. The preferred width of the occlusal rim in the anterior region is 4mm, premolar region 5mm and molar region 6mm. Wax rims are positioned buccolingually in the same place as the lost teeth, according to the amount of resorption that has taken place. The occlusal surface of the lower rim passes posteriorly from its anterior edge to a point 2/3 up the retromolar pads. The upper rim usually passes posteriorly parallel to the surface of the maxillary ridge. The arch form of the mandibular ridge dictates the future arch of the denture.

Mounting and setting up

The registration blocks are mounted on a semi-adjustable or average value articulator (according to clinical requirements), preferably using the split cast technique. After noting the prescription for tooth arrangement, the maxillary anterior teeth are set up in accordance with the marked central line, always conforming to the contour of the wax rim. Unless the prescription says otherwise, or a neutral zone technique has been used, the mandibular posterior teeth are placed to conform to the buccal contour of the wax rim. It is wise, particularly with flat lower ridges, to avoid the most posterior tooth being positioned over an inclined plane, and to achieve this the last tooth should be at the posterior extremity of the horizontal part of the ridge. The teeth are adjusted to allow balanced articulation in lateral and protrusive excursions. Any part of the try-in base removed to facilitate registration is replaced unless this interferes with occlusal balance.

Processing and finishing

While in occlusion on the articulator, the try-in is sealed to the casts with wax around the denture periphery. Following processing, the dentures (still on casts) should be replaced on the articulator, by means of the split cast, and any processing errors removed by occlusal adjustment. Finishing and polishing is carried out carefully to preserve the recorded periphery. Apart from the removal of imperfections, the fitting surface remains untouched. The completed dentures should be stored in clean water (with antiseptic as appropriate) after removal of traces of polishing material. Denture identification is a desirable option with complete dentures.

31

Complete denture treatment policy

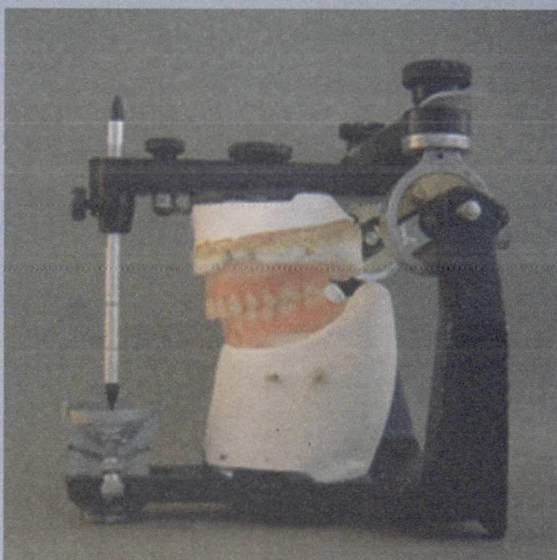

There are many right things which can be practiced but every clinic should have a policy to declare the technique they follow.

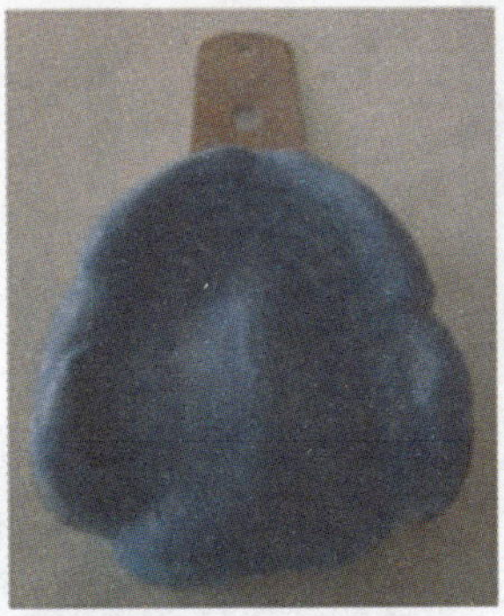

Fig. 31.1 Primary impression made with addition reaction vinyl siloxane putty consistency impression material and lined with addition reaction vinyl siloxane - light body - Maxillary

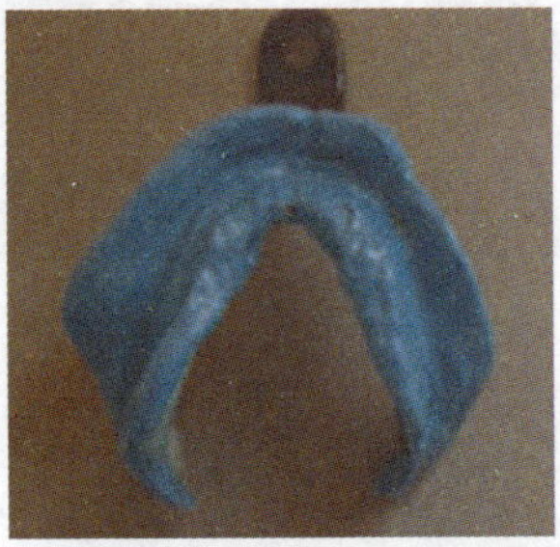

Fig. 31.2 Primary impression made with addition reaction vinyl siloxane putty consistency impression material and lined with addition reaction vinyl siloxane - light body - Mandibular

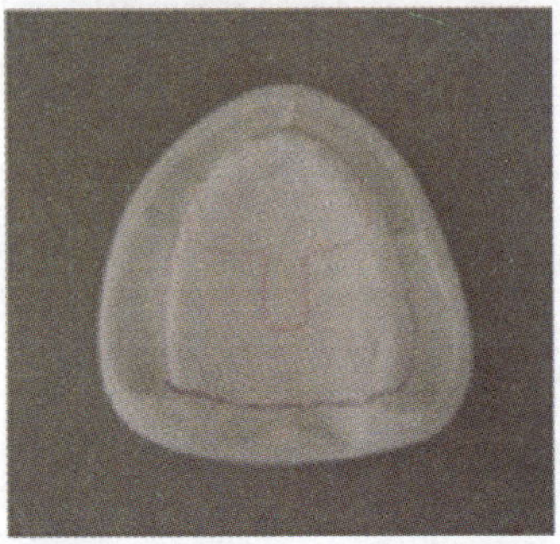

Fig. 31.3 Primary cast prepared in dental plaster - Maxillary
Thickness of base – measured from deepest portion of palate – 10mm
Red line – Extent of Spacer
Blue line – Extent of special tray

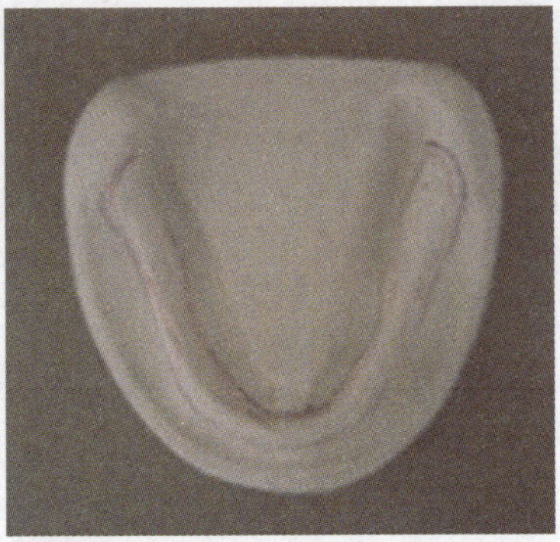

Fig. 31.4 Primary cast prepared in dental plaster – Mandibular
Thickness of base – measured from deepest portion of lingua l sulcus – 10mm
Red line – Extent of Spacer
Blue line – Extent of special tray

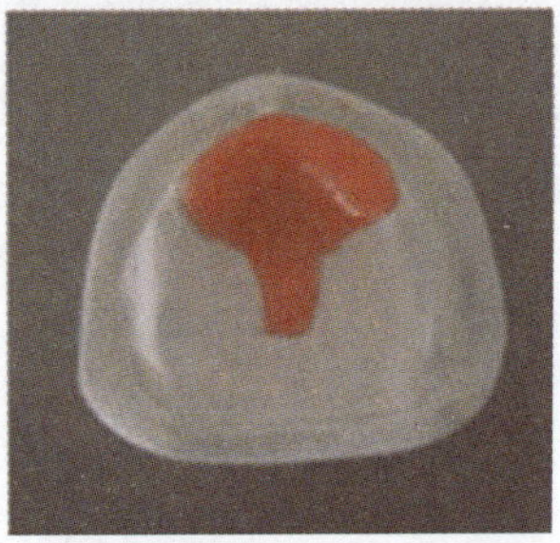

Fig. 31.5 Spacer design - Maxillary

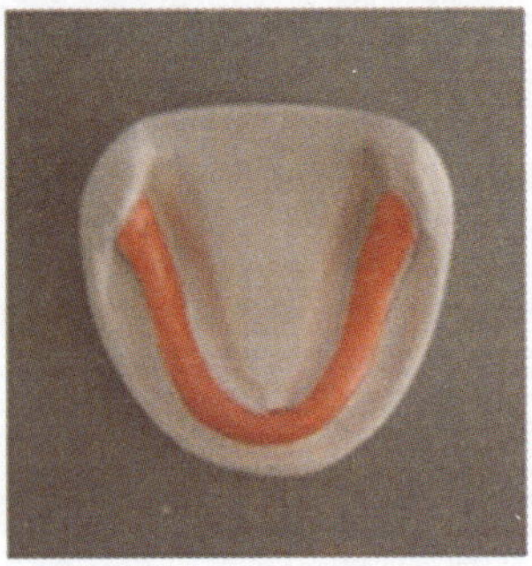

Fig. 31.6 Spacer design – Mandibular
All areas covered except for the buccal shelf area.

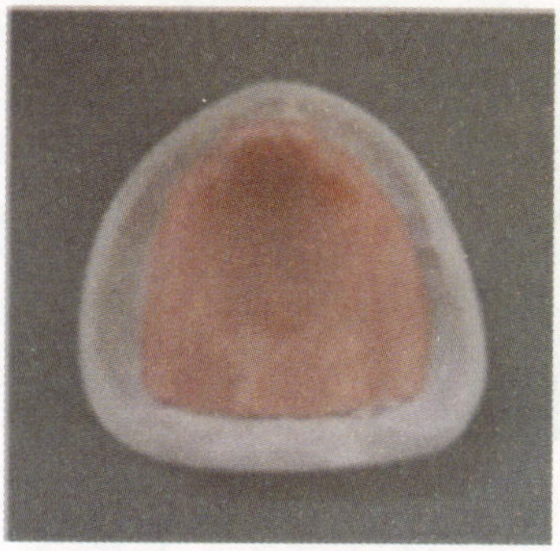

Fig. 31.7 Acrylic special tray prepared in autopolymerising acrylic resin – Maxillary.

Extent – 2 mm short of the fornix of labial and buccal sulci

Handle – min. 12mm wide and 25 mm length. Labiopalatal dimension 4mm and angulation of 15°

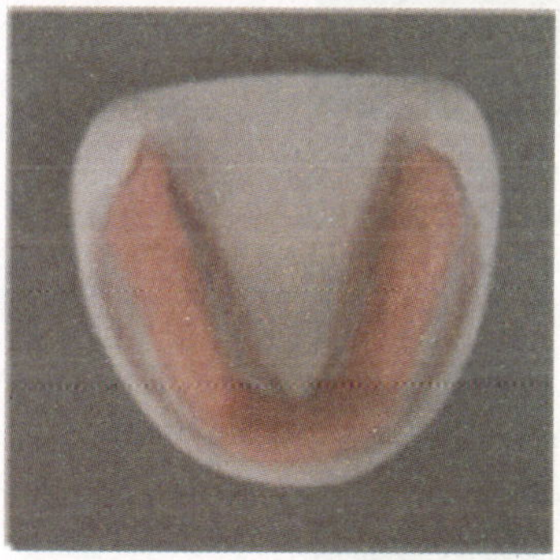

Fig. 31.8 Acrylic special tray prepared in autopolymerising acrylic resin – Mandibular.

Handle – mesiodistal width of four insiors and 4mm thick Height – 20 mm measured from sulcus. No labial angualtion. Bialteral finger rests – in the form of a rim extending from 1st premolar to 1st molar. Width – 4mm. This can be continuation of handle.

This form of finger rests keeps the operators' fingers sufficiently away from sulcus and thereby preventing possible distortion of sulcular impression especially in compromised ridges

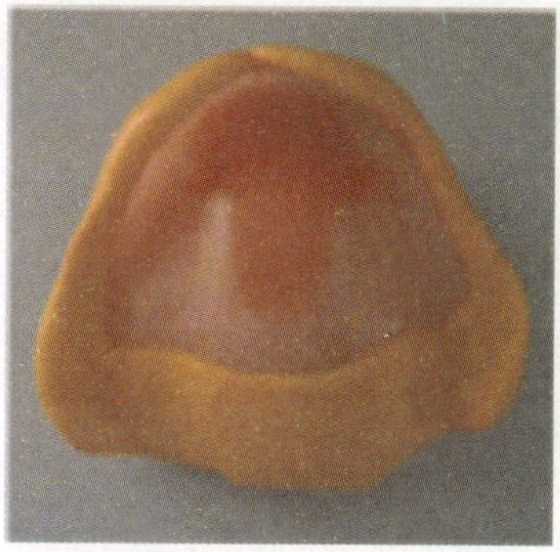

Fig. 31.9 Border molding done with addition reaction vinyl siloxane putty consistency impression material – Maxillary

Equal volumes of base paste and catalyst paste mixed thoroughly. Vaseline is incorporated in to each component separately and made in to a rope.

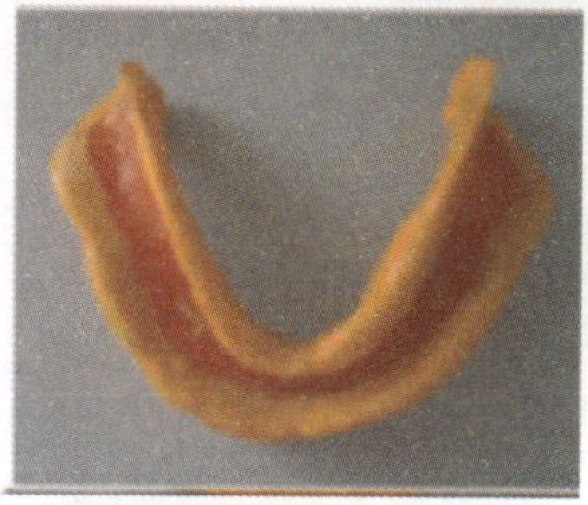

Fig. 31.10 Border molding done with addition reaction vinyl siloxane putty consistency impression material – Mandibular

Equal volumes of base paste and catalyst paste mixed thoroughly . Vaseline is incorporated in to each component separately and made in to a rope.

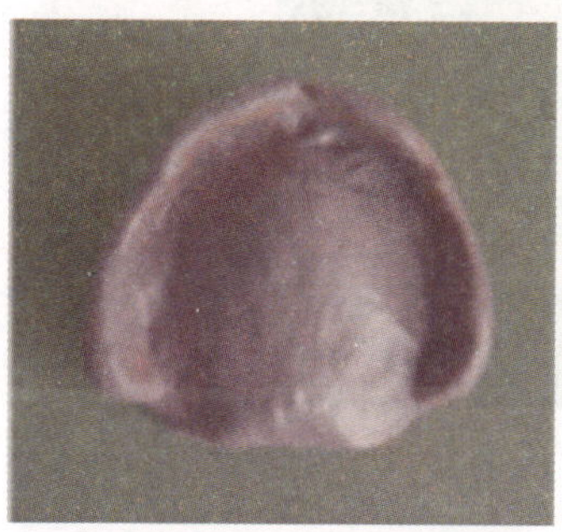

Fig. 31.11 Final impression made with addition reaction vinyl siloxane - light body - Maxillary

1 relief hole in palatal slope.

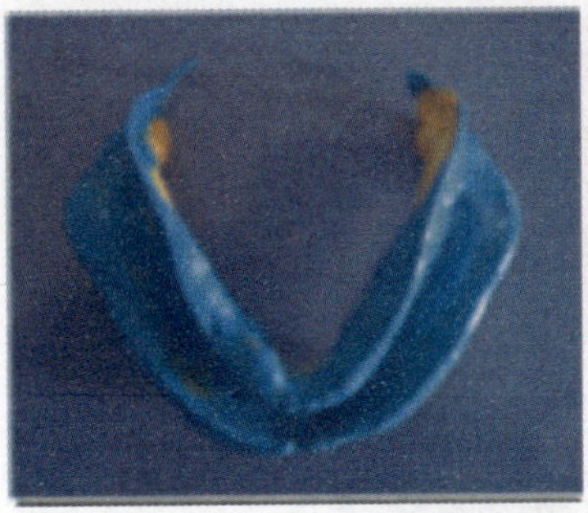

Fig. 31.12 Final impression with addition reaction vinyl siloxane - light body – Mandibular.
No relief hole.

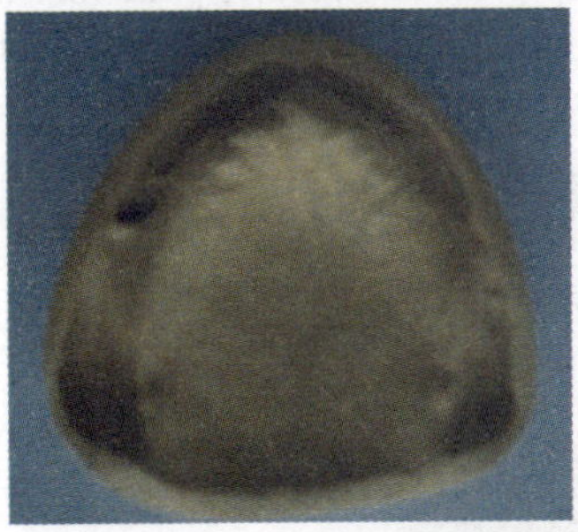

Fig. 31.13 Master cast prepared from dental stone – Maxillary.
Thickness of base – measured from deepest portion of palate – 10mm.
Land area – 3mm.

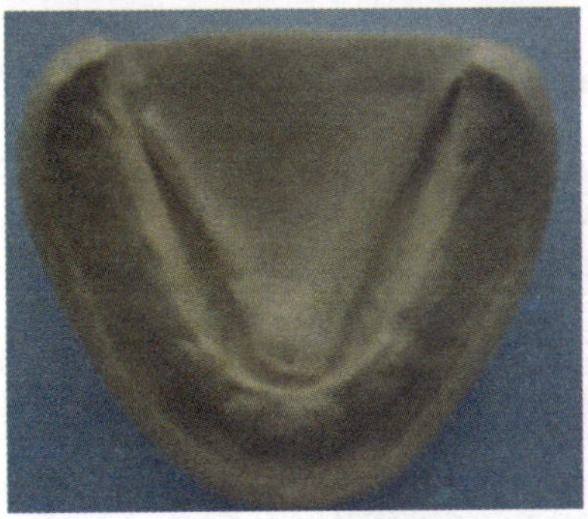

Fig. 31.14 Master cast prepared from dental stone – Mandibular
Thickness of base – measured from deepest portion of palveololingual sulcus – 10mm.
Land area – 3mm.

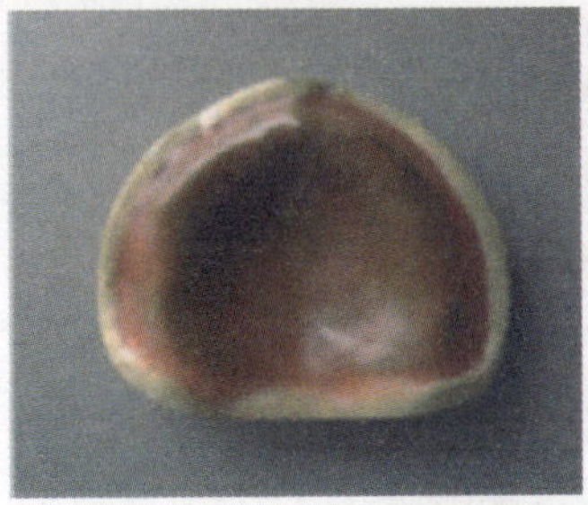

Fig. 31.15 Wax up for permanent record base - Maxillary.

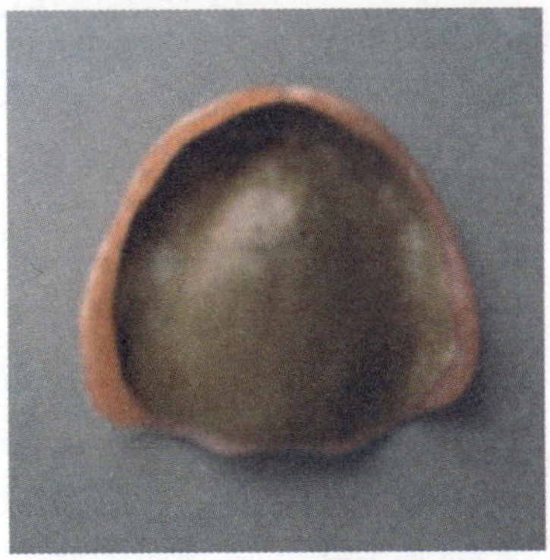

Fig. 31.16 Wax up for permanent record base – tissue surface - Maxillary

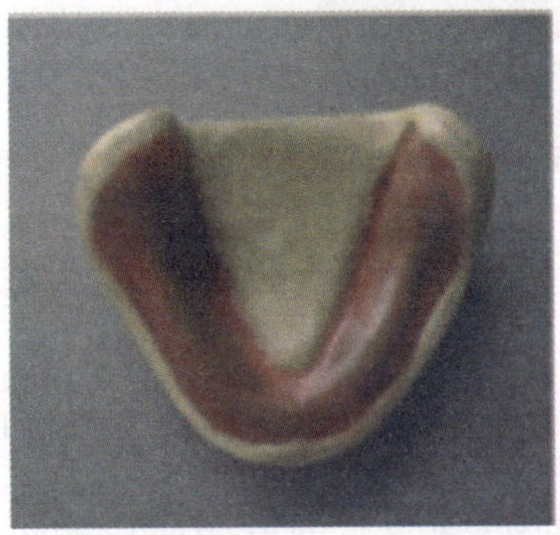

Fig. 31.17 Wax up for permanent record base - Mandibular

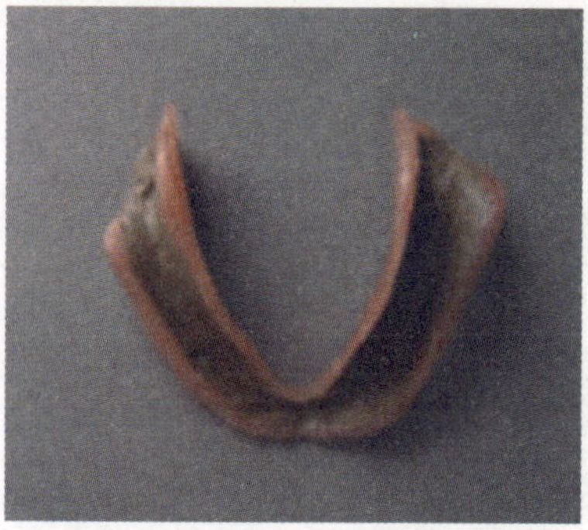

Fig. 31.18 Wax up for permanent record base – tissue surface - Mandibular

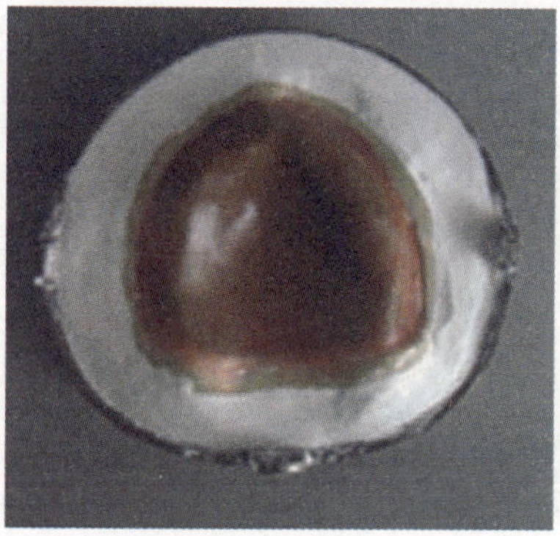

Fig. 31.19 Flasking done – for permanent record base - Maxillary

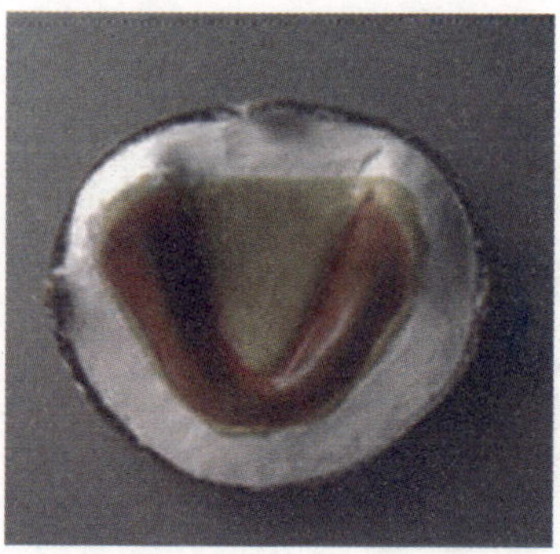

Fig. 31.20 Flasking done – for permanent record base – Mandibular

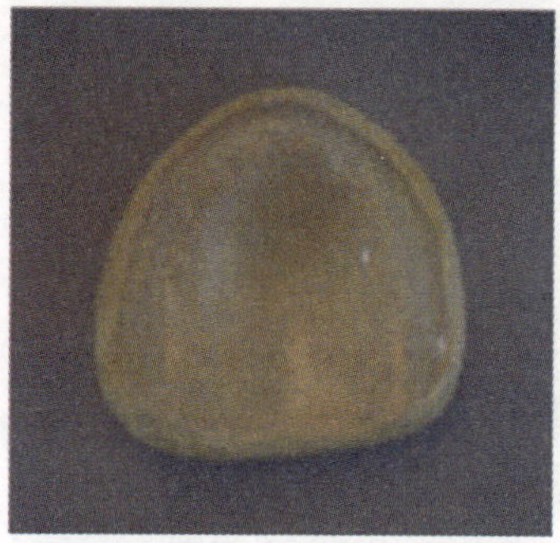

Fig. 31.21 Permanent record base prepared from heat cure clear acrylic – Maxillary
Cast prepared from permanent record base and made of dental stone

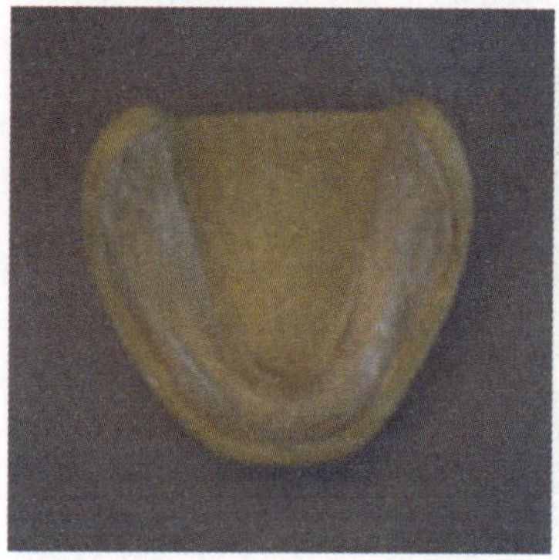

Fig. 31.22 Permanent record base prepared from heat cure clear acrylic – Mandibular
Cast prepared from permanent record base and made of dental stone

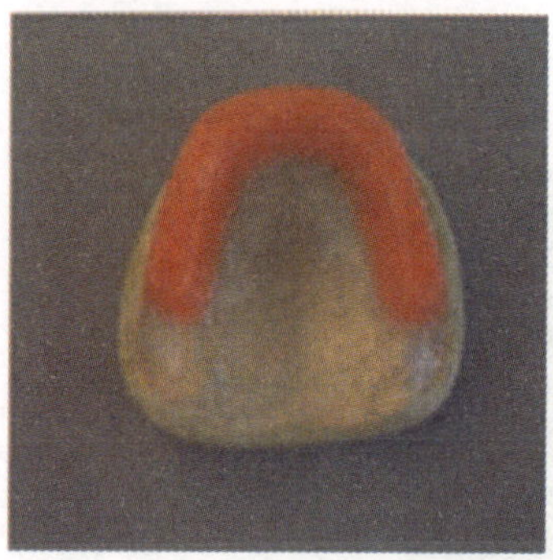

Fig. 31.23 Occlusal rim prepared from modelling wax – Maxillary
Width – incisal region – 4 mm, premolar region – 5mm and first molar region – 6mm.
Posterior terminal rounded and inclined.

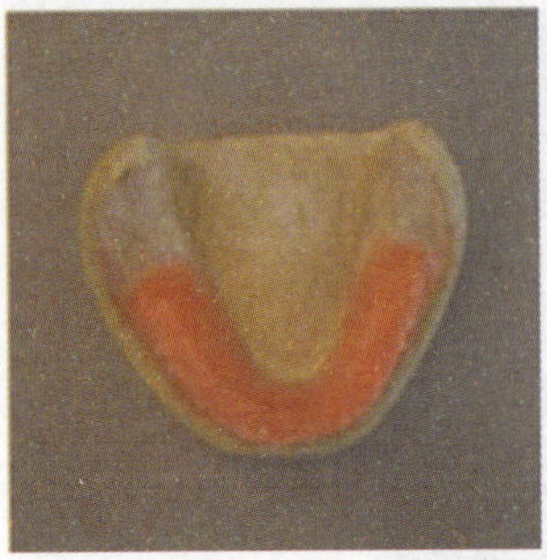

Fig. 31.24 Occlusal rim prepared from modelling wax – Mandibular
Width – incisal region – 4 mm, premolar region – 5mm and first molar region – 6mm.

Posterior terminal rounded and inclined. Posteriorly height maintained at middle third of retromolar pad.

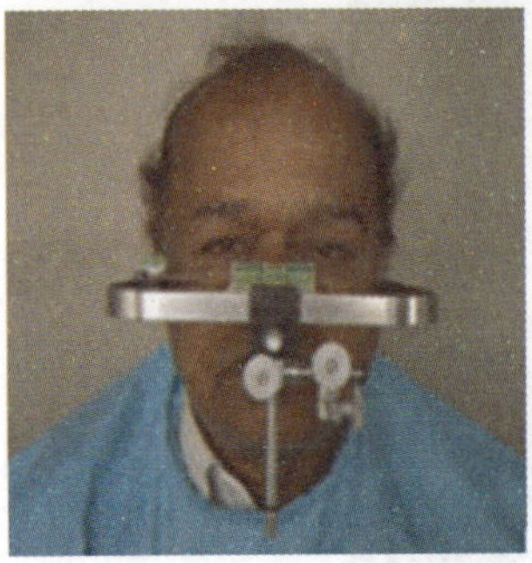

Fig. 31.25 Face bow transfer using Hanau Spring Bow with horizontal level marker.

The fork is fixed 3 mm above the occlusal surface on the occlusal rim and the midline of the fork coinciding with the patient's midline. The fork should be parallel to occlusal plane orientation.

Lower cast related to the upper in centric relation

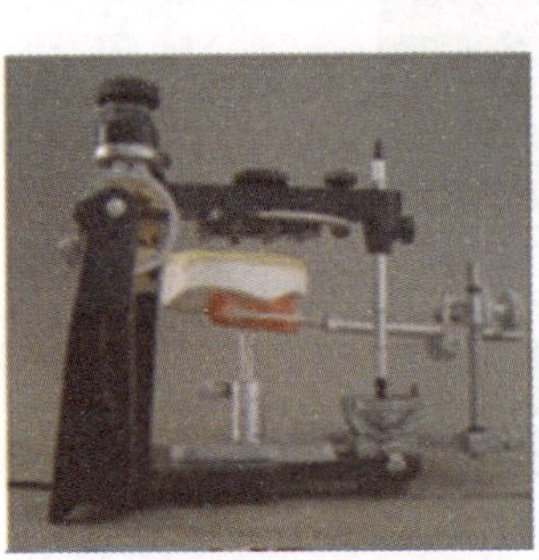

Fig. 31.26 Face bow transfer on Hanau Wide Veu arcon type semiadjustable articulator with transfer jig.

Split cast measuring 3mm in thickness is prepared from die stone

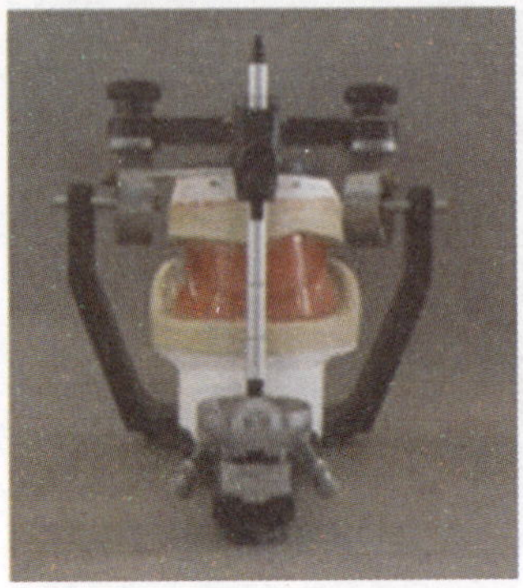

Fig. 31.27 Mandibular cast related to maxillary using tentative centric relation.

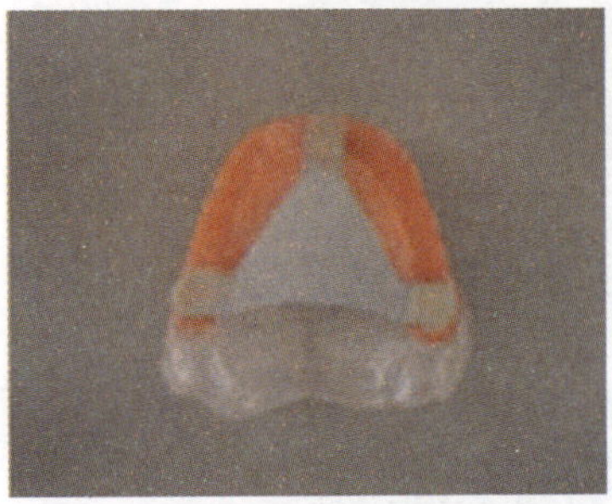

Fig. 31.28 Central bearing plate attached by recessing the occlusal rim and fixed using sticky wax - Maxillary

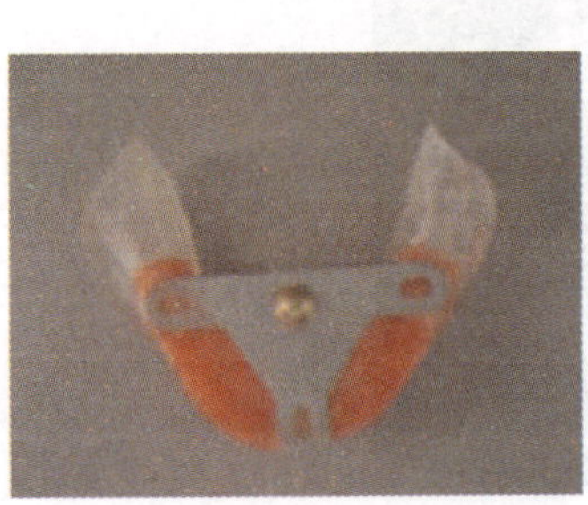

Fig. 31.29 The mandibular occlusal rim is first reduced by 3mm to accommodate for the central bearing plate and point.

Central bearing device attached by recessing the occlusal rim and fixed using sticky wax – Mandibular.

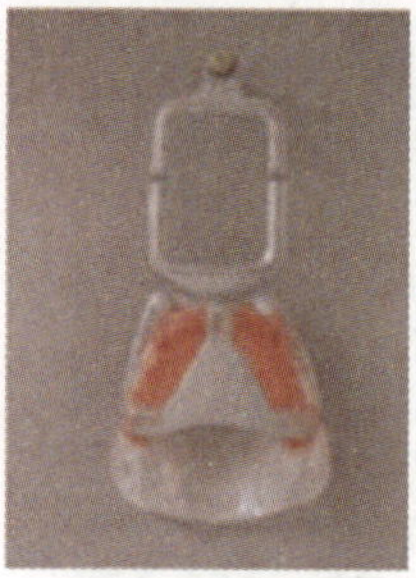

Fig. 31.30 Central bearing plate and tracer attached to occlusal rim - Maxillary

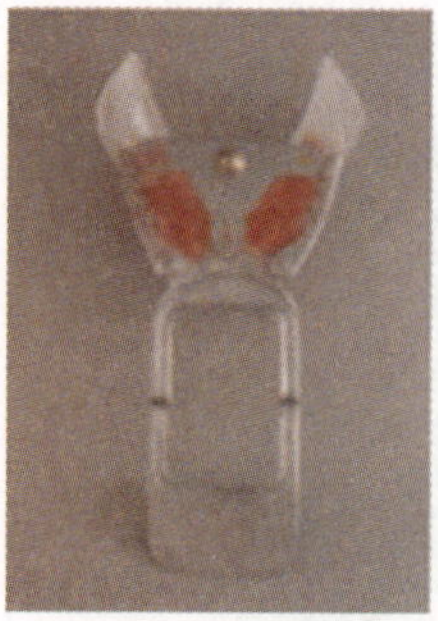

Fig. 31.31 Central bearing device and tracing plate attached to occlusal rim - Mandibular

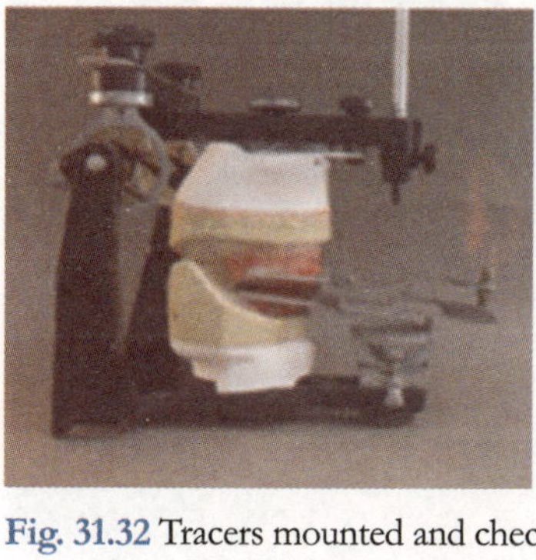

Fig. 31.32 Tracers mounted and checked for uniform space and parallelism. The arms of the tracers should be closer and parallel to each other. If the orientation of the occlusal plane demands, then the tracers are stepped up.

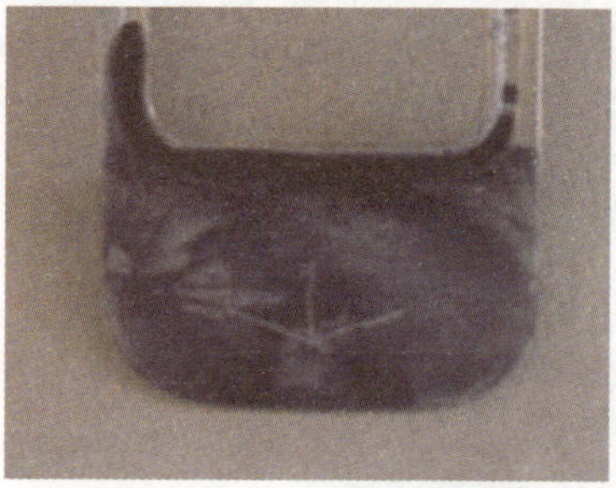

Fig. 31.33 Gothic arch tracing obtained on contrasting wax medium. 6 mm dimension marked with caliper.

Plastic sheet is fixed with sticky wax and points are drilled and interocclsual records obtained.

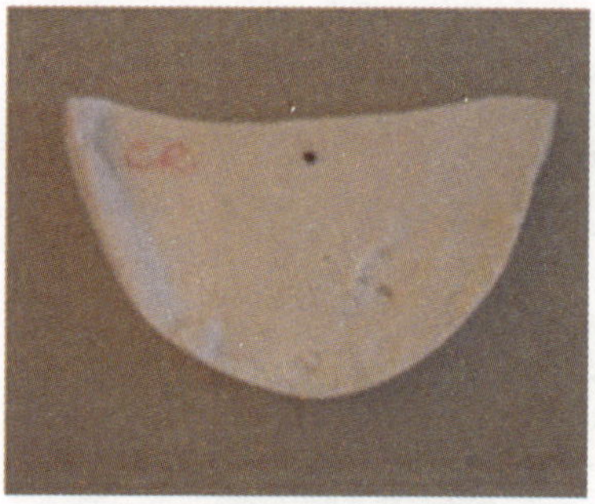

Fig. 31.34 Interocclusal record made from dental plaster – centric relation

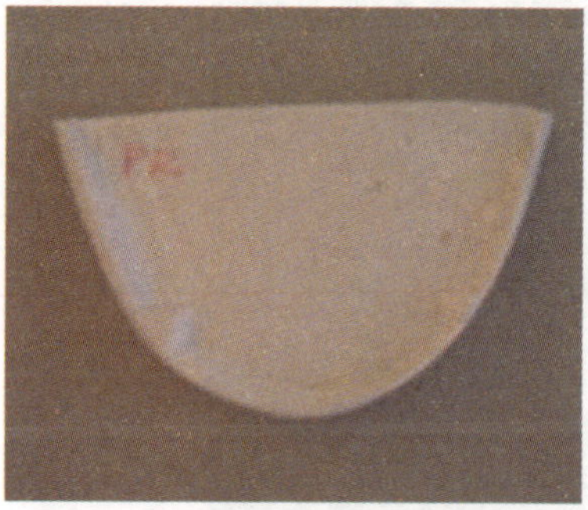

Fig. 31.35 Interocclusal record made from dental plaster – protrusive relation

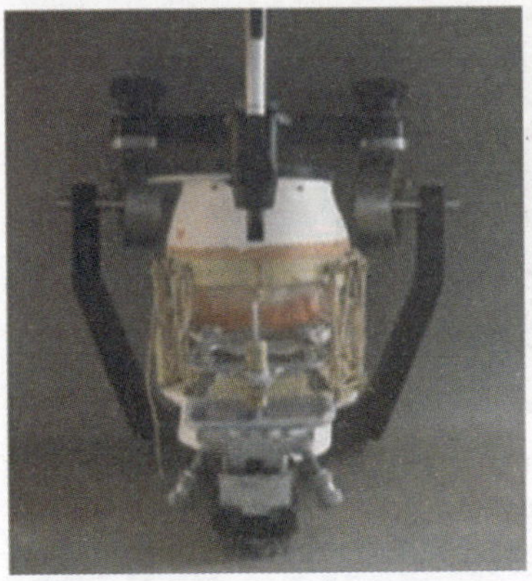

Fig. 31.36 Tentative centric relation verified with centric relation record.

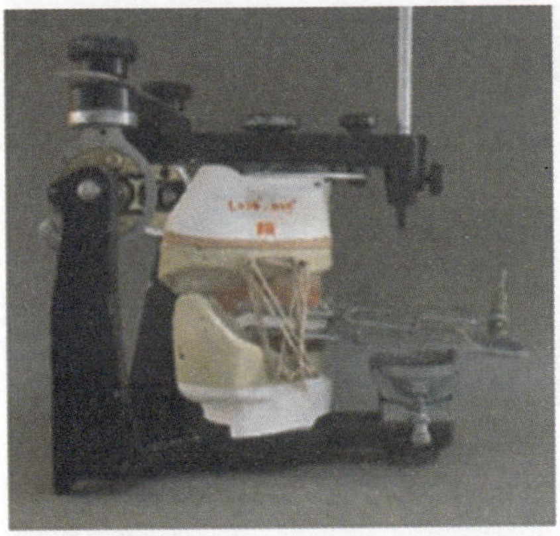

Fig. 31.37 Programming Done – Lateral And Horizontal Condylar Guidances Set Using Protrusive Record.

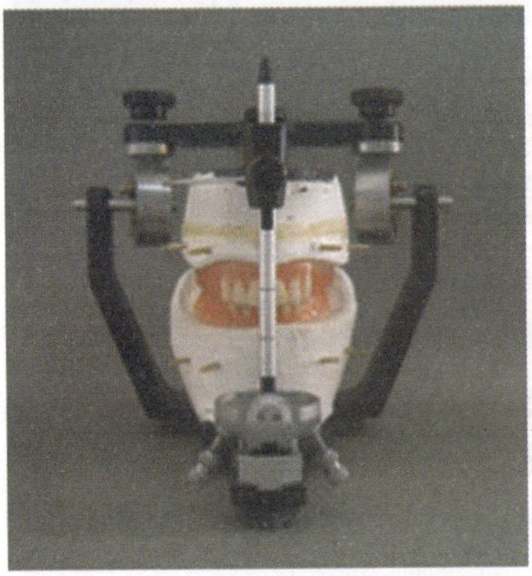

Fig. 31.38 Anterior teeth arranged for trial

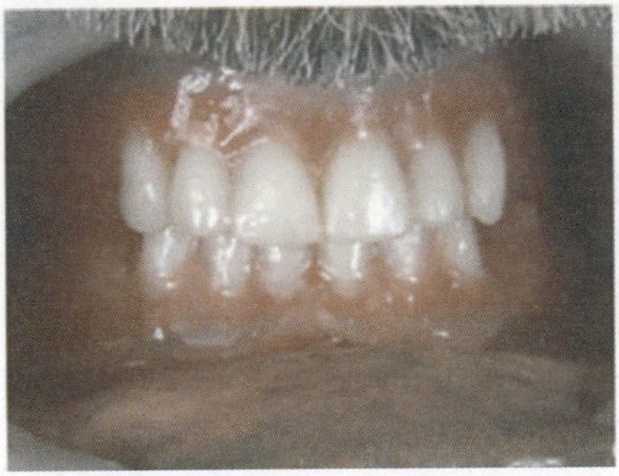

Fig. 31.39 Anterior trial

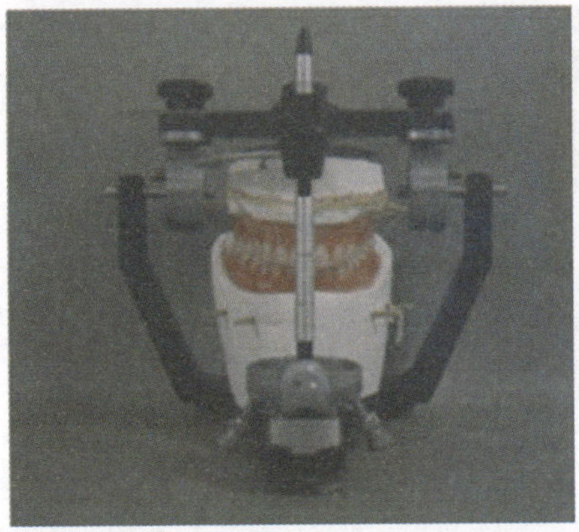

Fig. 31.40 Posterior teeth arranged for trial.
In case of space constraint, second molar is eliminated.

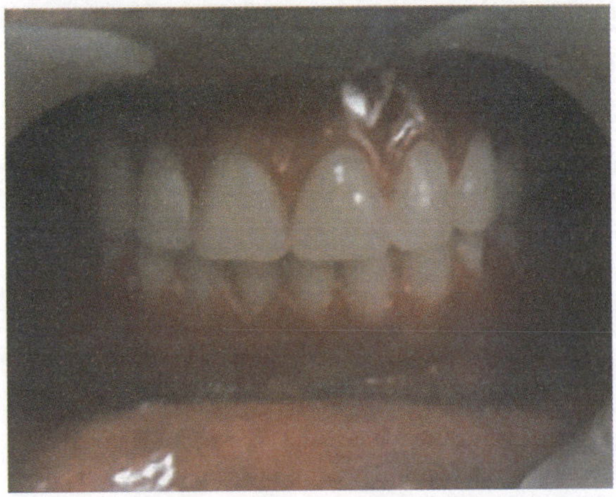

Fig. 31.41 Posterior trial

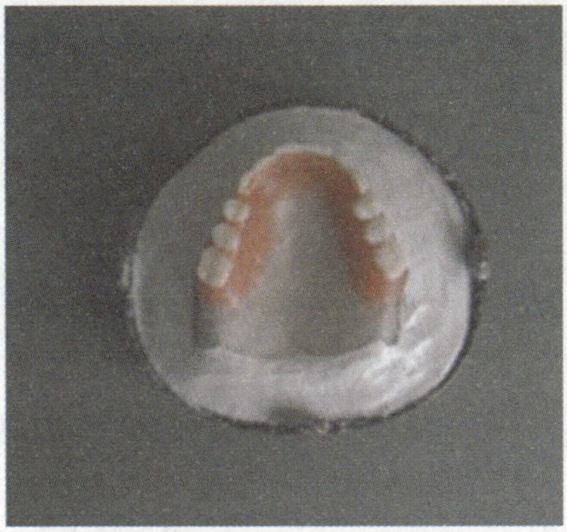

Fig. 31.42 Flasking done - Maxillary

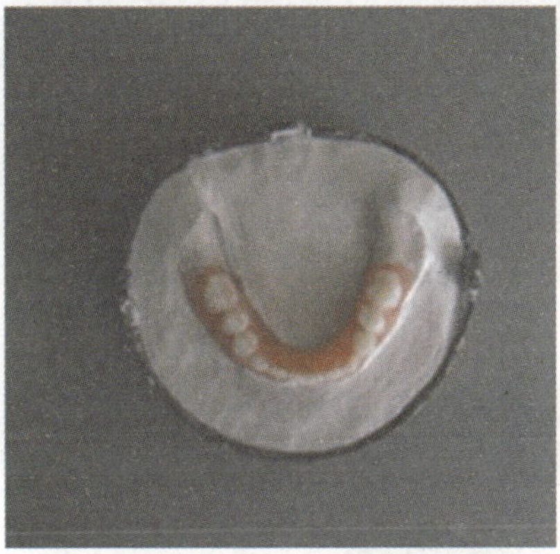

Fig. 31.43 Flasking done - Mandibular

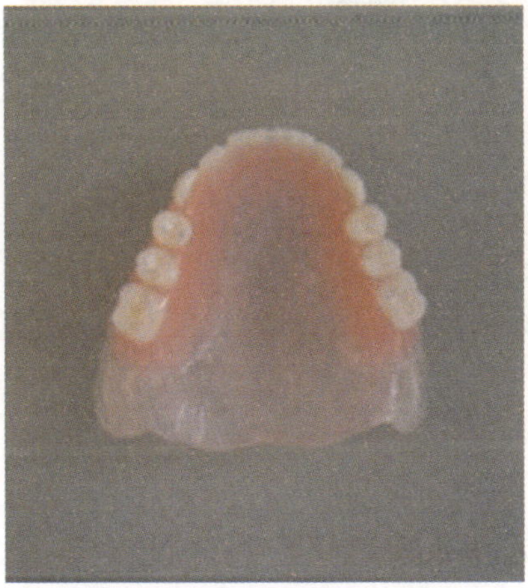

Fig. 31.44 Denture - Maxillary

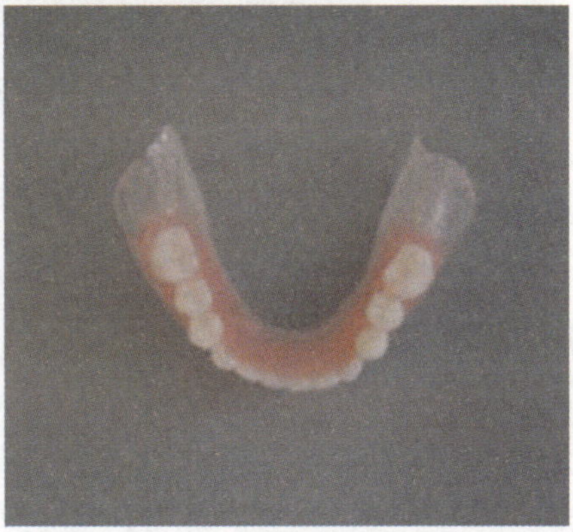

Fig. 31.45 Denture - Mandibular

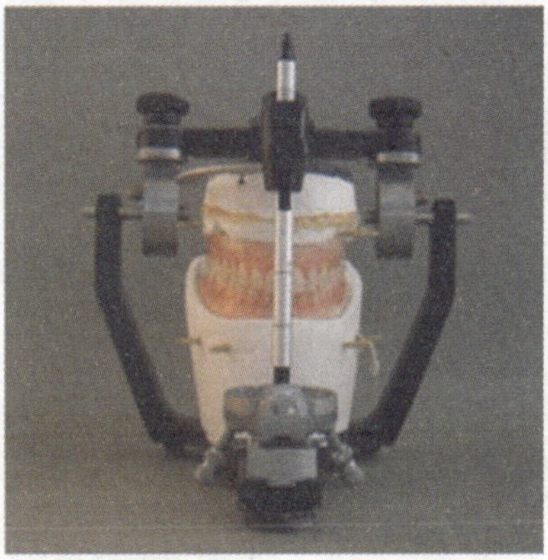

Fig. 31.46 Lab remounting done – frontal view

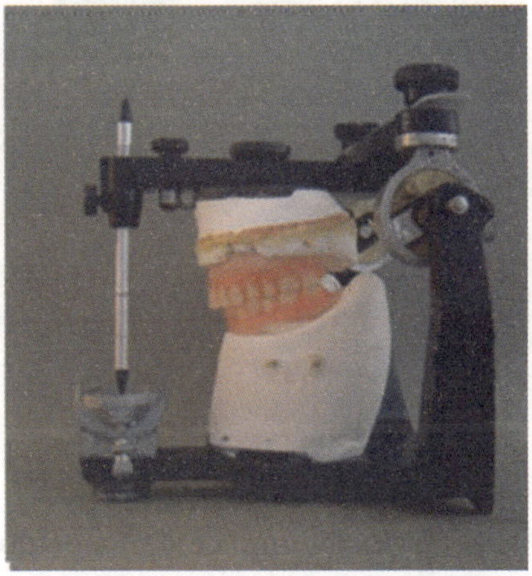

Fig. 31.47 Lab remounting done – lateral view

32

Denture duplication

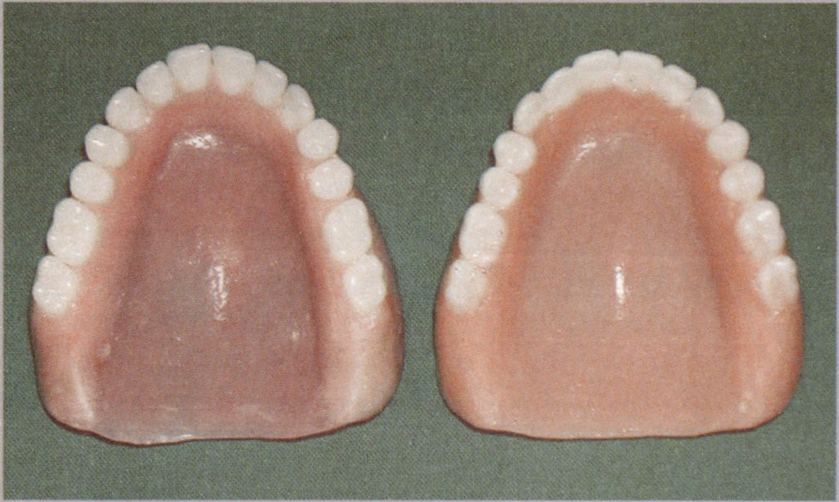

Exact duplicate of a denture that is in use can be made for regular or as a template

Wearing of complete dentures is a skill that is learnt subconsciously over a period of time. The oral muscles learn how best to stabilize a particular shape of denture. For a person who has to wear the denture for the second time, adaptation is much quicker, if the denture is similar to the previous one. A duplicate denture is indicated in this condition. When a denture is broken accidentally, no one would like to leave the denture with the dentist and go edentulous. Duplicate denture is an answer for this also. Recently implant treatment also uses duplicated denture to serve as templates.

Technique

1. Modify a denture flask to have a window. A rigid plastic box can also be used for this purpose
2. If the denture to be duplicated has thin areas, add wax to the exterior surface to avoid deficiency of flow
3. Make two wax sprues of 10 mm diameter and 75 mm length
4. Attach the sprues to the lingual surface of the heels of the mandibular denture or the palatal surface of the tuberosity region of the maxillary denture
5. Mix silicone putty or thick mix of alginate and fill the base of the flask with it. The denture is then placed on the impression material with the fitting surface towards the impression matcrial. Care should be taken to cover the borders for about 3 mm.
6. Trim away the excess impression material and create a regular surface which is to be smeared with oil.
7. Place the upper portion of the flask and fill the space with thin mix of alginate.
8. Once the alginate is set, separate the flask and gently remove the denture and sprues.
9. The alginate portions of the mould thus prepared must be protected with damp cloth.
10. The tooth indentations of the alginate mould is dried with tissue paper and gentle air flow.
11. Add tooth colored auto polymerizing acrylic resin by sprinkle or paint on method in different sections. The material should be restricted to the cervical borders of the teeth. Once the material is cured, the teeth can be removed and the excess can be trimmed off.
12. Reassemble the flask and secure it by adhesive tape.
13. Make a pourable mix of pink self cure resin and pour it through one sprue of the mould till the excess material comes out through the other sprue.
14. Rock the flask gently while pouring the resin.
15. Keep the flask in cold water and wait till the resin is cured.
16. The flask is separated and the duplicate denture is removed.
17. The sprues are cut off and the denture is polished.

Duplicating used Dentures

While duplicating a used denture, decision should be made on the features that are to be duplicated.

1. Shape of polished surfaces.
2. Occlusal face height or a controlled modification of it.
3. Occlusal plane.
4. Anterior tooth size, position and arrangement.
5. Posterior tooth size and position.
6. Occlusal surface.
7. Area and size of fitting surface.

The technique in this situation is of two different types – One uses a wax or resin duplicate of the existing denture as a starting point and the second uses the model of the previous denture as a guide to assist the setting up of the new denture.

Technique

- Modification of the existing dentures

  Minor extensions on the borders may be done using silicon putty. Aberrations in centric relation may be adjusted using fresh registration. If the occlusal height is to be increased, wax occlusal rim has to be prepared over the existing teeth. It is desirable to augment the height in self cure resin and allow the patient to use for a few weeks. The vertical height has to be determined using clinical parameters. If gross changes are to be made on the impression surface, tissue conditioner relining is to be done before duplication.

- The corrected denture is then duplicated.
- Duplication is done as in the previous technique.
- Base plate can be adapted on the tissue surface of the silicon putty cast over which wax can be poured to make a full fledged model.
- Old dentures can be returned to the patient at this stage.
- The wax duplicate can now be related to an articulator.
- Wax teeth can now be replaced one by one with new denture teeth.
- Trial is performed.
- Lining impressions are taken and stone casts are poured.
- Dentures are processed.

Different stages of denture duplication are shown in the following figures.

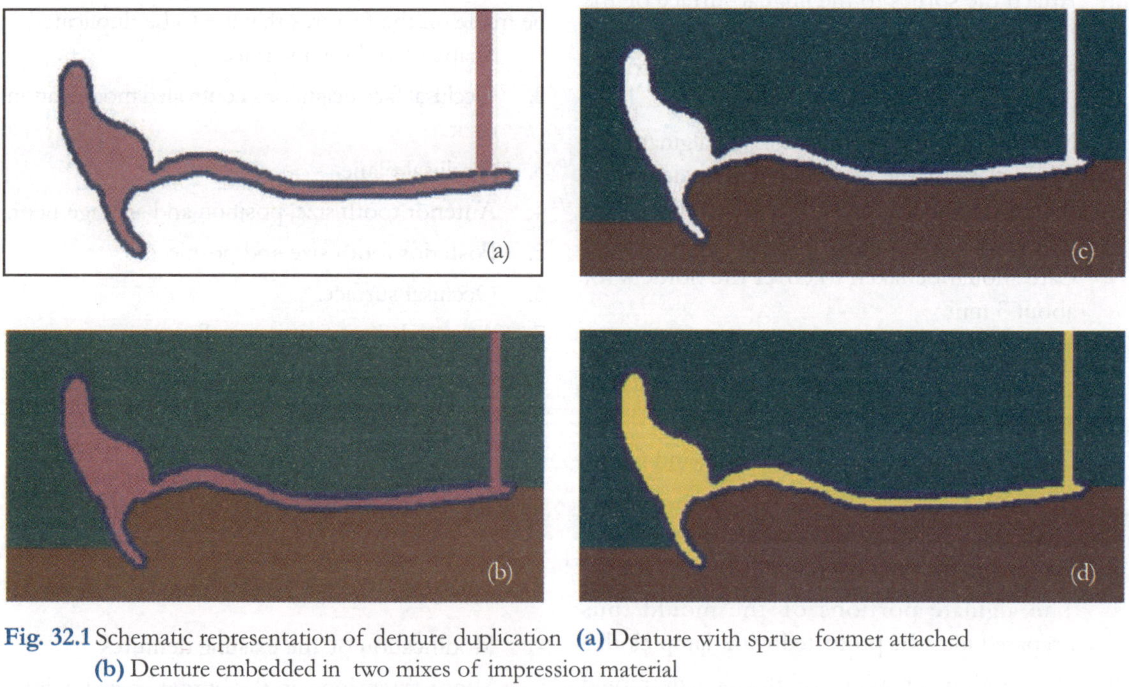

Fig. 32.1 Schematic representation of denture duplication **(a)** Denture with sprue former attached **(b)** Denture embedded in two mixes of impression material **(c)** Mould **(d)** Mould space filled with resin to make the duplicate denture

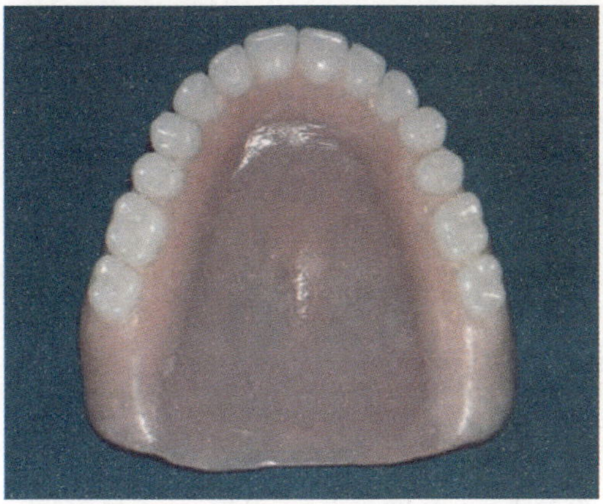

Fig. 32.2 Denture to be duplicated

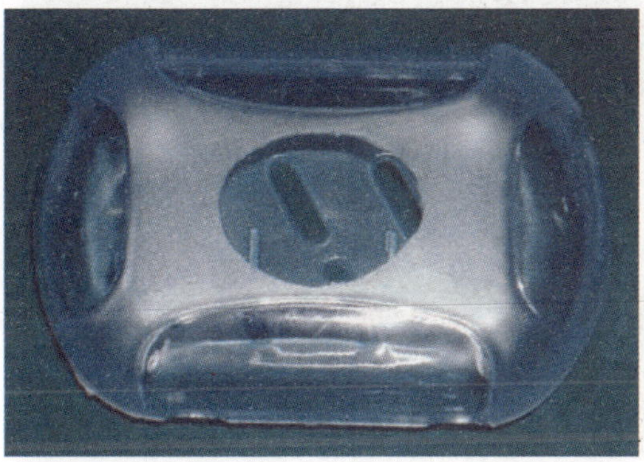

Fig. 32.3 Flak made out of a soap box. Large opening to pour impression material

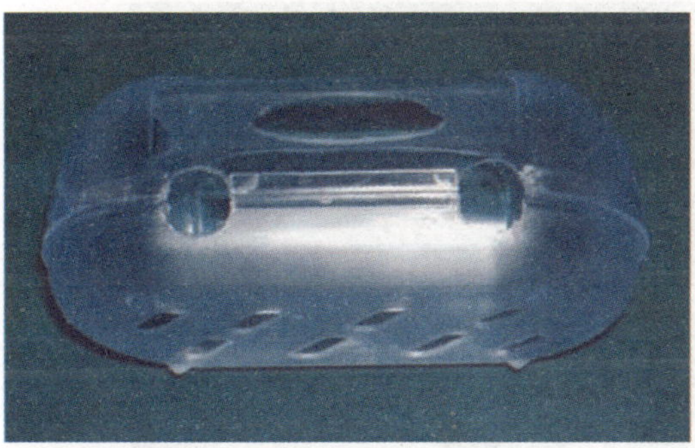

Fig. 32.4 Side view. Openings to accomodate sprue formers

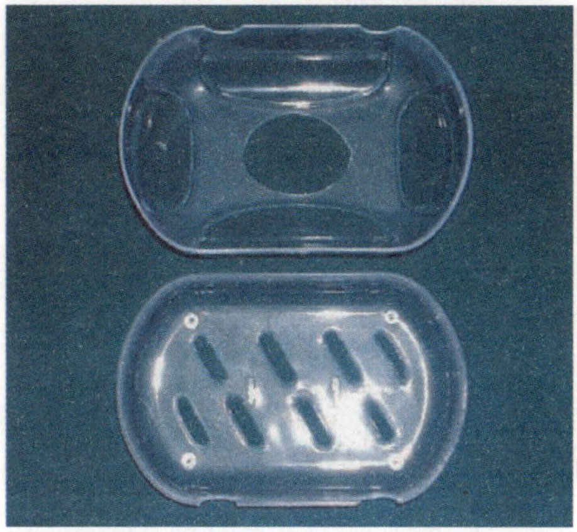

Fig. 32.5 Upper and lower portions of the flask

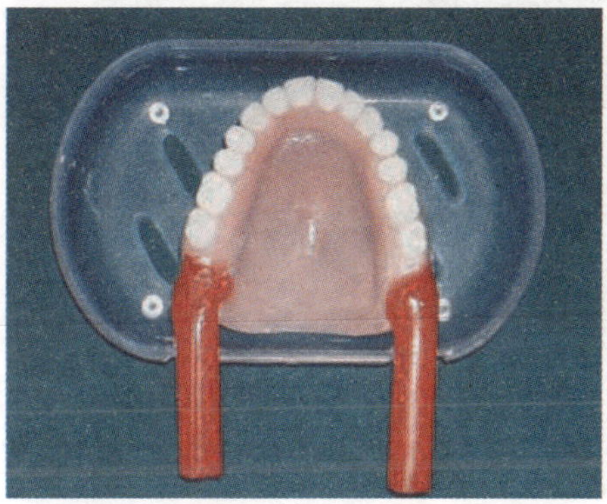

Fig. 32.6 Denture with wax sprue formers attached

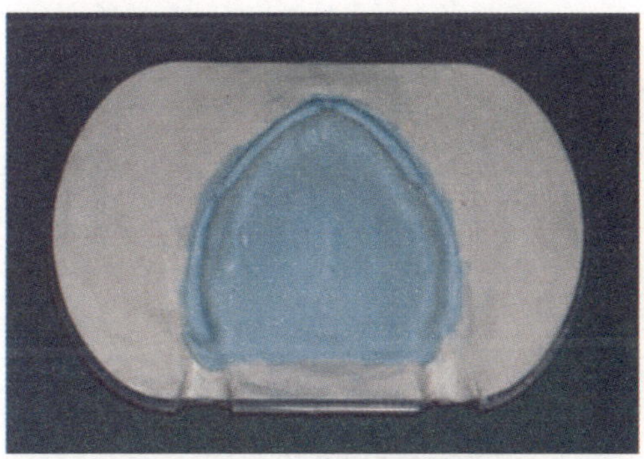

Fig. 32.7 Lower portion of the mould consisting of putty cast and plaster investment

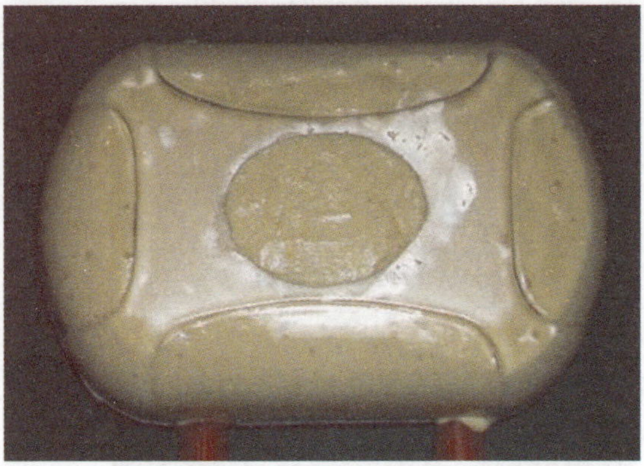

Fig. 32.8 Lower half of mould prepared in silicone putty

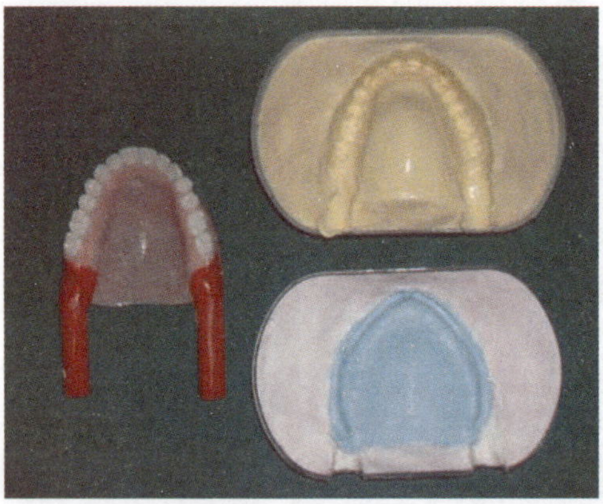

Fig. 32.9 Both the halves of the mould with the denture

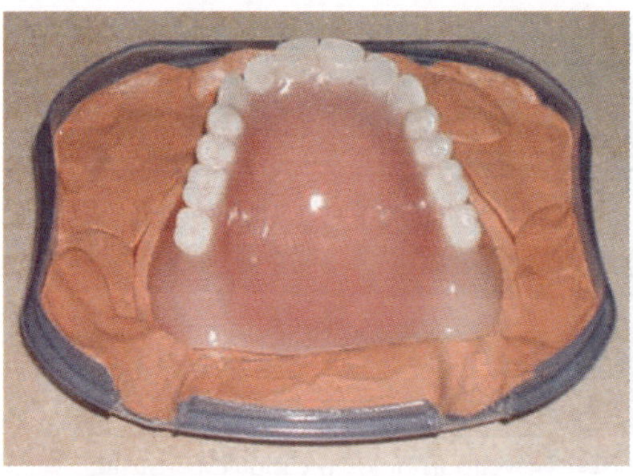

Fig. 32.10 Lower half of mould prepared in silicone putty

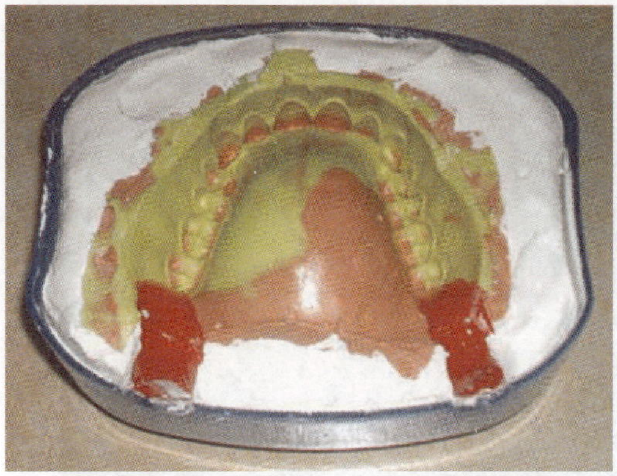

Fig. 32.11 Upper half of the mould prepared in putty and light body. Tooth portion is filled with tooth coloured acrylic

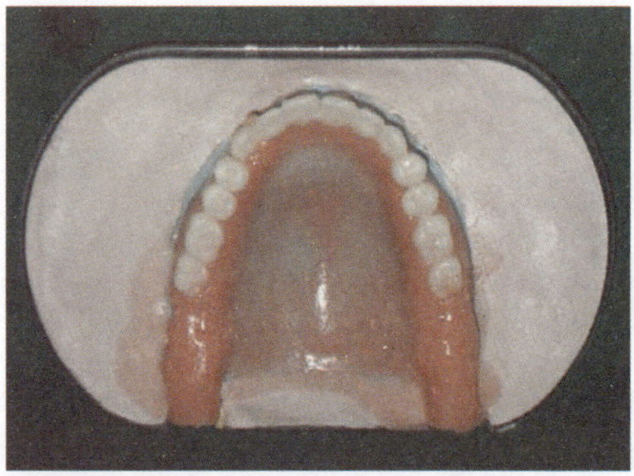

Fig. 32.12 Duplicated denture in the mould

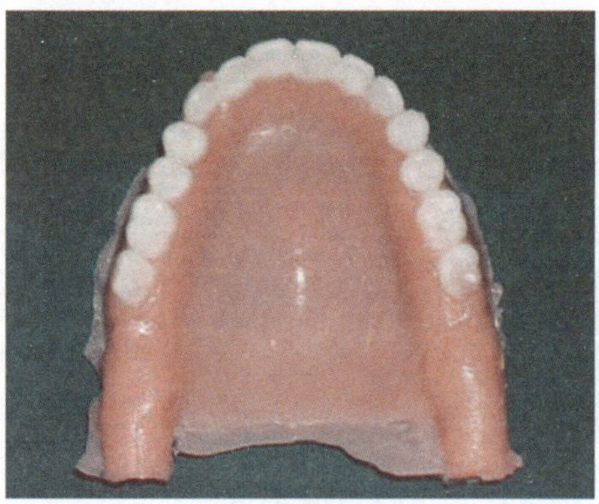

Fig. 32.13 Duplicate denture separated from the mould

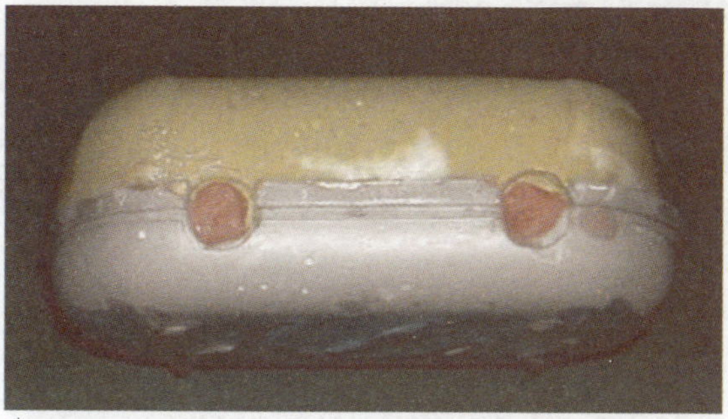

Fig. 32.14 Both the halves of the mould assembled and self cure acrylic is poured through one sprue

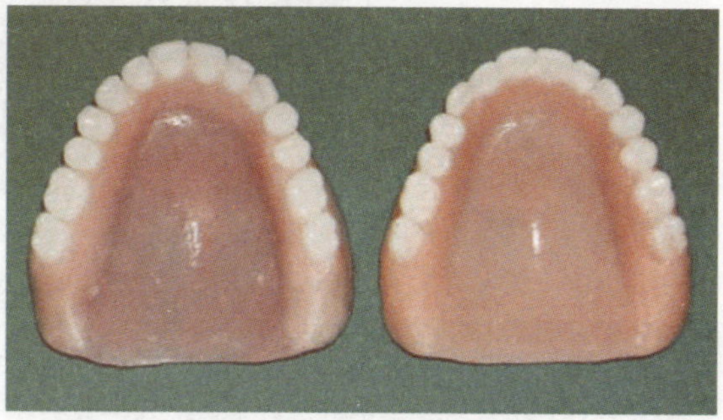

Fig. 32.15 Original and duplicated dentures

Suggested Reading

1. P. Azarmehr, H.H. Azarmehr: T*echnique for duplicating a denture.* J Prosthet Dent 1974; 31: 329-334.
2. G.L. Polyzois, G.A. Staurakis, and P.P. Demcrtrou: *Dimensional accuracy of duplicate dentures prepared by different methods.* J Prosthet Dent 1986; 55: 513-517.
3. C. E. Adam: *Technique for duplicating an acrylic resin denture.* J Prosthet Dent 1958; 8: 406-410.
4. D. R. Shaw: *Duplicate immediate dentures.* J Prosthet Dent 1962; 12: 47-57.
5. S. G. Manoli, T.P. Griffin: *Duplicate denture technique.* J Prosthet Dent 1969; 21: 104-107.
6. R. H. Boos, H.O. Carpenter, Jr.: *Technique for duplicating a denture.* J Prosthet Dent 1974; 31: 329-334.
7. J. Nassif, R. Jumbelic: *Duplicating maxillary complete dentures.* J Prosthet Dent 1984; 52: 755-759.
8. J. S. Cooper, A.C. Watkinson: *Duplication of full dentures.* Brit Dent J 1976; 141: 344-348
9. N. Duthie, F. Lyon, K.C. Sturrock, and R. Yemm: *A copying technique for replacement of complete dentures.* Brit Dent J 1978;144: 248-252.
10. A. Wagner: *Making duplicate dentures for use as final impression trays.* J Prosthet Dent 1970; 24: 111-113.
11. R. S. Krug: *Ceramic flask technique for duplication a complete denture.* J Prosthet Dent 1984; 52: 698-899.
12. J. R. Heath, J.C. Davenport: *A modification of the copy denture technique.* Brit Dent J 1982; 153: 300-302.

33

I believe, my denture is like this

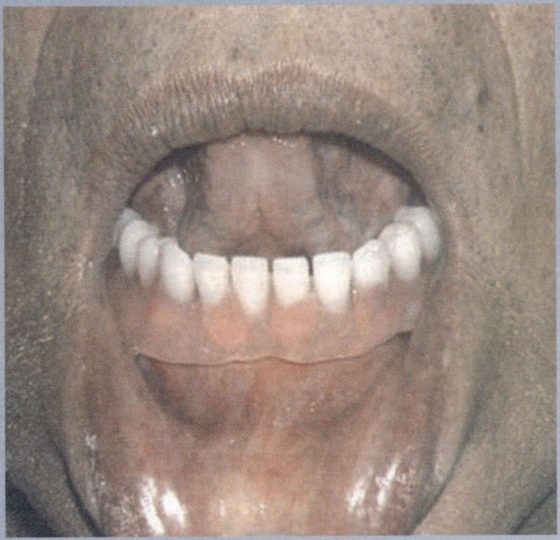

Understand patient's beliefs and expectations on dentures and help them land on realities.

Denture wearers entertain a number of myths. Unfortunately, many of the common misconceptions about dentures have prevented people from achieving their best health, appearance and self-confidence. The myths and answers are given in non technical terms so that the matter can be passed on to the patients effectively.

Dentures once made will last for ever

It is true that modern dentures are durable but they are not permanent. Dropping them can break a tooth or the denture base. Even with conscientious care, denture teeth can lose their natural appearance and chewing ability due to the cumulative effect of chewing, brushing and age. The way dentures are cared can also alter their fit. Dentures can warp if placed in hot water. If they become dried out, they may change shape. When dentures are removed at night, they have to be placed in a container of denture-cleaning solution or water. Also, it's best to use a brush designed for dentures as well as a denture cleaner rather than toothpaste, because some dentifrices may be too abrasive for dentures. It has to be considered that oral tissue change over a period of time and make the dentures loose. Dentures get discoloured by stains and calculus mainly due to oral fluids. Life of dentures can be considered as five years.

I have no complaint about the dentures, should I visit the dentist

This is probably the most common myth about dentures. Denture wearer should see the dentist regularly for an oral examination, because oral tissues continuously change. Mouth tissue can reveal signs of diseases, such as diabetes, that first manifest themselves in the mouth. Besides checking the dentures, the dentist will check the mouth for signs of oral cancer, and examine residual ridges, tongue and joints.

Denture look is a reality; dentures will not appear natural

No one wants a denture that looks like a "denture." Unlike old-fashioned dentures, today's denture can be made natural, allowing one to look and feel better without anyone knowing the presence of the denture. Many of the signs of dentures - clicking or slipping, unpleasant odor or stains - are actually signs of poor fit or improper home maintenance. Regular professional examinations and following the dentist's instructions on home care are essential steps in assuring a natural appearance. Confidence in wearing dentures comes from the realization that one has taken a positive step towards improving the health and appearance. Dentures help the wearer to lose the sunken look at the lower face, as well as the wrinkles around the mouth. Protecting oral health with properly fitting dentures is a smart move and it will make one look younger and smile very often.

Denture wearers can't eat or speak properly

Majority of denture-wearers discover that they can once again eat the food they love. While all denture wearers cannot eat everything they would like, many have few restrictions in their diets. Properly fitting dentures may actually encourage one to eat and chew more thoroughly, varied and well-balanced diet, further improving overall health. Good nutrition is important for mature adults as it is for younger individuals. Denture wearers can also enjoy the social benefits that make dining with friends a pleasant experience.

The ability to speak clearly depends on subtle interactions involving tongue, teeth, lips, cheeks and the palate. A denture that's properly fitted allows all the above components to work together properly.

Dentures have to be fixed with adhesives always

Dentures are made to fit precisely and usually do not require regular use of an adhesive. People with properly fitting dentures may find an adhesive product providing extra security and peace of mind, especially for important occasions. Adhesives may increase the performance of the best-fitting dentures. However, if the dentures begin to feel loose or cause pronounced discomfort, it is better to see the dentist immediately. Prolonged use of adhesive can mask infections and cause bone loss if the denture is unstable. Denture hygiene plays an extremely important role in preventing problems when adhesives are used for longer duration. However it is not a crime to use denture adhesives.

Dentures are not like natural teeth; they're not affected by medications

Drugs can affect fit of denture and wear ability. For example, certain medications like anti hypertensives can reduce the quantity of saliva, making it difficult to swallow or chew. Denture wearers should make the dentist aware of the drugs taken regularly or even occasionally.

Regular dental care is too expensive

Before deciding that oral examinations and denture care is too expensive, the situation can be discussed with the dentist. Be frank. Ask about charges for denture adjustments, repairs and possible replacement. Keep in mind that if you are in your 60s, you could have twenty more years of talking, eating and smiling. Your oral health is a vital part of your total health. Most dental professionals have a heart for the senior citizen.

I repair my dentures if it is necessary

Never try to make your own denture repairs. Denture self-repair can cause irreparable damage and may result in the need for a new denture. Even do-it-yourself reliners can be bulky, causing increased pressure on the jaw and more rapid loss of jawbone, and they can irritate the soft tissues of the mouth. . The common worry is "I'll be without teeth for days if I take my denture to the dentist for a refitting or repair." Advances in modern dentistry have made it possible for the dentist to reline or repair dentures quickly - often right in the office. If you let your dentist know that you are in need of a denture repair, the correction can frequently be made on the same day.

I know I should have my denture replaced, but I just don't want to go through a long adjustment period again

Don't avoid replacing your denture just because you don't want to go through another long adjustment period. With your first denture, you learned the basics – from eating and speaking with it to simply wearing it. While there will be a period of adjustment with a replacement denture, it is usually shorter – and easier – than the first time. Regardless, it's important that you do it. Prolonged use of ill-fitting dentures can irritate the gums, tongue and cheek, and even cause the ridges of your mouth to shrink to the point where it is almost impossible to fit you with normal dentures. Your ability to chew may decrease and your face may acquire deep aging lines and wrinkles. When you look at the big picture, the temporary adjustment period is a small price to pay.

All dentures are the same, go for the cheapest

All dentures are not created equal. If you look for the lowest price, you'll get what you pay for. Before prescribing a denture, a dental professional will review your health history, perform a thorough oral examination and carefully measure and prepare your mouth for your dentures. Dentists work closely with reputable dental laboratories, where trained technicians make your dentures to match your dental professional's specifications. And remember, you get what you pay for. Self-fitting dentures, which are sometimes offered for "discount" prices, may not fit as well, or be as well prepared, and therefore can lead to serious health problems. A dental professional and lab will make sure your denture features premium long-wearing, low-staining teeth and high impact acrylic denture base. So see your dentist and ask for these premium quality denture materials

34

Common prosthodontic terms

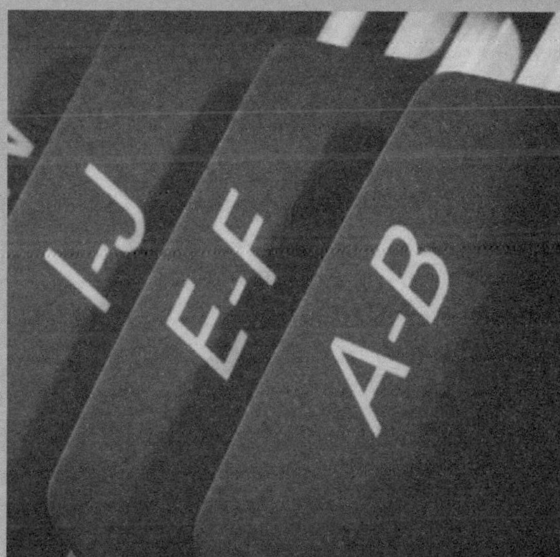

Use of uniform jargon will reduce difficulty in communication with different category of people working in the speciality

A universal acceptance of a standard terminology is essential for the clear understanding of any subject. Agreed formal glossaries are now part of the literature of prosthetic dentistry. Specialist societies have participated in the preparation of the glossaries as they appreciate that communication is impossible without generally agreed scientific terminology. Most commonly used term are listed below.

Terms	**Definitions**
Abutment.	A tooth, root, or portion of an implant used for the support or anchorage of a fixed or removable prosthesis.
Adhesion.	The physical force that attracts certain dissimilar molecules when in close approximation.
Adjustable axis facebow/ Hinge axis locating facebow.	A device, with adjustable side arms, that is attached to the mandible and used to locate the retruded hinge axis. Mandibular opening and closing movements are made in retruded jaw relation and the condyle pointers are adjusted until they rotate without translation.
Acrylic polymer/Acrylic resin.	A general term for synthetic polymers in which the repeating unit is a derivative of acrylic acid, usually rnethyl methacrylate. Polymerization is effected by a free radical mechanism which may be produced by heat energy, light energy, or chemical means. Systems using chemical means include those known as autopolymerizing, cold-curing, rapid-curing. The principal use is in the fabrication of dentures and synthetic resin teeth.
Agar impression material.	A reversible hydrocolloid impression material consisting of an aqueous agar gel. It liquefies when heated and returns to the gel state on cooling.
AIa-tragal line/ Camper's plane.	The line running from the inferior border of the ala of the nose to the superior border of the tragus of the ear.
Alginate impression material.	An irreversible hydrocolloid impression material in which a powder, consisting of soluble alginates and additives, is mixed with water and which on setting forms a gel. Gel formation is achieved by the precipitation of an insoluble calcium salt.
Arrow-point tracing/ Gothic arch tracing.	A horizontal tracing which resembles an arrowhead or a gothic arch, made by a tracer, and representing the posterior border movement of the mandible.
Articulating paper.	A strip of paper or cellulose acetate sheet coated with pigment used for marking areas of contact between opposing teeth.
Attachment.	A colloquial synonym for precision attachment.
Autopolymerizing Self-cure / Cold-cure.	Any resin that will polymerize with an activator and initiator but without the use of external heat.
Balanced occlusion.	Simultaneous contacts of the occluding surfaces on both sides of the mouth, in various jaw positions.
Baseplate.	The foundation on which an occlusal rim is built or on which a trial denture is set up.
Bennett angle.	The angle between the sagittal plane and the path of the advancing condyle during lateral mandibular movement, as viewed along the horizontal plane.
Bennett movement.	The lateral translation of the rnandible during lateral exertion.
Bite registration material.	A material used to register occlusion between opposing faces of maxillary and mandibular teeth. Occlusal indicator wax. Bite wax. It is usually in the form of a wax or a paste.
Bonwill triangle.	A 4-inch (102 mm) equilateral triangle postulated by Bonwill, formed by the medial contact of the mandibular central incisors and the centres of the condyles.

Border moulding.	The shaping of an impression material by the manipulation or activity of the soft tissues adjacent to the borders of an impression.
Border movement.	A movement of the mandible along the extremity of its range, in any direction.
Border seal.	The contact between the denture border and the adjacent tissues which prevents the passage air.
Boxing.	Of an impression. The provision of a wall, usually in wax, attached to the perimeter of an impression, in order to contain the cast material until it is set.
Boxing wax.	A wax that will adhere to impression material and is used to form a mould into which laboratory plaster or dental stone can be poured.
Bracing arm.	See reciprocating arm.
Cast.	(1) (Noun). A reproduction of the surface form of oral or facial tissuesobtained from an impression (2) (Verb). To form a cast from an impression or to form a casting in a mould.
Casting.	An object, usually of metal, formed in a mould.
Christiansen's phenomenon.	The development of a gap between the posterior ends of opposite flat occlusal rims, which occurs when the mandible is protruded.
Cohesion.	The property of a material by which its constituent molecules are attracted to each other and resist separation.
Compensating curve.	The curvature of the occlusal plane of dentures, created to permit balanced occlusion. The curve compensates for the effects of Christiansen's phenomenon.
Condylar angle.	The angle between the sagittal projection of the condylar path and the Frankfurt plane.
Condylar guide.	That part of an articulator which guides its condylar element,approximately as the mandibular joint guides the condyle.
Condylar guide angle.	The angle of inclination of the condylar guide to the horizontal plane or other reference plane.
Condylar path.	Any path travelled by the mandibular condyle during the various mandibular movements.
Copy dentures/ Replica dentures Duplicate dentures.	Copies of the patient's dentures that are used in the construction of new dentures.
Coronal plane.	Any plane passing longitudinally through the body from side to side, at right angles to the mid-sagittal plane, and dividing the body into front and back parts.
Curve of Monson. Monson's curve.	The curve of occlusion of natural teeth, described by Monson in which each cusp and incisal edge touches or conforms to a segment of the surface of a sphere 4 inches (102mm) in radius with its centre in the region of the glabella.*Note.* It is commonly assumed that this curve is an arch viewed from the front of the mouth.
Curve of Spee.	An arch of a circle of 65 mm to 70 mm radius, described by Spee, that touches the tips of all the mandibular teeth when the skull is viewed laterally. When continued, it touches the anterior surface of the condyles.
Cusp angle.	An angle made by the slopes of the cusp with the plane perpendicular to the long axis of the tooth.
Dental articulation/Articulation.	The close approximation of, or contact between, opposing teeth that occurs while the mandible is moving.
Denture base.	That part of the denture that rests on the denture bearing area of the oral mucosa.
Denture base material.	A material, usually composed of an acrylic polymer bead and acrylic monomer, used in the construction of dentures and other appliances by a dough-moulding technique.
Diagnostic cast/Study cast.	A cast as an aid to diagnosis and treatment planning.

Direct retainer.	A component of a partial denture that resists dislodgement along the path of withdrawal.
Direct retention.	The retention obtained in a partial denture by the use of direct retainers.
Doughing time.	That part of the working time measured from the end of the mixing time until the time a material is ready for manipulation. It is generallyused in connection with denture base resins and acrylic resin teeth.
Duplicating material/ Agar duplicating material.	A material used in the dental laboratory to duplicate accurately models, casts or other items. It is usually based on a hydrocolloid impression such as agar or alginate.
Eccentric jaw relation.	Any jaw relation that is lateral or protrusive to the retruded jaw relation.
Eccentric occlusion.	Any occlusion that is not the intercuspal occlusion.
Elastomeric impression material.	An impression material based on a non-aqueous polymeric system which exhibits rubber-like behaviour. The most important types are based on silicones, polysulphides and polyethers.
Endosteal implant. Endosseus implant.	An implant, usually made of metal, which is inserted into the edentulous alveolar bone so that part protrudes into the month. The protruding end is used as an attachment for a prosthesis.
Envelope of movement.	This three-dimensional space circumscribed by border movements of a given point in the mandible (or a device rigidly attached to it).
Extracoronal attachment.	A precision attachment joined to a restoration and situated outside the coronal contour.
Extra-oral tracing.	An arrow-point tracing made outside the oral cavity.
Facebow.	An instrument used to record the relation of the maxilla to the hinge axis of rotation of the mandible. It enables a similar relation to be established between the maxillary casts and the hinge axis of the articulator.
Final impression / Master impression.	The impression that is used for making the master cast. **Note.** 'Second impression' refers specifically to the final impression.There is no such term as third, etc., impression.
Working impression/ Second impression	
Flask.	(1) (Noun). A sectional metal case that contains and supports the mould in which dentures are formed.(2) (Verb). To invest the pattern in the flask.
Frankfurt plane.	A plane passing through the lowest point in the floor of left orbit, and the highest point in the margin of each external auditory meatus of the skull. It approximates to the horizontal when the head is in a normal upright position.
Functional impression.	An impression that during its formation is modified by masticatoryloads and adjacent muscular activity. **Note.** See also mucodisplacement impression.
Gingivally approaching clasp/Roach clasp.	A clasp, whose terminal point approaches a tooth from the direction of the gingivae.
Gnathodynamometer.	An instrument for measuring the force exerted in closing the jaws.
Grinding-in.	Occlusal correction of artificial teeth by grinding.
Guide plane.	Two or more paralleled surfaces of abutment teeth prepared to limit the path of insertion and improve the stability of a removable prosthesis.
High-impact denture base material.	A denture base material formulated to have higher resistance to fracture by impact or fatigue.
High lip-line.	The greatest height to which the upper lip is normally raised in function.
Hinge axis.	A horizontal axis in the region of the condyles about which the mandible can rotate without translatory movement of the condyles.
Horizontal overlap/ Overjet.	A projection of the maxillary teeth beyond the mandibular teeth in the horizontal plane.

Hydrocolloid impression material.	A general term used to refer to alginate and agar impression materials. Chemically, these are colloidal materials with water initially as the dispersing phase. After gelation, water becomes the disperse phase.
Impression compound/ Compound.	A thermoplastic material used to take impressions, comprising natural and synthetic resins, fillers and plasticizers, in the form of sticks, sheets and cones. It is softened to a working consistency byimmersion in hot water or by warming over a flame.
Impression plaster.	Finely ground plaster of Paris containing additives (e.g. potassium sulphate and borax) that minimise setting expansion and control the setting time.
Incisal angle.	The angle formed with the horizontal plane by drawing a line in the sagittal plane between the incisal edges of the maxillary and mandibular central incisors when the teeth are in intercuspal occlusion.
Incisal guidance.	The guidance provided by the surfaces of the maxillary incisors in lateral movement of the mandible.
Incisal guide/Incisal table.	That part of an articulator which maintains the incisal angle.
Incisal guide angle.	The angle to which the incisal guide is set.
Indirect retention.	The retention obtained by the extension of a partial denture base to provide the fulcrum of a class II lever. The retainer(s) providing direct retention between the fulcrum and that part of the denture which is subject to the displacing force.
Infra-orbital pointer/ Infra-orbital indicator.	The component of a facebow that records infra-orbital notch positionand thereby aligns it with the Frankfurt plane.
Interalveolar distance/ Inter-ridge distance.	The vertical distance between specified positions on the maxillary and mandibular alveolar ridges at the vertical dimension of occlusion.
Intercuspal occlusion/ Centric occlusion.	Maximal contact between opposing teeth.
Intercuspal position.	The position of the mandible when the teeth are in intercuspal occlusion.
Intercuspation.	The interdigitation of cusps of opposing teeth.
Interocclusal.	Between opposing occlusal surfaces.
Interocclusal space / Freeway space.	The space between the maxillary and mandibular occluding surfaceswhen the mandible is in the rest position.
Interocclusal record.	A record of any relation of opposing occlusal surfaces.*Note.* It is essential to specify the type of record, e.g. inter-cuspal,retrusive, protrusive or lateral, and contact or pre-contact.
Intracoronal attachment.	A precision attachment, one part of which is totally embedded in a restoration.
Master cast/Final cast	The cast produced from the final impression.
Modelling wax.	A blend of waxes, usually pink, red or orange in colour, that is adaptable at ambient temperature. The softening temperature range varies according to the intended use.
Mucodisplacement impression.	An impression made with the intention of displacing soft tissues.*Note.* See also functional impression.
Mucostatic impression.	An impression made with the intention of minimising mucosaldisplacement.
Neutral zone.	A term used to describe a zone in which the opposing forces of the cheeks/lips and tongue are said to be in equilibrium.
Non-working side/Balancing side/Contralateral side.	The side opposite the working side.
Non-working side contacts. Balancing contacts.	The contacts between maxillary and mandibular teeth, or denture bases on the non working side, or posteriorly in a protrusive occlusion.
Occlusal plane. Plane of occlusion.	An imaginary surface that touches the incisal surfaces of the maxillary incisors and the tips of the cusps of the posterior teeth. This surface is usually curved and is not strictly a plane.

Occlusal rim. Occlusion rim.	An occluding surface formed of mouldable material which is attached to a temporary or permanent denture base, for the purpose of recording jaw relations and indicating tooth positions.
Occlusal vertical dimension Occlusal face height.	Any vertical dimension when the teeth or occlusal rims are in contact.
Occlusally-approaching clasp.	A clasp originating from the occlusal side of the survey line.
Occlusion.	Any contact between teeth of opposing dental arches, usually referring to contact between the occlusal surface.
Packing.	The act of filling a mould with a plastic material in order to construct a dental prosthesis.
Pantograph.	A complex of tracing devices attached to the mandible and maxilla which enables records of mandibular movements to be made in threeplanes.
Path of insertion/withdrawal.	The path followed by the denture from its first contact with the supporting tissues until it is fully seated.
Polished surface.	The surface of the denture, usually polished, which is in contact with the lips, cheeks and tongue, excluding the occlusal surfaces.
Polyether impression material.	An impression material based on an organic polymer in which the repeating unit contains an ether linkage. Setting is achieved by the cross-linking reaction of pendant ethyleneimino groups, activated by acidic catalysts.
Poly(methylmethacrylate) (PMMA).	An acrylic polymer, formed by the polymerisation of methyl methacrylate and widely used for the fabrication of denture bases and acrylic resin teeth, by the dough technique.
Polysulphide impression material.	An impression material based on an organic polymer in which the repeating units are linked by disulphide groups. They are often referred to as mercaptans or thiokols. Setting is commonly achieved by increase in chain length and cross-linking.
Posterior palatal seal.	The seal at the posterior border of a maxillary denture.
Post-dam.	A ridge of denture base material on the posterior border of the maxillary denture impression surface which displaces the supporting soft tissues in order to create a seal.
Precision attachment.	A prefabricated interlocking device, one component of which is fixed to an abutment while the other is integrated into a denture or bridge in order to support and/or retain it.
Process Cure.	A procedure whereby denture base resin is polymerized in a mould.
Pourable denture base material/Pour resin/Pourable resin/Pour-type resin.	A denture base material specially formulated to allow it to flow under gravity to fill a mould.
Radio-opaque denture base material.	A denture base material rendered opaque to X-rays by the inclusion of a radio opaque material to facilitate location in human tissues.
Rebase.	The removal and replacement of the denture base.
Reciprocal arm.	A component of a partial denture used to prevent displacement of a tooth by a direct retainer.
Rest jaw relation.	The relation of the mandible to the maxilla when the mandible is in the rest position.
Retruded jaw relation. Centric jaw relation/ Centric relation.	Any position of the mandible on its retruded arc of closure.
Sectional impression.	An impression built up in the mouth from two or more parts which are then removed separately and reassembled.

Selective grinding/ Spot grinding.	The planned adjustment of the occlusal forms of teeth by grinding with a stone.
Separating medium.	A material used to facilitate the separation of a plaster surface from another surface of plaster, or other material (notably impression materials and denture base resins), and prevent or reduce the transfer of moisture. Alginates are the most widely-used materials for this purpose.
Silicone impression material.	An impression material based on an organo-siloxane polymer, with silicon-oxygen links from the basic structure. Setting is achieved by cross linking induced by various catalyst systems.
Soft liner/Resilient liner.	A soft, polymeric material used on the fitting surfaces of dentures to reduce trauma to the soft supporting tissues. They are generally synthetic elastomers or plasticized acrylic polymers.
Special tray/Custom tray.	An impression tray made specifically for an individual patient by means of which the impression material may be accurately controlled.
Split mounting.	A method of mounting the cast on an articulator to facilitate removal and accurate replacement. It may also be used for checking the accuracy of jaw relation records.
Sticky wax.	A blend of waxes that, when heated, melts and adheres to the surfaces to which it is applied. Its primary purpose is to hold components together prior to fixation.
Synthetic resin/Acrylic resin teeth.	Artificial teeth fabricated from synthetic resin. The most commonly used is poly(methylmethacrylate).
Tissue conditioner.	A specialised type of soft liner, used for short duration, which is intended to improve the condition of the soft tissues supporting the prosthesis. It is usually a highly plasticized acrylic polymer.
Tracing stick.	An impression compound in stick form, having a low softening point and used mainly for adapting the margins of impression trays, or for taking inlay/crown impressions.
Trial denture/Try-in.	The arrangement of teeth in wax for trial insertion prior to completion of the denture.
Tray adhesive.	A material for ensuring adhesion between the impression material and the containing tray. These are often specific to the type of impression material concerned, e.g. polysulphide adhesive.
Veined denture base material.	A denture base material to which short threads made of nylon, or other suitable organic filaments are added to simulate the appearance of blood vessels.
Working time.	The period of time, measured from the start of mixing, during which it is possible to manipulate a dental material without an adverse effect on its properties. Working time comprises mixing time, doughing time (when appropriate) and manipulation time. *Note.* This is the "normal" definition. Variations do exist in certain standards.
Zinc oxide-eugenol paste.	An impression paste obtained by mixing two pastes, one containing zinc oxide together with an oil such as liquid paraffin and an accelerator such as zinc acetate, and the other containing a resin such as colophony dissolved in eugenol.

35

Declaration of Helsinki
Declaration of Geneva

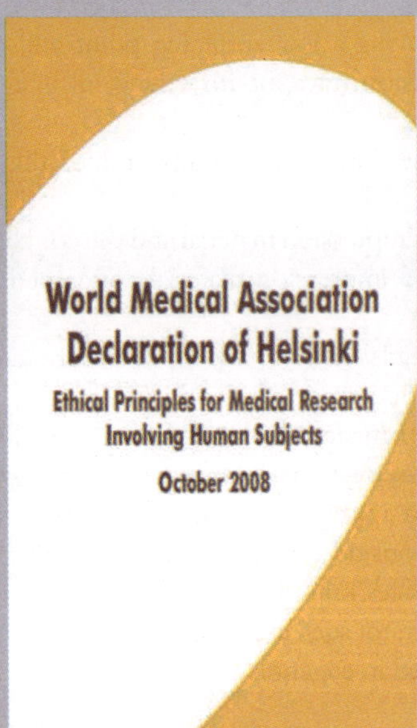
World Medical Association
Declaration of Helsinki
Ethical Principles for Medical Research
Involving Human Subjects
October 2008

Researchers of Prosthodontics should be aware of the Helsinki declaration

World Medical Association Declaration of Helsinki

Ethical Principles for Medical Research Involving Human Subjects Adopted by the 18th WMA General Assembly Helsinki, Finland, June 1964 and amended by the 29th WMA General Assembly, Tokyo, Japan, October 1975 35th WMA General Assembly, Venice, Italy, October 1983 41st WMA General Assembly, Hong Kong, September 1989 48th WMA General Assembly, Somerset West, Republic of South Africa, October 1996 52nd WMA General Assembly, Edinburgh, Scotland, October 2000

A. Introduction

The World Medical Association has developed the Declaration of Helsinki as a statement of ethical principles to provide guidance to physicians and other participants in medical research involving human subjects.

Medical research involving human subjects includes research on identifiable human material or identifiable data.

It is the duty of the physician to promote and safeguard the health of the people. The physician's knowledge and conscience are dedicated to the fulfillment of this duty.

The Declaration of Geneva of the World Medical Association binds the physician with the words, "The health of my patient will be my first consideration," and the International Code of Medical Ethics declares that, "A physician shall act only in the patient's interest when providing medical care which might have the effect of weakening the physical and mental condition of the patient."

Medical progress is based on research which ultimately must rest in part on experimentation involving human subjects.

In medical research on human subjects, considerations related to the well-being of the human subject should take precedence over the interests of science and society.

The primary purpose of medical research involving human subjects is to improve prophylactic, diagnostic and therapeutic procedures and the understanding of the aetiology and pathogenesis of disease. Even the best proven prophylactic, diagnostic, and therapeutic methods must continuously be challenged through research for their effectiveness, efficiency, accessibility and quality.

In current medical practice and in medical research, most prophylactic, diagnostic and therapeutic procedures involve risks and burdens.

Medical research is subject to ethical standards that promote respect for all human beings and protect their health and rights. Some research populations are vulnerable and need special protection. The particular needs of the economically and medically disadvantaged must be recognized. Special attention is also required for those who cannot give or refuse consent for themselves, for those who may be subject to giving consent under duress, for those who will not benefit personally from the research and for those for whom the research is combined with care.

Research Investigators should be aware of the ethical, legal and regulatory requirements for research on human subjects in their own countries as well as applicable international requirements. No national ethical, legal or regulatory requirement should be allowed to reduce or eliminate any of the protections for human subjects set forth in this Declaration.

B. Basic principles for all medical research

It is the duty of the physician in medical research to protect the life, health, privacy, and dignity of the human subject.

Medical research involving human subjects must conform to generally accepted scientific principles, be based on a thorough knowledge of the scientific literature, other relevant sources of information, and on adequate laboratory and, where appropriate, animal experimentation.

Appropriate caution must be exercised in the conduct

of research which may affect the environment, and the welfare of animals used for research must be respected.

The design and performance of each experimental procedure involving human subjects should be clearly formulated in an experimental protocol.

This protocol should be submitted for consideration, comment, guidance, and where appropriate, approval to a specially appointed ethical review committee, which must be independent of the investigator, the sponsor or any other kind of undue influence. This independent committee should be in conformity with the laws and regulations of the country in which the research experiment is performed. The committee has the right to monitor ongoing trials. The researcher has the obligation to provide monitoring information to the committee, especially any serious adverse events. The researcher should also submit to the committee, for review, information regarding funding, sponsors, institutional affiliations, other potential conflicts of interest and incentives for subjects.

The research protocol should always contain a statement of the ethical considerations involved and should indicate that there is compliance with the principles enunciated in this Declaration.

Medical research involving human subjects should be conducted only by scientifically qualified persons and under the supervision of a clinically competent medical person. The responsibility for the human subject must always rest with a medically qualified person and never rest on the subject of the research, even though the subject has given consent.

Every medical research project involving human subjects should be preceded by careful assessment of predictable risks and burdens in comparison with foreseeable benefits to the subject or to others. This does not preclude the participation of healthy volunteers in medical research. The design of all studies should be publicly available.

Physicians should abstain from engaging in research projects involving human subjects unless they are confident that the risks involved have been adequately assessed and can be satisfactorily managed. Physicians should cease any investigation if the risks are found to outweigh the potential benefits or if there is conclusive proof of positive and beneficial results.

Medical research involving human subjects should only be conducted if the importance of the objective outweighs the inherent risks and burdens to the subject. This is especially important when the human subjects are healthy volunteers.

Medical research is only justified if there is a reasonable likelihood that the populations in which the research is carried out stand to benefit from the results of the research.

The subjects must be volunteers and informed participants in the research project.

The right of research subjects to safeguard their integrity must always be respected. Every precaution should be taken to respect the privacy of the subject, the confidentiality of the patient's information and to minimize the impact of the study on the subject's physical and mental integrity and on the personality of the subject.

In any research on human beings, each potential subject must be adequately informed of the aims, methods, sources of funding, any possible conflicts of interest, institutional affiliations of the researcher, the anticipated benefits and potential risks of the study and the discomfort it may entail. The subject should be informed of the right to abstain from participation in the study or to withdraw consent to participate at any time without reprisal. After ensuring that the subject has understood the information, the physician should then obtain the subject's freely-given informed consent, preferably in writing. If the consent cannot be obtained in writing, the non-written consent must be formally documented and witnessed.

When obtaining informed consent for the research project the physician should be particularly cautious if the subject is in a dependent relationship with the physician or may consent under duress. In that case the informed consent should be obtained by a well-informed physician who is not engaged in the investigation and who is completely independent of this relationship.

For a research subject who is legally incompetent, physically or mentally incapable of giving consent or is a legally incompetent minor, the investigator must obtain informed consent from the legally authorized representative in accordance with applicable law. These groups should not be included in research unless the research is necessary to promote the health of the population represented and this research cannot instead be performed on legally competent persons.

When a subject deemed legally incompetent, such as a minor child, is able to give assent to decisions about participation in research, the investigator must obtain that assent in addition to the consent of the legally authorized representative.

Research on individuals from whom it is not possible to obtain consent, including proxy or advance consent, should be done only if the physical/ mental condition that prevents obtaining informed consent is a necessary characteristic of the research population. The specific reasons for involving research subjects with a condition that renders them unable to give informed consent should be stated in the experimental protocol for consideration and approval of the review committee. The protocol should state that consent to remain in the research should be obtained as soon as possible from the individual or a legally authorized surrogate.

Both authors and publishers have ethical obligations. In publication of the results of research, the investigators are obliged to preserve the accuracy of the results. Negative as well as positive results should be published or otherwise publicly available. Sources of funding, institutional affiliations and any possible conflicts of interest should be declared in the publication. Reports of experimentation not in accordance with the principles laid down in this Declaration should not be accepted for publication.

C. Additional principles for medical research combined with medical care

The physician may combine medical research with medical care, only to the extent that the research is justified by its potential prophylactic, diagnostic or therapeutic value. When medical research is combined with medical care, additional standards apply to protect the patients who are research subjects.

The benefits, risks, burdens and effectiveness of a new method should be tested against those of the best current prophylactic, diagnostic, and therapeutic methods. This does not exclude the use of placebo, or no treatment, in studies where no proven prophylactic, diagnostic or therapeutic method exists.

At the conclusion of the study, every patient entered into the study should be assured of access to the best proven prophylactic, diagnostic and therapeutic methods identified by the study.

The physician should fully inform the patient which aspects of the care are related to the research. The refusal of a patient to participate in a study must never interfere with the patient-physician relationship.

In the treatment of a patient, where proven prophylactic, diagnostic and therapeutic methods do not exist or have been ineffective, the physician, with informed consent from the patient, must be free to use unproven or new prophylactic, diagnostic and therapeutic measures, if in the physician's judgement it offers hope of saving life, re-establishing health or alleviating suffering. Where possible, these measures should be made the object of research, designed to evaluate their safety and efficacy. In all cases, new information should be recorded and, where appropriate, published. The other relevant guidelines of this declaration should be followed.

Declaration of Geneva

At the time of being admitted as a member of the medical profession:

I solemnly pledge to consecrate my life to the service of humanity;

I will give to my teachers the respect and gratitude that is their due;

I will practise my profession with conscience and dignity;

The health of my patient will be my first consideration;

I will respect the secrets that are confided in me, even after the patient has died;

I will maintain, by all the means in my power, the honour and the noble traditions of the medical profession;

My colleagues will be my sisters and brothers;

I will not permit considerations of age, disease or disability, creed, ethnic origin, gender, nationality, political affiliation, race, sexual orientation, social standing or any other factor to intervene between my duty and my patient;

I will maintain the utmost respect for human life;

I will not use my medical knowledge to violate human rights and civil liberties, even under threat;

I make these promises solemnly, freely and upon my honour.

36

Write an essay to success

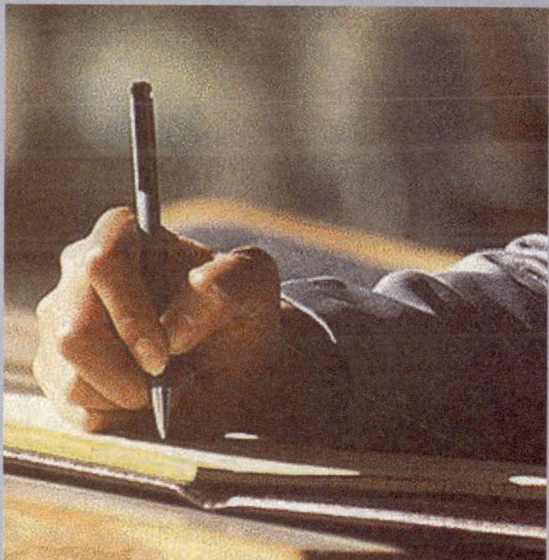

A well written essay will assess the overall standards of a candidate

A student of dentistry is trained to become knowledgeable, skillful in various clinical processes, laboratory procedures and communication and the student should develop a positive attitude to patients, colleagues and to the society at large which is befitting to a professional. Essay question is an essential tool used to evaluate the knowledge of a student of dentistry. In a class examination or the final qualifying examination essay is asked to evaluate the knowledge of the student. Very often it is used as a part of an assignment given to the student. Essay allows the student free expression and organization of thoughts. Essay gives an insight into the **depth of knowledge**; to be precise from a mere recall of facts to understanding and to application. The following examples will give an insight into "the depth of knowledge"

- List five commonly used impression materials (recall)
- Classify impression materials into elastic and non elastic based on the physical state of the set material. (understanding)
- Select an appropriate impression material to be used in a partially edentulous situation (application)

The first question can be answered if you learn by heart a list of impression materials. As such this will not be asked as an essay question but it can form part of an essay question. To answer the second question, the knowledge base must be broad and systematized. To answer the third question you should have the capability of reasoning and intelligence.

The expression of the question should be understood first. There will be a verb in the question which will decide precisely what the question is intended for. A few of such verbs are listed below:

Analyse – various components of a concept is identified and the inter relationship is described

Compare – describe the similarities of two or more things

Contrast – describe the differences of two or more things

Define/Describe – give the definition and describe the components of the topic

Discuss – different aspects of a problem are presented and a conclusion is drawn

Enumerate – give a listing of the topics asked and briefly describe each

Justify – your point of view presented must be argued

Outline – provide the main points of a topic

Summarise – outline the main points briefly

State – present the points clearly

Outline of the essay: Before answering the essay question, an outline of the essay must be made and it would indicate all the major points included in the essay. By doing this, the thoughts will be organized and no major point will be missed. The answering becomes fast and even if the answering is not complete, some credit will be given for the points given in the outline. Between two answers sufficient space should be given so that at a later stage you can come back and more points can be added if necessary and if there is time. While starting the answer, immediately get to the point asked for. If the question asked is on vertical dimension, start with a statement on vertical dimension.

Components of an essay: There are three main components for an essay:

- introduction
- main body
- conclusion

Introduction is generally begun with a general issue on the topic asked and then narrowed down to the specifics that are discussed in the essay. Background information is given in the introduction which will make the subject content of the essay more relevant. A statement is also included on what you understand from the question. If possible a restatement of the question can be made with an outline of what is going to be discussed in the body of the essay.

The body should be arranged logically from a focal point and should contain a series of paragraphs which are packages of information. Each paragraph starts with a topic defining sentence which is expanded with details, examples and illustrations. There must be an uninterrupted flow of thought. Unnecessary statements which do not have relevance should be avoided because it is going to affect the time management.

Information in the conclusion moves from the specifics to the general and summarizes the content of the body. It provides a generalized answer to the question but new points cannot be made. Always devote some time to write the conclusion. Abrupt endings are never relished by the readers.

In the introduction you state what you are going to say, in the body state what you have to and in the conclusion state what you have already said.

Time management: Effective time management is essential in exams or else you will find it difficult to complete the answering of all the required questions. Familiarize with the scheme of the examination and find out the marks for each question. Accordingly the time can be allocated for each question in a realistic fashion. Before answering, read the question carefully three times and this will give you clarity on what is asked. Make the outline and note down the key points and prioritize them. If the time allocated for one question is exhausted, leave it with some space to come back later if you get a chance to. Plan the time in such a way that at least five minutes are left at the end for correction of errors and to make a revisit to the questions which are not completed.

Strategic approach: Questions can be categorized as follows:

- questions you definitely know and you can work out – these are the questions to be attempted first
- questions you think you know and you could guess – read these questions repeatedly and select logical answers without losing control over the time
- questions you are not sure of and have no clue about – read and reread the questions and think of the answers without making wild guesses and losing control over the time

On the previous night

- Confirm the time table and exam centre
- Organise pen, pencils, rulers etc
- Refer the revision notes; not the texts
- Go to sleep early
- Practise yoga if you can
- Think of a time plan based on previous question papers

On the exam day

- Get up reasonably early
- To get energy for the exam, have a good break fast
- Briefly go through your notes
- Reach the exam centre early; never rush
- To avoid distress do not talk too much on your preparation
- After reading the question do not look around to see other's reaction, every one will be stressed but that will be covered up by a smile and this smile might distress you
- Be positive; you can do it
- Remain as calm as possible

Helpful tips

- Write clearly, concisely and legibly
- Answer the questions in the order of your preference unless specified but remember to put the number clearly
- The first five marks are easier to get than the last five marks
- Draw relevant figures; it is equivalent to hundred words and more conspicuous
- Answer to the point. Writing more will not fetch more marks
- Do not get stuck to tough questions. Leave them and try later
- If you run short of time and cannot come back, complete the sub headings without describing the details
- Leave some space at the end of the answer

- If you get a point as a flash, immediately jot it down somewhere or else you may forget it
- After the exam do not hang around and discuss

Exam panic

- Once you read the question paper, you may suffer from exam panic which is manifested by some or all of the following:
  - Nausea
  - Sweaty palms
  - Hot and cold feeling
  - Quick shallow breathing
  - Stomach churning
  - Lack of concentration
  - Rushing in of thoughts
  - Writer's block
  - Blank memory
- If you feel exam panic set aside 5 minutes to deal with it
- Concentrate on breathing
- Consciously relax the muscles
- Try tackling an easy question first
- If nothing works, switch off your mind for a while
- Think of something pleasant, pray God
- Come back to the question

In short

- Answer all the parts of the question
- Make an outline
- Define relevant terms in the question
- Cite examples, references
- Avoid incorrect observations
- Read the question paper thoroughly
- If the question is ambiguous, write your interpretation
- Prioritize the points
- Remember to put the question number
- Give space between answers
- Manage the time

Appendix

List of text books in Complete Denture Prosthodontics

1. Essentials of Complete Denture Prosthodontics – Second edition -Sheldon Winkler
2. Prosthodontic treatment for edentulous patients – twelfth edition – Zarb Bolender
3. Complete Denture Prosthodontics – John J Sharry
4. Dental Lab Procedures – Complete Dentures – Volume I – Rudd and Morrow
5. Complete Prosthodontics – Problems, Diagnosis and Management – Alan A Grant, J R Heath and J Fraser McCord
6. Syllabus of complete denture –Heartwell-3ed
7. Complete dentures - Swenson 4ed
8. Dental prosthesis – complete dentures- Sears
9. Principles of denture prosthesis – Wlfred Fish
10. The complete denture clinical pathway – Mac Entee
11. Removable complete dentures – Phillips

Seminar Topics on complete dentures

1. Patient examination, diagnosis, treatment plan
2. The concepts and technique of denture impression
3. Posterior palatal seal
4. Reduction of residual ridge
5. Retention , stability and support in complete dentures
6. Horizontal jaw relation
7. Vertical and orientation relation
8. Articulators in complete dentures
9. Complete denture occlusion, laws of articulation
10. Selection of anterior teeth
11. Posterior teeth selection
12. Denture insertion/ patient education/ maintenance
13. Complaints
14. Repair,relining,rebase
15. Over denture
16. Single dentures
17. Immediate dentures
18. Denture duplication

Faculty / PG Student / Others

Postgraduate Department of Prosthodontics

AECS Maaruti College of Dental Sciences, Bangalore

Evaluation of Seminar Presentation

Title...

....

Presenter...

Sl.no.	Item for observation	Poor	Below average	Average	Good	Very good
		0	1	2	3	4
1.	Relevant publications consulted	0	1	2	3	4
2.	Cross references consulted	0	1	2	3	4
3.	Completeness of preparation	0	1	2	3	4
4.	Clarity of presentation	0	1	2	3	4
5.	Explanation	0	1	2	3	4
6.	Response to questions	0	1	2	3	4
7.	Use of AV aids	0	1	2	3	4
8.	Audibility	0	1	2	3	4
9.	Eye contact	0	1	2	3	4
10.	Confidence	0	1	2	3	4
11.	Fluency	0	1	2	3	4
12.	Time management	0	1	2	3	4
13.	Body language	0	1	2	3	4
14.	Understanding of the subject	0	1	2	3	4

Total Score:.....................

Postgraduate Department of Prosthodontics

AECS Maaruti College of Dental Sciences, Bangalore

Resource articles for seminars

1. Engelmeier RL; Phoenix RD; Patient evaluation and treatment planning for complete denture therapy; Dental Clinics of North America; 1996;40(1):1 - 17
2. Gamer.S, M.M House classification revisited, J Prosthet dent 2003;89:297-300
3. Perezous F Letecia, Colonisation of candida species in denture wearers with emphasis on HIV infection : A literature review. J Prosthet dent 2005; 93: 288-93
4. Fitzpatrick Brian ,Standard of care for the edentulous mandible: A systematic review, J Prosthet dent 2006; 95:71-8
5. Christensen J Gordan, Treatment of the edentulous mandible. J Am Dent Assoc 2001; 132:231-33
6. Huang Pei - Sheng et al, The proportion of 3 classes of lateral throat form. Int J Prosthodont 2007; 20: 640-42.
7. Friedman, N, Landesman, H.M. & Wexler, M. The influence of fear, anxiety and depression on the patient's adaptive response to complete dentures. Part I. J Prosthet dent 1987; 58: 687-693.
8. Friedman, N., Landesman, H.M. & Wexler, M. The influence of fear, anxiety and depression on the patient's adaptive response to complete dentures. Part II. J Prosthet dent 1988; 59: 45-8.
9. Friedman, N., Landesman, H.M. & Wexler, M. The influence of fear, anxiety and depression on the patient's adaptive response to complete dentures. Part III. J Prosthet dent 1988; 59: 169-73.
10. Devan MM. Basic principles in impression making. J Prosthet Dent 1952;2:26-35.
11. McCord J F, Tyson K W, A conservative prosthodontic option for the treatment of edentulous patients with atrophic (flat) madibular ridges , Br Dent J 1997; 182(12): 469-72
12. Tyson K W, McCord J F, Chairside options for the treatment of complete denture problems associated with the atrophic (flat) mandibular ridge , Br Dent J 2000; 188: 10-14
13. Lynch C D and Allen P F, Management of the flabby ridge : using contemporary materials to solve an old problem. Br Dent J 2006; 200: 258-61
14. Crawford W I and Walmsley, A review of prosthodontic management of fibrous ridges. Br Dent J 2005; 199: 715-19
15. Hasanreisoglu Ufuk et al, Evaluation of reproducibility of the peripheral tissues in edentulous patients. Tr.J. of Medical sciences 1998; 28: 291-94
16. Shetty Sanath et al, The selective pressure maxillary impression: A review of the techniques and presentation of an alternate custom tray design, J Indian Prosthodontic Society 2007; 7(1):8-11
17. Komiyama Osamu et al, effects of relief space and escape holes on pressure characteristics of maxillary edentulous impressions, J Prosthet dent 2004; 91:570-6
18. Al-Ahmad Adel et al, Pressure generated on a simulated mandibular oral analog by impression materials in custom trays of different design. J Prosthdont 2006;15:95-101
19. Duncan P Jacqueline et al, A selective impression technique for the edentulous maxilla, J Prosthet Dent 2004; 92:299-301
20. Smith Dale et al, One step border molding of complete denture impressions using a polyether impression material, J Prosthet Dent 1979; 41 : 347-51

21. Irving R Hardy, Krishan K Kapur, Posterior border seal-Its Rationale and Importance. J Prosthet Dent 1958; 8: 386-397

22. Atwood D.reduction of residual ridges : A major oral disease entity, J Prosthet Dent 1971;26:266-279

23. Tallgren A.The continuing reduction of the residual alveolar ridges in complete denture wearers a mix longitudinal study covering 25 years J Prosthet dent 1972;27:120-132

24. Kapur Krishnan and Shklar Gerald, the effect of complete dentures on alveolar mucosa J Prosthet Dent 1963;13(6): 1030-37

25. Carlsson E Gunnar and Odont, Clinical morbidity and sequelae of treatment with complete dentures, J Prosthet dent, 1997; 79: 17-23

26. Jacobson, T. E. and Krol, A. J, A contemporary review of the factors involved in complete denture retention, stability, and support.Part I.J Prosthet Dent 1983 49:5-15.

27. Jacobson, T. E. and Krol, A contemporary review of the factors involved in complete retention , stability, and support Part II J Prosthet Dent 1983 ;49: 165-172 .

28. Jacobson, T. E. and Krol, A contemporary review of the factors involved in complete retention , stability, and support PartI III J Prosthet Dent 1983;49:306-313.

29. Darvell B.W The physical mechanisms of complete denture retention, Br Dent J 2000;189:248-252

30. Riley A Melissa, Magnets in prosthetic dentistry, J Prosthet Dent 2001;86:137-42

31. Lindstrom et al, Physical –chemical aspects of denture retention and stability: A review of literature, J Prosthet Dent 1979;42(4):371- 75

32. Granger.E.R. Centric relation, J Prosthet Dent 1953;2(2):160-177

33. Cohen.R, Hinge axis and its practical application in the determination of centric relation,J Prosthet Dent 1960;20(2):248-257

34. Martin E. Kantor, Sidney I. Silverman and Lawrence Garfinkel Centric- relation recording techniques-a comparative investigation, J Prosthet Dent 1972;28(6):59-63

35. James Hart long, An instrument for locating centric relation ,J Prosthet Dent 1973;30(1):50-52

36. William E. Avant , Using the term "centric", J Prosthet Dent 1971;25(1):12-15

37. Yurkstas Albert, Kapur Krishnan, Factors influencing centris relation records in edentulous mouths, J Prosthet Dent 1964;14(6):1054- 64

38. EGR Solomon, Craniomandibular relations – determinant II- Centric jaw relation , Journal of Indian Prosthodontic Society, 2001;1(3): 6-16

39. Keshvad A, Winstanley R B, An appraisal on the literature of centric relation. Part II, J Oral Rahabil, 2000; 27: 1013-23

40. Keshvad A, Winstanley R B, An appraisal on the literature of centric relation. Part III, J Oral Rahabil, 2001; 28: 55-63

41. Villa Honorato, Gothic arch tracing, J Prosthet Dent 1959; 9(4): 624 - 28

42. Lauritzen G Arne, Occlusal relationships: The split cast method for articulator techniques,J Prosthet Dent 1964;14(2): 256-65

43. Wilkie Noel, The anterior point of reference, J Prosthet Dent 1979;41(5): 488 – 96

44. E G R Solomon, The morphology of tragus Part 1: The confusion about tragus terminology, Journal of Indian Prosthodontic Society, April 2000; 11(1): 11-15

45. E G R Solomon, Part 2: the reliability of tragus morphology and its reference to establish Camper's plane, Journal of Indian Prosthodontic Society, April 2000;11(1): 16-22

46. E G R Solomon, Part 3: Definability of tragus morphology as a reference landmark in edentulous subjects, Journal of Indian Prosthodontic Society, April 2000; 11(1): 23-26

47. Wognsen Brandrup Thure, The facebow – its significance and its application, J Prosthet dent 1953; 3(5): 618-30

48. E G R Solomon, Craniomandibular relations, Journal of Indian Prosthodontic Society, April 2001; 1(2):6-16

49. E G R Solomon,Rest vertical heihjt of the jaws with and without occlusal rims , Journal of Indian Prosthodontic Society, April 2001; 1(2):17-20

50. Fayz Farhad, Eslami Ahmad, determination of occlsual vertical dimension: A literature review, J Prosthet Dent, 1988 ;59(3):321-23

51. Bissasu Majid, Preextratcion records for complete denture fabrication : a literature review , J Prosthet Dent 2004; 91(1):55-58

52. Watt D M, Durran C M, Adenubi, Biometric guides to the design of complete maxillary dentures,Dent Mag Oral Top 1967 Jun ;84(3):109-11

53. A.Rihani, Classification of articulators, J Prosthet Dent 1980;43:344-347

54. Bennet G Norman, A contribution to the study of the movements of the mandible ,J Prosthet Dent , 1958;8 (1) :41-54

55. Edward.J.Mehringer,Function of steep cusps in mastication with complete dentures ,J Prosthet Dent 1973;30(4):367-372

56. Edward.J.Mehringer, Physiologically generated occlusion, J Prosthet Dent 1973; 30(4):373-379

57. Finn Tengs Christensen, Divided incisal guidance, J Prosthet Dent 1973;30(2): 147-150

58. William E. Elkins, Gold occlusal surfaces and organic occlusion in denture construction ,J Prosthet Dent 1973;30(1):94-98

59. Nimmo. A. and Frank J. Kratochvil, Balancing ramps in nonanatomic complete denture occlusion 1985;53:431-433

60. S. Davies and R. M. J. Gray, What is occlusion? Br Dent J 2001;191(5):236-245

61. S. J. Davies, R. M. J. Gray and J. F. McCord,Good occlusal practice in removable prosthodontics, Br Dent J 2001;191(9): 491-502

62. Ash M. Occlusion: Reflections on science and clinical reality. J Prosthet Dent 2003; 90:373-84.

63. Levin Bernard, A reevaluation of Hanau's Laws of articulation and the Hanau quint 1978; 39(3): 254- 58

64. Mitchell Donald, Wilkie Donald, Articluators through the years. Part I. Upto 1940, J Prosthet dent 1978;39(3): 330-38

65. Mitchell Donald, Wilkie Donald, Articluators through the years. Part II. From 1940, J Prosthet dent 1978; 39(4): 451-58

66. FrushJ.P And Fischer R.D, Introduction To Dentogenic Restoration J Prosthet Dent 1955 ;5:586-595

67. Frush.J.P, Fisher R.D, The dyesthetic interpretation of dentogenic concept JProsthet Dent, 1958; 8 : 558-581

68. Mccord J.F. Registration :Stage III selection of teeth, Br Dent J 2006;188:660-666

69. George Murell,Complete denture esthetics, Dent Clin N Am, 1996;40(1):71-84

70. Mc Cord, Firestone, Grant , Phonetic determinants of tooth placement in complete dentures, Quintessence Inetrnational, 1994; 25(5): 341-45

71. Murell George, Phonetics, function and anterior occlusion, J Prosthet dent, 1974; 32(1):23-31

72. Driscoll Carl, Masri M Radi, Single maxiallry complete denture ,Dent Clin N Am, 2004; 48: 567-83

73. Madan Nishta, Datta Kusum, Combination syndrome, Journal of Indian Prosthodontic Society, 2006;6(1):10-13

74. Miller Ernst, Clinical management of denture induced inflammation, J Prosthet Dent 1977; 38 (4): 362-65.

75. Palmer John, Structural changes for speech improvement In complete denture fabrication,J Prosthet Dent 1979; 41(5): 507-10

76. Jeganathan S, Payne J A, Common faults in complete dentures : A review Quintessence International 1993; 24(7): 483-87

77. Morstad A T, Peterson A D, Post insertion denture problems. J Prosthet dent 1968; 19(2): 126-131

78. Seo S Rosangala et al, Factors affecting the strength of denture repairs,J Prosthodontics, 2007; 16(4): 302-10

Reading List

1. Abelson, D.C. Denture plaque and denture cleansers: Review of the literature, Gerodontics 1985, 1: 202-6.

2. Adell, R., Lekholm, U., Rockler, B and Branemark, P.I. A 15-year study of osseointegrated implants in the treatment of the edentulous jaw. Int. J. Oral Surg. 1981;10: 387-416.

3. Arendorf, T.M. & Walker, D.M. Denture stomatitis: a review. J of Oral Rehabil. 1987;14: 217-227.

4. Atwood, D.A. Reduction of residual ridges: a major oral disease entity. J Prosthet Dent. 1971; 26: 266-79

5. Atwood, D.A. A cephalometric study of the clinical rest position of the mandible. Part I. J of Prosthet Dent 1956; 6: 504-19. Part II. J Prosthet Dent 1957;7: 544-552. Part III. J Prosthetic Dent 1958;8: 693-708.

6. Basker, R.M., Davenport, J.C. & Tomlin, H.R. Prosthetic Treatment of the Edentulous Patient. Macmillan Press, London, 1983.

7. Bates, J.F., Stafford, G.D. & Harrison, A. Masticatory function -part 3. J Oral Rehabil 1976;3: 57-67.

8. Bates, J.F., Stafford, G.D. & Harrison, A. Masticatory function - a review of the literature (part 2). J Oral Rehabil 1975;2: 349-61.

9. Bates, J.F. & Harrison, A. A Survey of House Bound Persons in Cardiff with Special Reference to Dental Care. Public Health, London, 1975.

10. Beck, H.O. and Morrison, W. G. Investigation of the arcon articulator. J Prosthet Dent 1956;6: 359-372.

11. Beck, H.O. A clinical evaluation of the arcon concept of articulation. J Prosthet Dent 1959;9: 409-421.

12. Bergstrom, G. On the reproduction of dental articulation by means of articulators. Acta Odontologica Scandinavica 1950; 9: suppl 4.

13. Breustedt, A. Age induced changes in oral mucosa and their therapeutic consequences. Int. Dent. J. 1983; 33: 272-80.

14. Brill, N. Factors in the mechanism of full denture retention. Dental Practitioner 1967;18: 9-19.

15. Butz-Jorgensen, G. Effect of controlled oral hygiene in overdenture wearers. Int Journal of Prosthodont 1991;4: 226-231.

16. Cawood, J. and Howell, R. A classification of the edentulous jaws. Int. J. Oral Maxillofac. Surg. 1988;17: 232-236.

17. Chou, T.M. & Parmeijer, C.H. An investigation into the reproducibility of articulators. J Prosthet Dent 1987;58: 442-448.

18. Christensen, J. Introducing gerodontology to students in Denmark. Comm. Dent. Oral. Epid. 1987; 15: 137-40.

19. Drummond, J.R., Newton, J.P. and Yemm, R. Dentistry for the elderly: a review and assessment for the future. J.Dent. 1988; 16: 47-54.

20. Duthie, N., Lyon, J., Sturrock, K. and Yemm, R. A copying technique for the replacement of complete dentures. Br. Dent.J. 1978;144: 248-252,.

21. Edgar, W.M. & O'Mullane, D.M. Saliva and Dental Health. British Dental Association 1990.

22. Ekelund, R. Effectiveness of tooth and denture brushing in the disabled elderly in municipal old peoples' homes in Finland. Gerodontics 1988; 4: 63-5.

23. Exton-Smith, A.N. & Stanton, B.R. Report of an Investigation into the Dietary Intake of Elderly Women Living Alone. King Edward's Hospital Fund, London, 1965.

24. Faigenblum, M.J. Retching, its causes and management in prosthetic practice. Br Dent J 1968;125:485.

25. Fayz,, F. & Eslami, A. Determination of occlusal vertical dimension: a literature review. J. Prosthet. Dent. 1988; 59: 321-323.

26. Fish, S.F. Adaptation and habituation to full dentures. Br Dent J 1969;127:19.

27. Franks, A.S.T. & Hedegard, B. Geriatric Dentistry. Blackwell Scientific Publications, Oxford, 1973.

28. Friedman, N, Landesman, H.M. & Wexler, M. The influence of fear, anxiety and depression on the patient's adaptive response to complete dentures. Part I. J Prosthet dent 1987;58: 687-693.

29. Friedman, N., Landesman, H.M. & Wexler, M. The influence of fear, anxiety and depression on the patient's adaptive response to complete dentures. Part II. J Prosthet dent 1988;59: 45-8.

30. Friedman, N., Landesman, H.M. & Wexler, M. The influence of fear, anxiety and depression on the patient's adaptive response to complete dentures. Part III. J Prosthet dent 1988;59: 169-73.

31. Giles, D.L. and Murphy, W.M. Dental treatment of the elderly in-patient. J.Dent. 1980; 8(4): 341-48.

32. Gordon, S.R. Older Adults: Demographics and need for quality care. J.Prosthet. Dent. 1989; 61. 6: 737-41.

33. Grant, A.A., Heath, J.R. and McCord, J.F. Complete Prosthodontics: Diagnosis, Treatment and Management. Wolfe Publishing, London, 1994.

34. Haines, R.W. & Barrett, S.G. The structure of the mouth in the mandibular molar region. J Prosthet dent 1959;9: 962-974.

35. Heath, R. A study of the morphology of the denture space. Dental Practitioner 1970;21(4): 109- 117.

36. Hickey, J.C., Lundeen, H.C. and Bohannan, H.M. A new articulator for use in teaching and general dentistry. J Prosthet Dent 1967; 18: 425-437.

37. Hoad-Reddick, G. et al. The dental health of an elderly population in N.W. England: results of a survey undertaken in the Halton Health Authority. J.Dent. 1987; 15(4): 139-46.

38. Hoad-Reddick, G. et al. Knowledge of Dental Services provided: investigations in an elderly population. Comm. Dent. Oral Epid. 1987;15: 137-40.

39. Hoad-Reddick, G. A study to determine oral health needs of institutionalised elderly patients by non dental health care workers. Comm. Dent. Oral Epid. 1991.

40. Lauritzen, A.G. & Bodner, G.H. Variations in location of arbitrary and true hinge axis points. J Prosthet Dent 1961;11: 224-229.

41. Lawson, W.A. Current concepts and practice in complete dentures: impressions; principles and practice. J Dent 1978;6: 43-58.

42. Lawson, W.A. An analysis of the commonest causes of full denture failure. Dental Pract. Dent. Rec. 1959;10: 61-63.

43. Lee, J.H. Dental Aesthetics. John Wright & Sons, Bristol, 1962. Makila, E. & Honka, O. Clinical study of a heat-cured silicone soft lining material. J oral rehab 1979;6: 199-204.

44. Martone, A.L. & Edwards, L.F. Anatomy of the mouth and related structures. Part 1. The face. J Prosthet dent 1961;11: 1009-18. Part 2. Musculature of expression. J Prosthet dent 1962;12: 4-27. Part 3. Functional anatomic considerations. J Prosthet dent 1962;12: 206-19.

45. McCord, J.F., Grant, A.A. and Quayle, A.A. Treatment options for the edentulous mandible. Euro. J. Prosthodont. Rest. Dent. 1992 ; 1: 19-23.

46. McMillan, C.R. & McMillan, A.S. A comparison of habitual jaw movements and articulator function. Acta Odontologica Scandinavica 1986; 44: 291-299.

47. Mitchell, D.L. and Wilkie, N.D. Articulators through the years. Part 1: Up to 1940. J Prosthet dent39: 330-380, 1978. Part 2: From 1940. J Prosthet dent 1978;39: 451-458.

48. Monasky, G.E. Placement of overdenture attachments using a visible light-cured resin. Quintessence International 1989 ;19: 67-69.

49. Morgan, S.M., Malone, W.F.P. et al. Tissue management with dental impression materials. Am.J.Dent. 1989; 2: 279-284.

50. O'Brien, W.J. Base retention. Dental Clinics of North America 1980;24: 123-130. Osborne, J., Maddick, I, Gould, A. and Ward, D. Dental demands of old people in Hampshire. Br Dent J 1979; 146: 351-5.

51. Ritchie, G.M. A report of dental findings in a survey of geriatric patients. J Dent. 1973; 1: 106-12.

52. Santos, J.D. and Ash, M. A comparison of the equivalence of jaw and articulator movements. J Prosthet Dent 1988; 59: 36-42.

53. Scandrett, F.R. Essentials of Complete Denture Prosthodontics ed. S Winkler, W B Saunders Philadelphia, 1979, Ch.11, pp 216-262.

54. Schmidt, W.F., Smith, D.E. A six-year retrospective study of Molloplast-B-lined dentures. Part I: patient response. J Prosthet dent 1983;50: 308-13. Part II: liner serviceability. J Prosthet dent 1983; 50: 459-65.

55. Smith, J.M. and Sheiham, A. How dental conditions handicap the elderly. Comm. Dent. Oral Epid. 1979; 5: 22-8.

56. Tallgren, A. The effect of denture wearing on facial morphology - a 7-year study. Acta Odontologica Scandinavica 1967; 25: 563.

57. Tallgren, A. Changes in adult face height due to aging, wear, and loss of teeth, and prosthetic treatment. Acta Odontologica Scandinavica 15 (Supplement 24), 1957.

58. Tallgren, A., Lang, B.R. and Miller, R. Longitudinal study of soft-tissue profile changes in patients receiving immediate complete dentures. Int J Prosthodont 1991;4:9-16.

59. Wachtel, H.C. and Curtis, D.B. Limitations of semi-adjustable articulators. Part 1: Straight line articulators without setting for immediate side shift. J Prosthet dent 1987;58: 438-442. Part 2: Straight line articulators with provision for immediate side shift. J Prosthet dent 1987; 569-581.

60. Weinberg, L.A. Arcon principle in the condylar mechanism of adjustable articulators. J Prosthet dent 1963;13: 263-268.

61. Weinberg, L.A. An evaluation of basic articulators and their concepts: Part 1: Basic concepts. J Prosthet dent 1963;13:622-644; Part 2: Arbitrary, positional, semi-adjustable articulators. J Prosthet dent 1963;13: 645-

653.; Part 3: Fully adjustable articulators. J Prosthet dent 1963;13: 873-885. ; Part 4: Fully adjustable articulators. J Prosthet dent 1963; 13: 1038-1051.

62. Wilson, S.J. and Wilson, H.J. The effect of chlorinated disinfecting solutions on alginate impressions. Journal of Restorative Dentistry 1987;3: 86.

63. Wilson, H.J., Mansfield, M.A., Heath, J.R. and Spence, D. Dental Technology and Materials for Students 8th Ed. Blackwell Scientific Publications, Oxford, (UK), 1987.

64. Wilson, N.H.F., Dunne, S.M. and Gainsford, I.D. Current materials and techniques for direct restorations in posterior teeth. Part 2: Resin Composite Systems. Int Dent.J. 1997; 47: 185-193.

65. Winkler, S. (ed). Essentials for complete denture prosthodontics. W.B. Saunders. Philadelphia. 1989.

67. Wright, S.M. Prosthetic reproduction of gingival pigmentation. Br Dent J 1974;136: 367.

Classic articles

1. Ash M. Occlusion: Reflections on science and clinical reality. J Prosthet Dent 2003;90:373-84.

2. Bennett NG. A Contribution to the Study of the Movements of the Mandible. Proc R Soc Med; 1908; 1(Odontol Sect): 79–98.

3. Beresin VE. The neutral zone in complete dentures. J Prosthet Dent 1976; 36:357-67.

4. Bonwill WGA, The science of the articulation of artificial dentures. Dental Cosmos 1878;20(1): 321-324..

5. Boucher C. Complete denture prosthodontics—the state of the art. J Prosthet Dent 1975 ;34:372-83.

6. Boucher C. Method of recording functional movements of full-denture bases in three dimensions. J Dent. Res 1934;14(1): 39-47.

7. Campbell DD. Some fundamental factors in the construction of efficient dentures. J Dent Res 1927; 7(2):127-143.

8. Christensen C. The problem of the bite. Dental Cosmos 1905; 47(10): 1186-1195.

9. Dalbey WC. (I) How to Obtain Accurate Measurements in Artificial Denture Making. (II) Locating the Fundamental Lines Used in Anatomical Articulation. Dental Cosmos 1914; 56(3):269-275..

11. Devan MM. Basic principles in impression making. J Prosthet Dent 1952; 2: 26-35.

12. Fox F. The principles Involved in Full Upper and Lower Denture Construction. Dental Cosmos 1924;66(2)1:51-157.

13. Gysi A. The problem of articulation . Dental Cosmos 1910 ; 52(1)

14. Hardy IR. The developments in the occlusal patterns of artificial teeth. J Prosthet Dent 1951 ;1 (1-2):14-28.

15. Helkimo M. Studies on function and dysfunction of the masticatory system. Acta Odontologica Scandinavica 1974; 32(4): 255 - 267.

16. Henderson D. Occlusion in removable partial prosthodontics,J ProsthetDent 1972;27:151–9..

19. Hoff NS. Plate prosthesis. Dental Cosmos 1917; 59(2): 158-165.

20. Hoffman A. The Practical Measurements Involved in the Construction of Complete Dentures. Dental Cosmos 1916; 58(11): 1269-1278 .

21. How WS. Plaster Prosthetic Models. Dental Cosmos 1888; 30(9): 634-638.

22. How WS. New Bite-Taking Means and Methods. Dental Cosmos 1894; 36(9): 692-699.

23. Jacobson ET, Krol AJ. A contemporary review of the factors involved in complete denture retention, stability, and support. Part I: Retention. J Prosthet Dent 1983;49(1):5-15.

24. Jacobson ET, Krol AJ. A contemporary review of the factors involved in complete denture retention, stability, and support. Part II: stability. J Prosthet Dent 1983 ;49(2):165-172..

25. Jacobson ET, Krol AJ. A contemporary review of the factors involved in complete denture retention, stability, and support. Part III: Soport. J Prosthet Dent 1983;49(3):306-313..

26. Krishan K. Kapur, Sham Soman, Katherine Stone. The effect of denture factors on masticatory performance: Part I: Influence of denture base extension. J Prosthet Dent 1965; 15(1): 54-64.

27. Krishan K. Kapur, Sham Soman. The effect of denture factors on masticatory performance: Part II: Influence of the polished surface contour of denture base. J Prosthet Dent 1965; 15(2): 231-240

28. Krishan K. Kapur, Sham Soman, Katherine Stone. The effect of denture factors on masticatory performance: Part III. The location of food platforms. J Prosthet Dent 2006; 95(4): 265-334

29. Krishan K. Kapur, Sham Soman, Katherine Stone. The effect of denture factors on masticatory performance: Part IV. Influence of occlusal patterns. J Prosthet Dent 1965; 15(4): 662-670.

30. Krishan K. Kapur, Sham Soman, Katherine Stone. The effect of denture factors on masticatory performance: Part V. Food platform area and metal inserts. J Prosthet Dent 1965; 15(5): 857-866.

31. Kelly E. Changes caused by a mandibular removable partial denture opposing a maxillary complete denture. J Prosthet Dent 2003 ;90(3):213-219.

32. Lucia, V. O. A technique for recording centric relation, Journal of Prosthetic Dentistry, 1964;14: 492–505.

33. McCollum BB. The mandibular hinge axis and a method of locating it. J Prosthet Dent 1960;10(3): 428-435..

34. Monson GS. Applied mechanics to the theory of mandibular movements, Dental Cosmos 1932;74(11):1039–1053.

35. Payne SH. A comparative study of posterior occlusion. J Prosthet Dent 1952;2:661-6.

36. Paterson AH. Construction of artificial dentures, Dental Cosmos 1923;65(7):679–689.

37. Pendleton EC. The positive pressure technique for impression taking. Dental Cosmos 1931; 73(11): 1045-1056.

38. Posselt U. Hinge open axis of the mandibule, Acta Odont. Scand 1956;4(4):49-63 .

39. Posselt U. Range of movement of the mandible. J Am Dent Assoc;56: 10-13, 1958.

40. Preston JD. A reassessment of the mandibular transverse horizontal axis theory. J Prosthet Dent 1979;41:605-13.

41. Sears VH. Occlusal refinements on completed dentures. J Am Dent Assoc 1959;59:1250-2,

42. Sears VH. Balanced Occlusions. J Am Dent Assoc 1925; 12:1448.

43. Sears VH. Occlusal pivots. J Prosthet Dent 1956;6:332-338.

44. Sears VH. Channel type posterior tooth forms. J Am Dent Assoc 1928;15:1111-1117.

45. Sears VH. Some fundamental factors in tooth articulation. J Dent Res 1928 ; 8(3): 339-352,

46. Sears VH. Thirty years of nonanatomic teeth. J Prosthet Dent 1953; 3(5):596-617.

47. Sears VH. The selection and management of posterior teeth. J Prosthet Dent 1957; 7(6): 723-737.

48. Sears VH. Jaw Relations and a Means of Recording the Most Important Articulator Adjustment. Dental Cosmos 1926; 68(11): 1047-1054.

49. Sears H. Indications for and Limitations of Alveolectomy with an Original Means of Control. Dental Cosmos 1926; 68(12): 1187-1190.

50. Shanahan TE. Physiologic jaw relations and occlusion of complete dentures. J Prosthet Dent 1955;5(3):319-324.

51. Shanaham TE. Physiologic vertical dimension and centric relation. J Prosthet Dent 1956;6(6): 741-747.

52. Silverman M. The speaking method in measuring vertical dimension. J Prosthet Dent 1953 ;3:193-99.

53. Silverman M. Determination of vertical dimension by phonetics. J Prosthet Dent 1956; 6(4):465-471.

54. Silverman M. Pre-extraction records to avoid premature aging of the denture patient. J Prosthet Dent 1955;(4):465-476.

55. Silverman M. Vertical dimension must not be increased. J Prosthet Dent 1952; 2(2):188-197.

56. Snow GB. The Philosophy of Mastication. Dental Cosmos 1900; 42(6): 531-535.

57. Snow GB. Articulation. Dental Cosmos 1900; 42(1): 51-55.

58. Spee FG. The condylar path of the mandible along the skull. Arch anat Physiol., 16: 285, 1890 (in German); J Amer Dent Assoc., 100: 670, 1980 (English translation).

59. Toolson LB, Smith DE. Clinical measurement and evaluation of vertical dimension. J Prosthet Dent 2006; 95(5): 335-406.

60. Turrel AJ. Clinical assessment of vertical dimension.J Prosthet Dent 1972;28:238-45.

61. Wadsworth F. A practical system of denture prosthesis including the restoration of anatomical articulation. Dental Cosmos 1925; 67(7): 670-682.

62. Walker WE. Dental Articulation and Occlusion. Dental Cosmos; 41(9): 92-898. 1899

63. Walker WE. Prosthetic Dentistry: the Glenoid Fossa; the Movements of the Mandible; the Cusps of the Teeth. Dental Cosmos 1896; 38(1): 34-43.

64. Washburn HB. History and evolution of the study of occlusion. Dental Cosmos;67(3):223-237.1925

65. Waugh DB. The Arrangement of Teeth in Natural and Artificial Dentures. Dental Cosmos 1936; 78(11): 1125-1135.

66. Williams JL. Original Communications; The Esthetic and Anatomical Basis of Dental Prosthesis. Dental Cosmos 1911; 53(1): 1-26.

67. Williams JL. Type vs. temperament in the selection of teeth. Dental Cosmos 1917; 59(11): 1126-1128 .

68. Willis FM. Features of the Face Involved in Full Denture Prosthesis. Dental Cosmos 1935; 77(9):851-854.

69. Wilson G. Some Phrases of Construction of Complete Artificial Dentures. Dental Cosmos 1908; 50(10):1045-1067.

70. Wright WH. Important factors of denture service; Dental Cosmos 1927; 69(6): 584-589..

71. Yurkstas AA, Kapur KK. Factors influencing centric relation records in edentulous mouths. J Prosthet Dent 1964;14:1054-65.

72. Felton et al, evidence based guidelines for the care and maintainance of complete dentures : A publication of the American College of Prosthodontists, J Am Dent Assoc 2011;142(2):1-20

A list of skills which are essential for a Prosthodontist

Clinical skills

Complete dentures

Patient examination

1. Extra oral examination
2. Intra oral examination/ investigations
3. Identification of conditions affecting CD
4. Selection of stock tray
5. Selection of impression material for preliminary Impression - alginate/ putty silicone
6. Manipulation of impression material for preliminary Impression
7. Selection of material for custom made tray
8. Selection of material for border moulding – putty silicone/ greenstick/Border moulding
9. Lining the impression- elastomer

Jaw relations

10. Lip support and lip fullness
11. Check for denture base retention and extension
12. Marking the midline on the rims
13. Orientation of the plane on maxillary and mandibular occlusion rims
14. Establishment of vertical dimension- identification of free way space, closest speaking space
15. Registration of centric relation (check bite method)

Face bow transfer

16. Identification of parts of face bow (spring bow)
17. Fixing the fork
18. Positioning the bow on the patient
19. To confirm horizontality using spirit level markers
20. Transferring the relation to semi adjustable articulator (Hanau wide vue)
21. Mounting the upper cast
22. Mounting the lower cast using tentative jaw relation

Verification of the centric using graphic method

23. Attachment of tracing units, space for plaster record, height maintenance by central bearing point
24. Tracing on the table and its analysis
25. Making inter occlusal records - centric/ protrusive
26. Verification of centric
27. Programming the articulator

Preparation of trial denture

28. Selection of anterior teeth
29. Selection of posterior teeth
30. Arrangement of teeth in balanced articulation (lingualised)
31. Factors to be checked during trial/ Characterization of teeth

Remount procedures

32. Check for balanced articulation and identify the interferences and eliminate

Denture evaluation

33. Check for esthetics, retention ,stability ,support vertical dimension , phonetics and balanced using articulating paper

Instructions and periodic evaluation

34. List of instructions given to the patient
35. Prescription containing denture brush, denture cleansers , denture adhesives, multivitamin tablets

Lab skills

CD

36. Pouring the cast, removal, trimming
37. Fabrication of special tray
38. Boxing the final impression
39. Making the cast
40. Making denture bases

41. Making the mould with denture flask
42. Compression moulding
43. Selection of curing cycle
44. Deflasking
45. Trimming and polishing of denture/bases
46. Occlusion rims
47. Mounting of cast on semi adjustable articulator
48. Teeth arrangement in balanced occlusion

Handling of equipments

49. Dental Chair
50. Airotors
51. Dental x ray/ RVG
52. Lap top/ Digital camera
53. Intra oral camera
54. Semi adjustable articulator/ face bow
55. Micromotor hand piece
56. Reduction gear hand piece

Communication skills

57. Preparation of case sheets
58. Viva voce skills
59. Lecture classes
60. Participating in group discussion
61. Summarizing ability
62. Scientific writing
63. Paper presentation
64. E mails
65. Internet skills and ethics
66. Inter personal skills
67. Patient interview

Hanau's Articulation Quint.

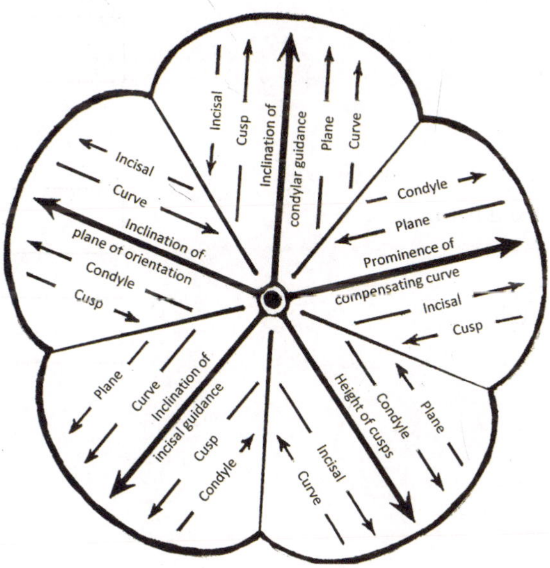

This figure diagramatically represent the five factors of the loss of articulation and their interrelationship. Direction of the arrow indicates increase and dicrease of the influence. The arrrows pointing away from the centre indicates and increase of the influence whereas arrows pointing towards the centre indicate the decrease of influence.

Postgraduate Department of Prosthodontics

AECS Maaruti College of Dental Sciences and Research Centre, Bangalore

Preclinical Exercises in Complete Dentures

1. Custom made trays in shellac base plate
   Maxillary (edentulous)
   Mandibular (edentulous)

2. Custom made trays in acrylic with spacers incorporated
   Maxillary (edentulous)
   Mandibular (edentulous)

3. Temporary (transfer) bases in acrylic
   Maxillary (edentulous)
   Mandibular (edentulous)

4. Occlusion rims
   Maxillary
   Mandibular

5. Mounting on articulator (fixed path)

6. Arrangement of anterior teeth

   Maxillary

   Mandibular

7. Arrangement of posterior teeth

   Maxillary
   Mandibular

8. Waxing up, carving, finishing

9. Processing

10. Laboratory remount/adjustments

11. Submission of dentures mounted in the articulator

12. Denture in Class I relationship (semi adjustable articulator)

13. Denture in Class II relationship (semi adjustable articulator)

14. Denture in Class III relationship (semi adjustable articulator)

15.Denture in Cross bite relationship (semi adjustable articulator)

On completion of 13 to 15 you are expected to familiarize with impression procedures, jaw relations including face bow transfer, graphic tracings and balanced articulation using semi adjustable articulator)

On submission of each exercise get the signature of the teacher with date as a sign of approval

Guidelines for the care and maintenance of dentures (American College of Prosthodontists)

1. Careful daily removal of the bacterial biofilm present in the oral cavity and on complete dentures is of paramount importance to minimize denture stomatitis and to help contribute to good oral and general health.
2. To reduce levels of biofilm and potentially harmful bacteria and fungi, patients who wear dentures should do the following: (a) Dentures should be cleaned daily by soaking and brushing with an effective, nonabrasive denture cleanser. (b) Denture cleansers should ONLY be used to clean dentures outside of the mouth. (c) Dentures should always be thoroughly rinsed after soaking and brushing with denture-cleansing solutions prior to reinsertion into the oral cavity. Always follow the product usage instructions.
3. Although the evidence is weak, dentures should be cleaned annually by a dentist or dental professional using ultrasonic cleansers to minimize biofilm accumulation over time.
4. Dentures should never be placed in boiling water.
5. Dentures should not be soaked in sodium hypochlorite bleach, or in products containing sodium hypochlorite, for periods that exceed 10 minutes. Placement of dentures in sodium hypochlorite solutions for periods longer than 10 minutes may damage dentures.
6. Dentures should be stored immersed in water after cleaning, when not replaced in the oral cavity, to avoid warping.
7. Denture adhesives, when properly used, can improve the retention and stability of dentures and help seal out the accumulation of food particles beneath the dentures, even in well-fitting dentures.
8. In a quality-of-life study patient ratings showed that denture adhesives may improve the denture wearer's perceptions in retention, stability, and quality of life; however, there is insufficient evidence that adhesives improve masticatory function.
9. Evidence regarding the effects of denture adhesives on the oral tissues when used for periods longer than 6 months is lacking. Thus, extended use of denture adhesives should not be considered without periodic assessment of denture quality and health of the supporting tissues by a dentist, prosthodontist, or dental professional.
10. Improper use of zinc-containing denture adhesives may have adverse systemic effects. Therefore, as a precautionary measure, zinc-containing denture adhesives should be avoided.
11. Denture adhesive should only be used in sufficient quantities (three or four pea-sized dollops) on each denture to provide sufficient added retention and stability to the prostheses.
12. Denture adhesives should be completely removed from the prosthesis and the oral cavity on a daily basis.
13. If increasing amounts of adhesives are required to achieve the same level of denture retention, the patient should see a dentist or dental professional to evaluate the fit and stability of the dentures.
14. While existing studies provide conflicting results, it is not recommended that dentures should be worn continuously (24 hours per day) in an effort to reduce or minimize denture stomatitis.
15. Patients who wear dentures should be checked annually by the dentist, prosthodontist, or dental professional for maintenance of optimum denture fit and function, for evaluation for oral lesions and bone loss, and for assessment of oral health status.

Young complete denture wearer

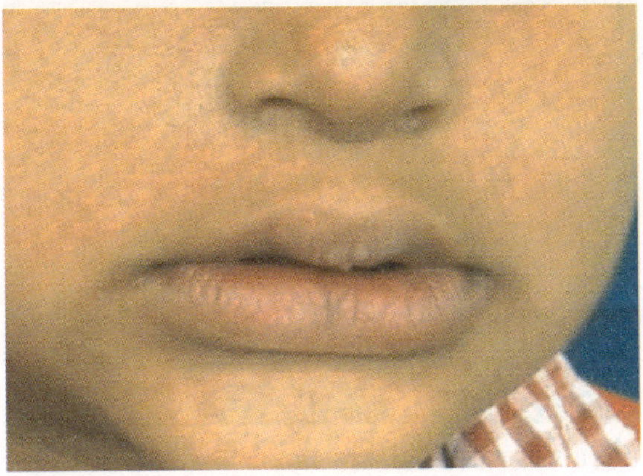

Fig. 1 Young(6) completely edentulous patient with hereditary ectodermal dysplasia

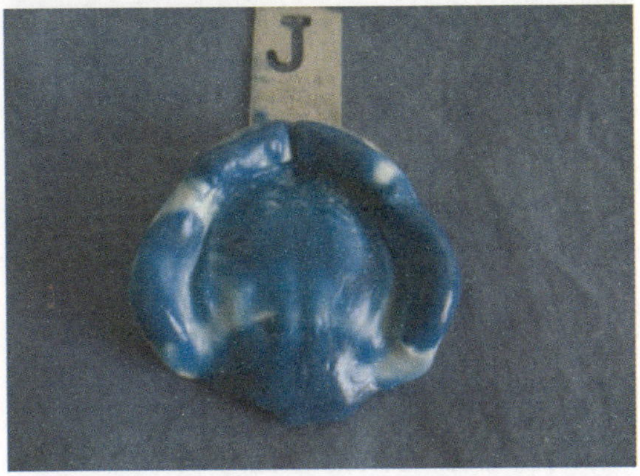

Fig. 2 Preliminary impression of maxillary ridge with putty and light body elastomer

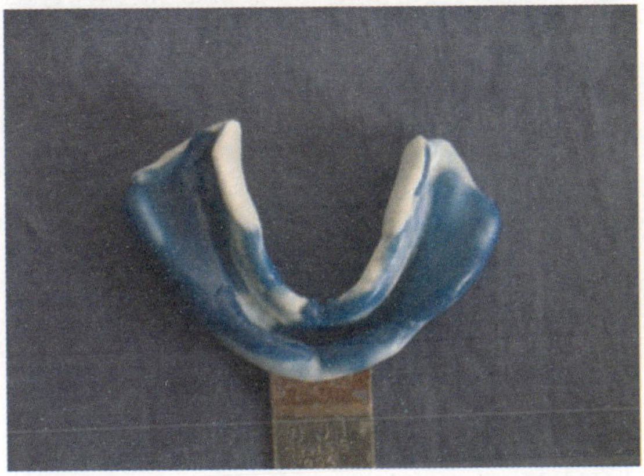

Fig. 3 Preliminary impression of mandibular ridge with putty and light body elastomer

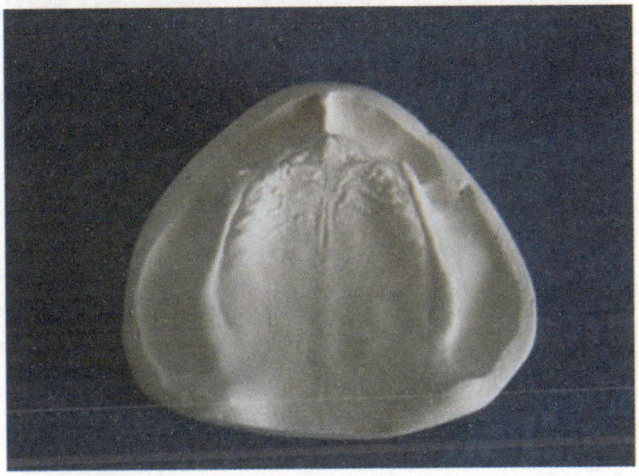

Fig. 4 Maxillary primary cast

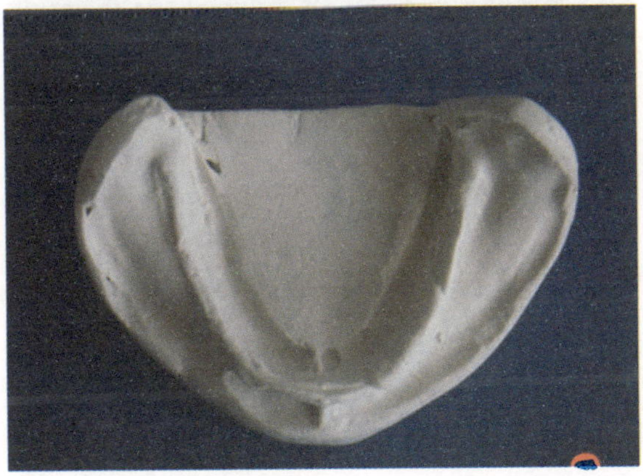

Fig. 5 Mandibular primary cast

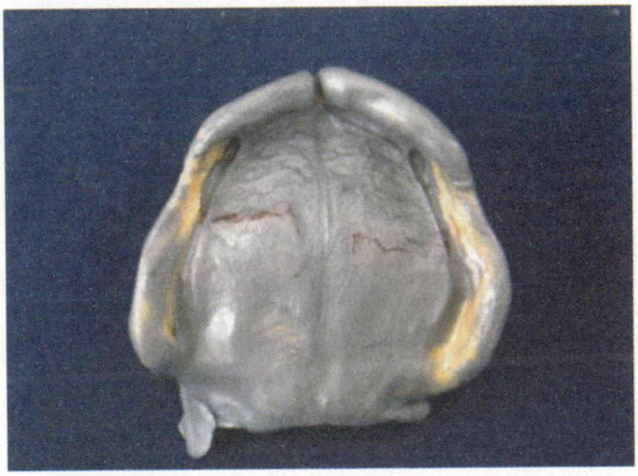

Fig. 6 Maxillary final impression

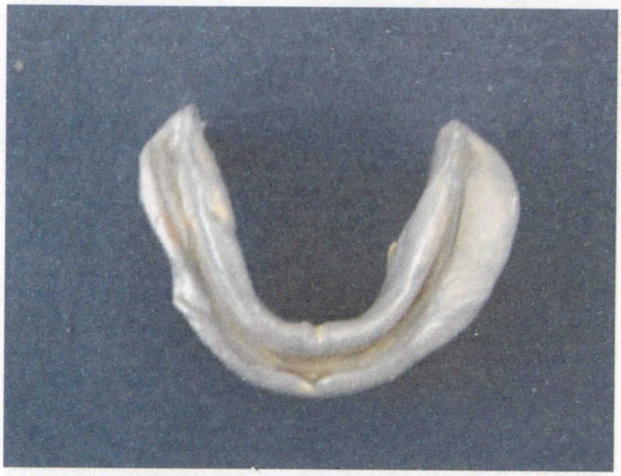

Fig. 7 Mandibular final impression

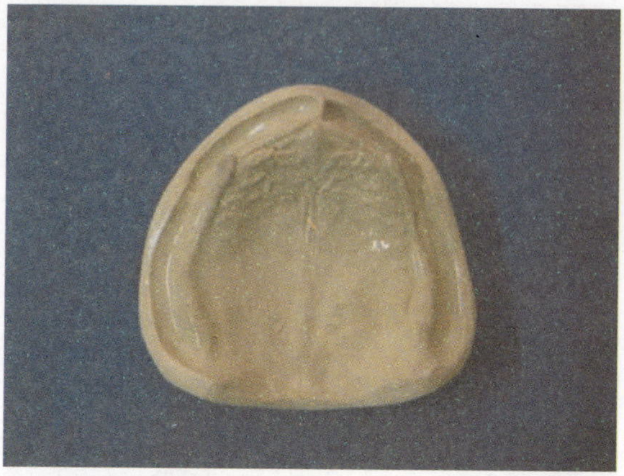

Fig. 8 Final maxillary cast

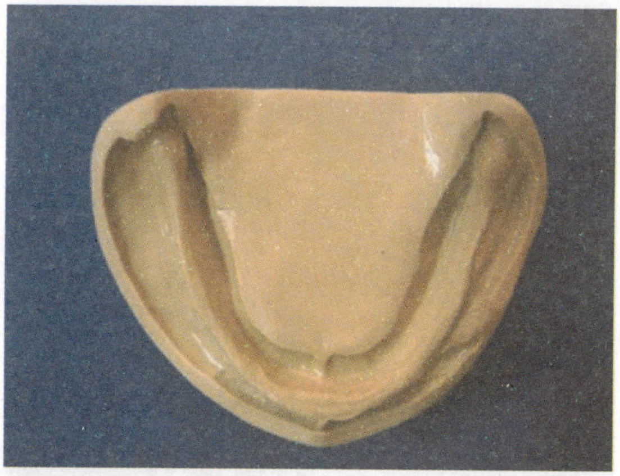

Fig. 9 Final mandibular cast

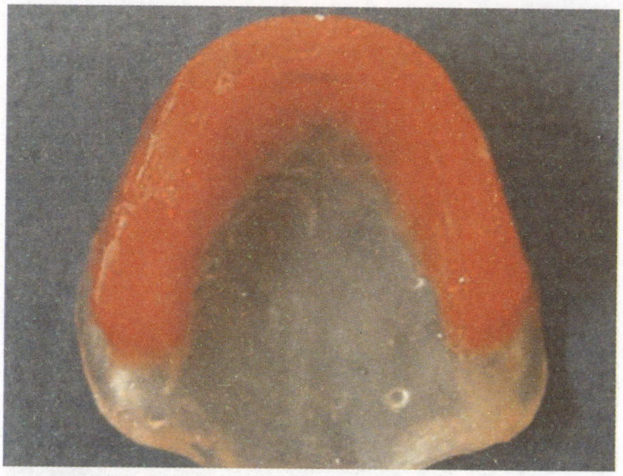

Fig. 10 Maxillary occlusion rim

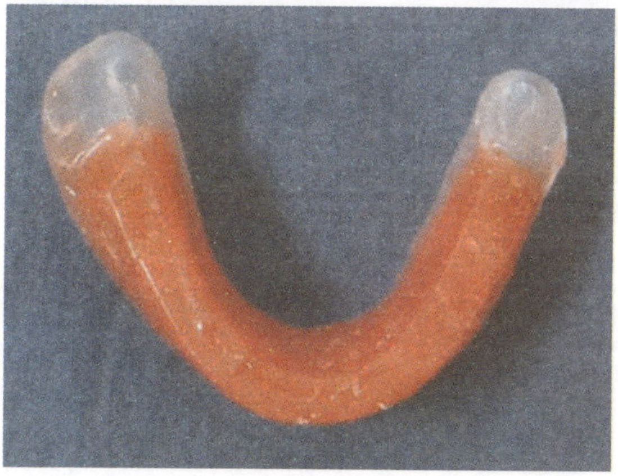

Fig. 11 Mandibular occlusion rim

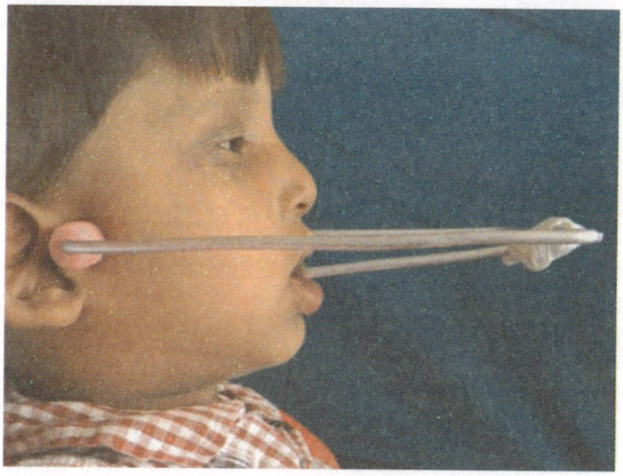

Fig. 12 Custom made face bow

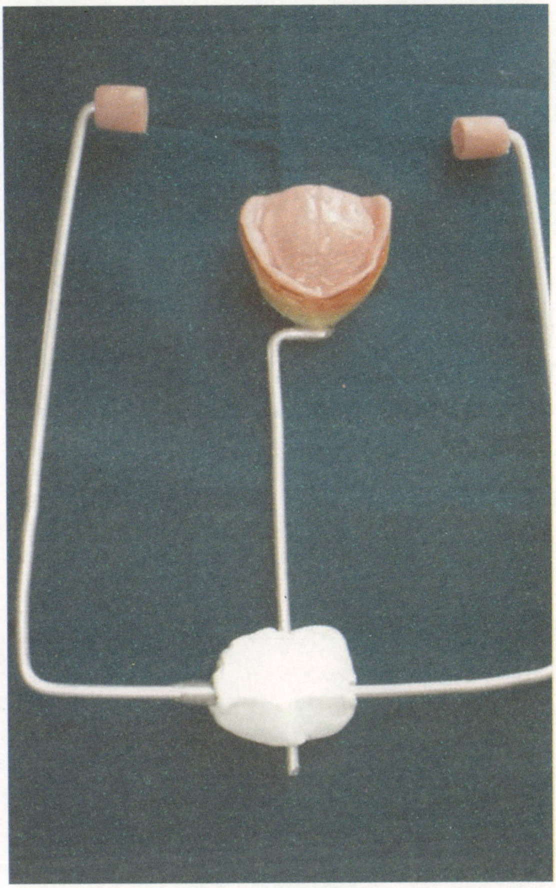

Fig. 13 Face bow assembly

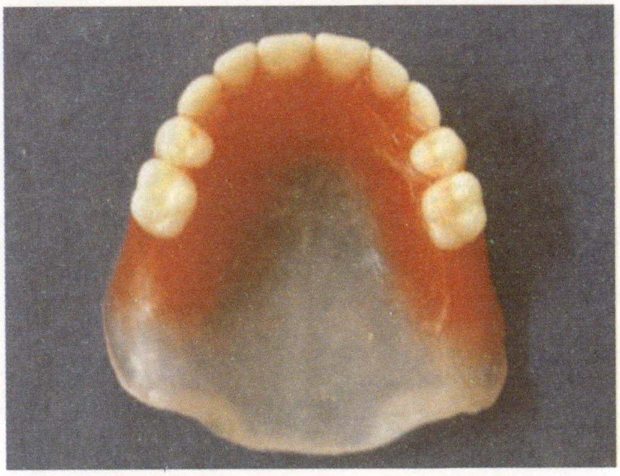

Fig. 15 Maxillary trial denture

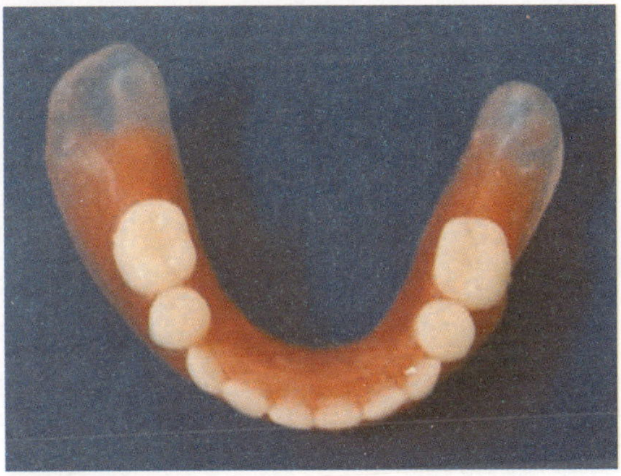

Fig. 16 Mandibular trial denture

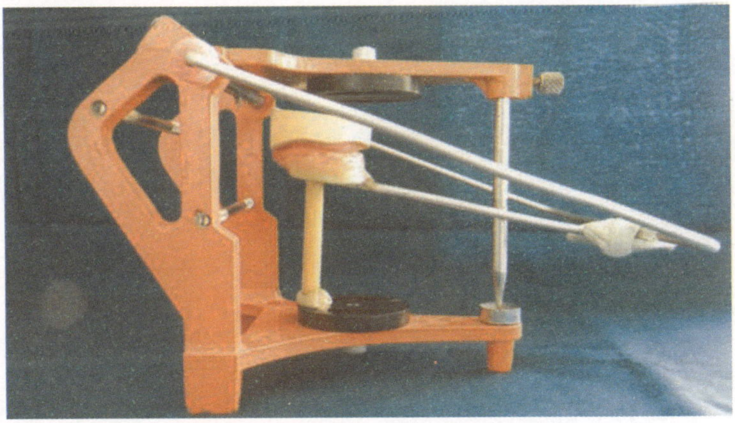

Fig. 14 Face bow transfer

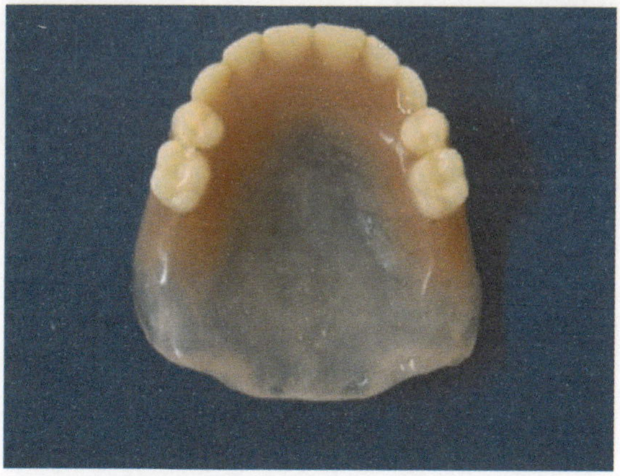

Fig. 17 Maxillary denture

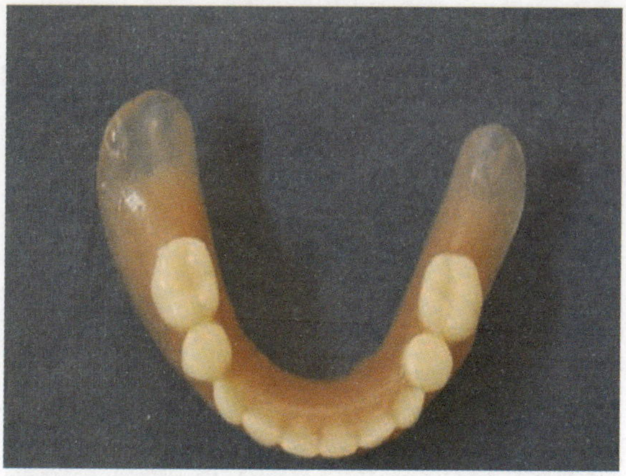

Fig. 18 Mandibular denture

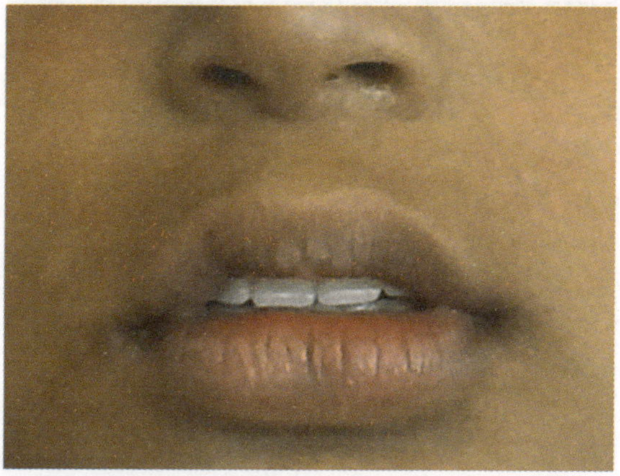

Fig. 19 Wearing the denture

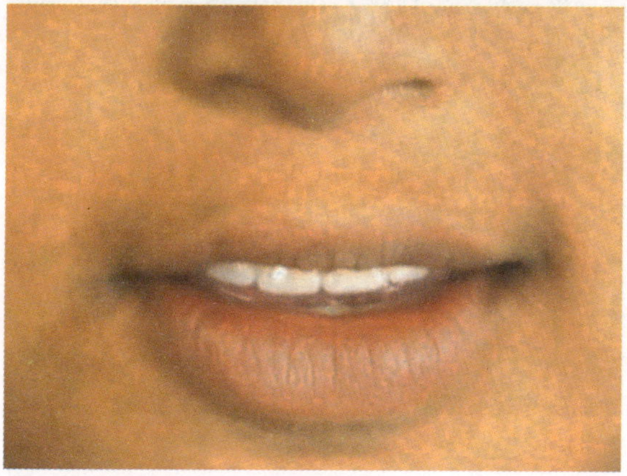

Fig. 20 Smile with the denture

Index